医学教学图谱

U0312262

人体系统解剖图谱

Atlas of
Human Systematic Anatomy

主编
陈金宝　刘　强

主审
王振宇

上海科学技术出版社

图书在版编目（CIP）数据

人体系统解剖图谱/陈金宝，刘强主编 . —— 上海：
上海科学技术出版社，2016.1
（医学教学图谱）
ISBN 978-7-5478-2673-7

Ⅰ.① 人… Ⅱ.① 陈… ② 刘… Ⅲ.① 人体解剖学 –
图谱 Ⅳ.① R322-64

中国版本图书馆 CIP 数据核字 (2015) 第 120695 号

人体系统解剖图谱

主编 陈金宝 刘 强

主审 王振宇

上海世纪出版股份有限公司
上 海 科 学 技 术 出 版 社 出版
（上海钦州南路 71 号 邮政编码 200235）
上海世纪出版股份有限公司发行中心发行
200001 上海福建中路 193 号 www.ewen.co
浙江新华印刷技术有限公司印刷
开本 787×1092 1/16 印张 21.5
字数：500 千字
2016 年 1 月第 1 版 2016 年 1 月第 1 次印刷
ISBN 978-7-5478-2673-7/R · 927
定价：98.00 元

内容提要

　　本书是为了适应我国高等医学教育改革和发展的需要，根据我国 5 年制高等医学院校学生的培养目标和临床需求而编写的教学图谱。全书采用汉英对照的形式，根据解剖学教学的要求，按照普通高等教育国家级规划教材《系统解剖学》的内容，从运动系统、内脏学、脉管系统、感觉器、神经系统、内分泌系统等对人体结构进行系统解剖，充分显示了人体的正常结构。

　　本图谱采取人工绘制和标本拍摄相结合的方式，人工绘制的图像色泽艳丽、结构清晰、边界明确、形态典型；标本拍摄的图像更直观、更真实、更实用。两者结合使用相互补充，相互对照，可为医学生、临床医生及解剖工作者更好地了解和掌握正常人体结构提供参考与指导。

编委名单

主　编
陈金宝　刘　强

主　审
王振宇

副主编
段坤昌　齐亚力　周艳芬　季雪芳　陆　宇

编　委
（按姓氏笔画排序）
刘　强　齐亚力　李　亮　杨　雄　陈金宝
季雪芳　周艳芬　段坤昌　傅　强

主编简介

陈金宝

1944 年生，山东单县人，1963 年考入中国医科大学医疗系学习，1969 年毕业。1994 年晋升为教授，2000 年获得国务院特殊津贴。一直在中国医科大学从事医学图像制作和医学图像处理的研究及资源库建设等工作。

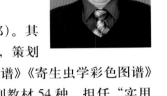

发表论文及出版

在国家级杂志发表的论文、编写出版的教材及专著共 140 余篇（部）。其中主编专著《医学摄影》，副主编《断面解剖与 MRI CT ECT 对照图谱》，策划并参加主编的医学彩色图谱《人体解剖学彩色图谱》《组织胚胎学彩色图谱》《寄生虫学彩色图谱》《病理解剖学彩色图谱》《实验诊断学彩色图谱》，策划并参加总主编系列教材 54 种。担任"实用人体解剖图谱"系列中头颈分册、概论与断面分册、躯干内脏分册、四肢分册的主编。

承担课题

国家"九五"重点攻关课题"人体解剖学课件""组织胚胎学课件" 2 项，国家新世纪网络建设工程课题"人体解剖学网络课程""组织胚胎学网络课程" 2 项，教育部重大研究课题子课题 1 项，"药理学"国家级优秀网络课程 1 项，辽宁省科委课题 1 项，辽宁省教育厅课题 1 项。

获得奖励

卫生部奖 6 项，教育部奖 1 项，美国医学电教学会（HESCA）奖 1 项。

辽宁省科技进步一等奖"现代医学教育资源库" 1 项，辽宁省优秀教学成果一等奖 1 项，辽宁省优秀教学成果二等奖 2 项，辽宁省优秀教学成果三等奖 1 项，辽宁省优秀课件一等奖 1 项，沈阳市科技进步三等奖 1 项。

曾任职务

中国医科大学教育技术中心主任，网络教育学院常务副院长。卫生部继续医学教育和乡村医生教育的视听教育专家，中华医学会教育技术分会委员、常务委员、副主任委员、主任委员、名誉主任委员，教育部高等医药院校现代教育技术与计算机教学指导委员会委员，中国电化教育协会理事、医学委员会主任委员，辽宁省高等院校电化教育研究会副理事长等职。

主编简介

刘 强

1975 年生，辽宁省丹东市人，1994 年考入中国医科大学日语临床医学专业学习，2000 年毕业，硕士学位。一直从事医学教育管理、教育技术研究、教学资源库建设等工作。

担任职务

中国医科大学网络教育学院院长，教育技术中心主任；中华医学会教育技术分会第七届委员会委员，虚拟仿真应用研究专业学组副组长；辽宁省医学会医学教育学分会第五届委员会教育技术与应用学组委员。

获得奖励

制作的《药理学》《护理学基础》课程获得国家级精品资源共享课程（网络教育），制作的《生活方式与健康》课程获得国家级精品视频公开课程，制作十余门辽宁省精品视频公开课和精品资源共享课等。

编写教材及专著

参与编写"成人高等教育基础医学教材""成人高等教育护理学专用教材""成人高等教育药学专用教材"，由上海科学技术出版社出版。担任"实用人体解剖图谱"系列中头颈分册、概论与断面分册、躯干内脏分册、四肢分册的副主编。

承担课题

2008 年教育部课题：继续教育改革和发展战略与政策研究行业继续教育子课题"乡村医生继续教育现状改革和发展研究"；2011 年辽宁省课题：中国医科大学临床医学本科综合改革试点专业建设立项子课题"优质教学资源建设与共享项目"。

前　言

　　人体解剖学是研究人体正常形态结构的科学，其任务在于理解和掌握人体各器官的形态与结构、位置和毗邻关系，为学习其他基础医学和临床医学课程奠定基础。人体解剖图谱是医学院校解剖学教学的重要辅助工具书，也是每个医学生学习和掌握人体正常形态结构必备的工具书。

　　本书的编纂参照本科系统解剖学教学大纲，与教材内容相配套。为了充分体现实用性原则，以系统解剖学内容展示人体器官的形态结构为主，并适当展示各器官局部的层次和毗邻关系。采取了系统解剖、局部解剖、影像解剖相结合的形式，充分展示人体的正常结构。系统解剖部分重点是展示骨骼、肌肉、血管和神经的有关内容。局部解剖部分按照内容的需要，进行逐层解剖，充分显示浅组织、筋膜、肌肉、骨骼、血管、神经的相互位置关系。此外，还采用了断面解剖和临床的一些影像，从不同侧面展示了人体的正常结构。

　　本图谱内容按总论、运动系统（骨学、关节学、肌学）、内脏学（消化系统、呼吸系统、泌尿系统、生殖系统、腹膜）、脉管系统（心血管系统、淋巴系统）、感觉器（视器、前庭蜗器）、神经系统与内分泌系统（神经系统总论、中枢神经系统、周围神经系统、神经系统传导通路、脑和脊髓的被膜、血管及脑脊液循环、内分泌系统）等编排。

　　在表现形式上，我们采取人工绘制和标本拍摄相结合的方式。人工绘制的图像色泽艳丽、结构清晰、边界明确、形态典型。标本拍摄的图像更直观、更真实、更实用。两者结合使用相互补充、相互对照，为读者掌握正常人体结构提供了方便。

　　在图谱的编绘过程中，参阅了国内外出版的图谱和专著。在此，对出版社和作者表示衷心的感谢。

　　由于作者的水平限制，本图谱难免存在不当或错误，敬请学界专家和读者给予批评指正。

陈金宝

2015 年 8 月

目 录

第一节

体 表

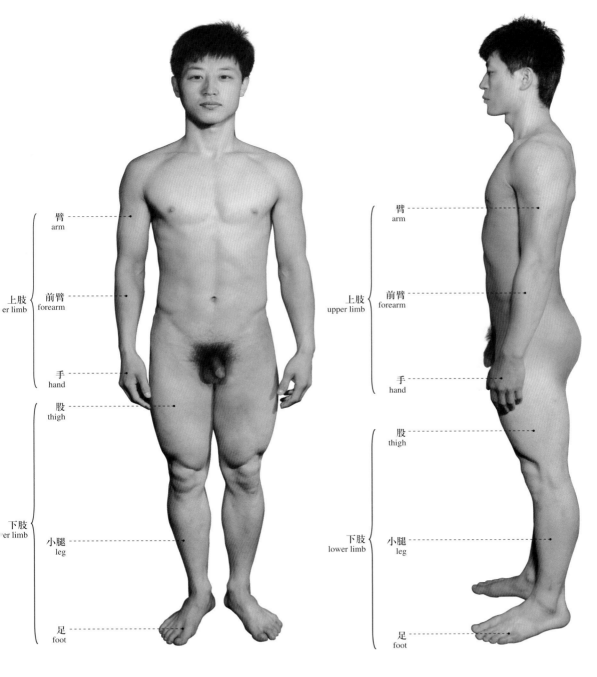

上肢
er limb

臂
arm

前臂
forearm

手
hand

股
thigh

下肢
er limb

小腿
leg

足
foot

上肢
upper limb

臂
arm

前臂
forearm

手
hand

下肢
lower limb

股
thigh

小腿
leg

足
foot

图 1　男性全身体表（前面观）
Surface of the male body (anterior aspect)

图 2　男性全身体表（侧面观）
Surface of the male body (lateral aspect)

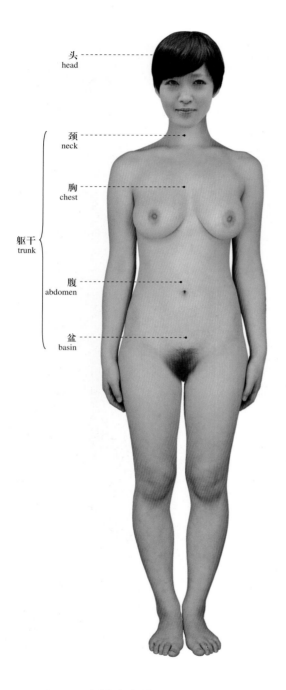

头
head

颈
neck

胸
chest

躯干
trunk

腹
abdomen

盆
basin

图 3　女性全身体表（前面观）
Surface of the female body (anterior aspect)

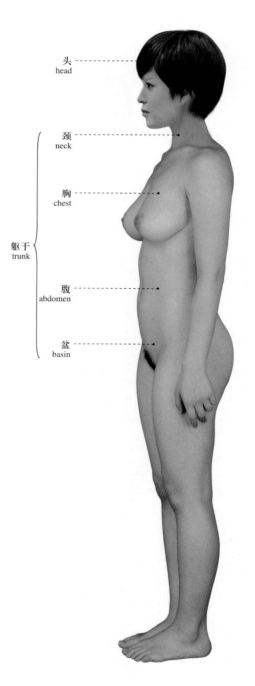

头
head

颈
neck

胸
chest

躯干
trunk

腹
abdomen

盆
basin

图 4　女性全身体表（侧面观）
Surface of the female body (lateral aspect)

第二节

人体的轴和面

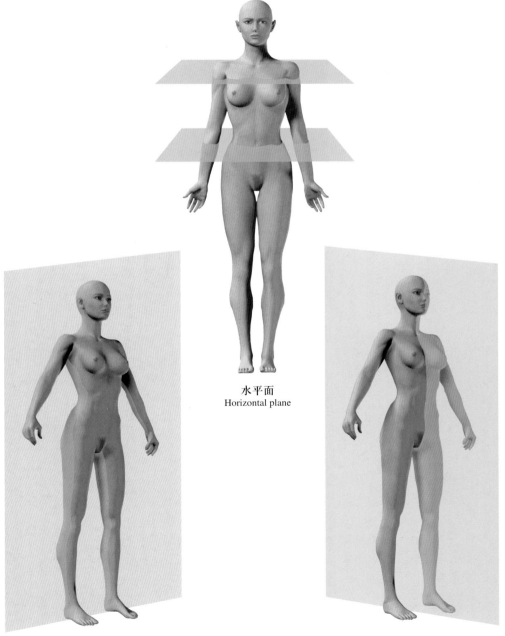

水平面
Horizontal plane

冠状面
Frontal plane

矢状面
Sagittal plane

图 5　人体的轴和面
Axis and plane of the human body

第一节

全身骨骼

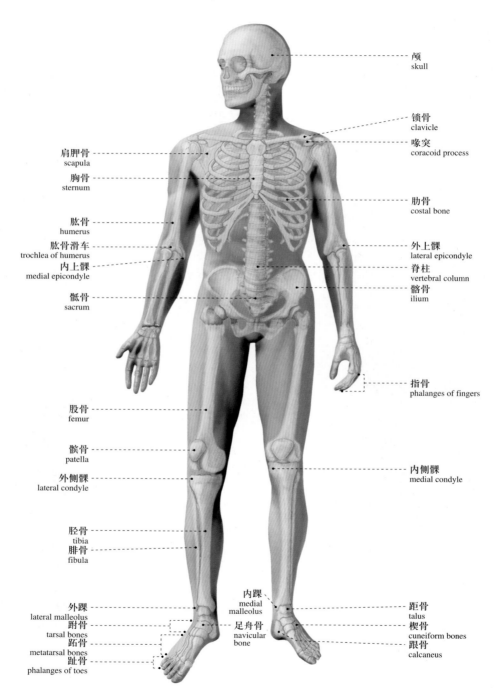

颅
skull

锁骨
clavicle

喙突
coracoid process

肩胛骨
scapula

胸骨
sternum

肋骨
costal bone

肱骨
humerus

肱骨滑车
trochlea of humerus

外上髁
lateral epicondyle

内上髁
medial epicondyle

脊柱
vertebral column

骶骨
sacrum

髂骨
ilium

指骨
phalanges of fingers

股骨
femur

髌骨
patella

外侧髁
lateral condyle

内侧髁
medial condyle

胫骨
tibia

腓骨
fibula

外踝
lateral malleolus

内踝
medial malleolus

距骨
talus

跗骨
tarsal bones

足舟骨
navicular bone

楔骨
cuneiform bones

跖骨
metatarsal bones

跟骨
calcaneus

趾骨
phalanges of toes

图 6　全身骨骼（前面观）

Skeleton (anterior aspect)

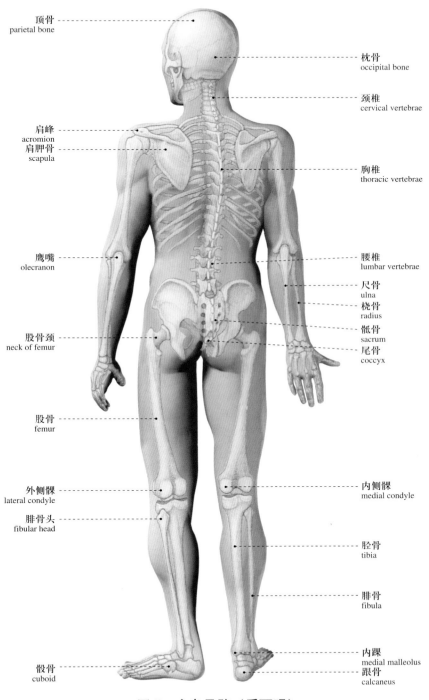

顶骨
parietal bone

枕骨
occipital bone

颈椎
cervical vertebrae

肩峰
acromion
肩胛骨
scapula

胸椎
thoracic vertebrae

鹰嘴
olecranon

腰椎
lumbar vertebrae

尺骨
ulna

桡骨
radius

骶骨
sacrum

尾骨
coccyx

股骨颈
neck of femur

股骨
femur

外侧髁
lateral condyle

内侧髁
medial condyle

腓骨头
fibular head

胫骨
tibia

腓骨
fibula

内踝
medial malleolus

骰骨
cuboid

跟骨
calcaneus

图 7   全身骨骼（后面观）

Skeleton (posterior aspect)

第二节

骨 的 构 造

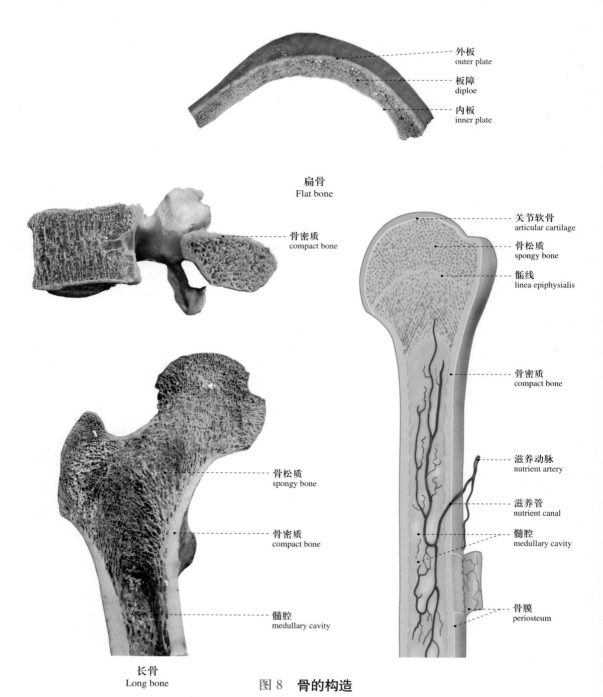

外板
outer plate

板障
diploe

内板
inner plate

扁骨
Flat bone

骨密质
compact bone

关节软骨
articular cartilage

骨松质
spongy bone

骺线
linea epiphysialis

骨密质
compact bone

滋养动脉
nutrient artery

滋养管
nutrient canal

骨松质
spongy bone

骨密质
compact bone

髓腔
medullary cavity

髓腔
medullary cavity

骨膜
periosteum

长骨
Long bone

图 8　骨的构造
Structure of the bones

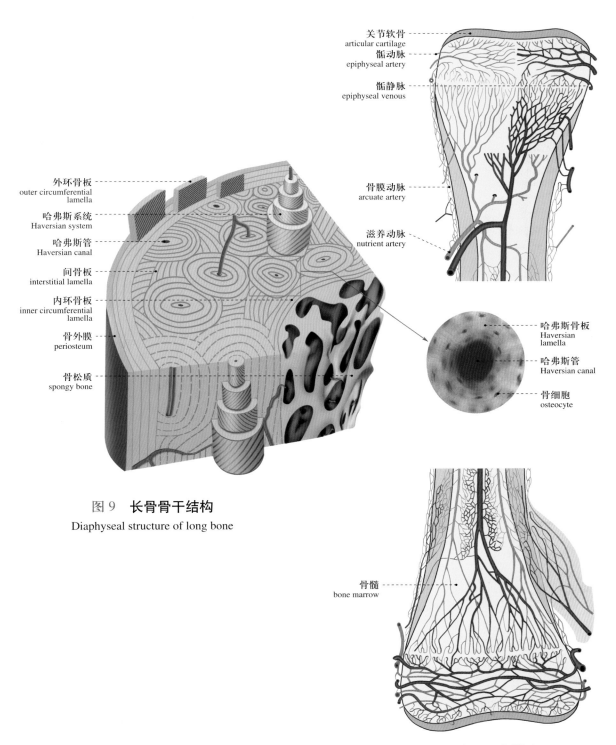

关节软骨
articular cartilage
骺动脉
epiphyseal artery
骺静脉
epiphyseal venous

骨膜动脉
arcuate artery

滋养动脉
nutrient artery

哈弗斯骨板
Haversian lamella
哈弗斯管
Haversian canal
骨细胞
osteocyte

外环骨板
outer circumferential lamella
哈弗斯系统
Haversian system
哈弗斯管
Haversian canal
间骨板
interstitial lamella
内环骨板
inner circumferential lamella
骨外膜
periosteum
骨松质
spongy bone

图 9　长骨骨干结构
Diaphyseal structure of long bone

骨髓
bone marrow

图 10　长骨血管神经分布模式图
Diagram of the distribution of the blood vessels and nerves of the long bone

第三节

中 轴 骨 骼

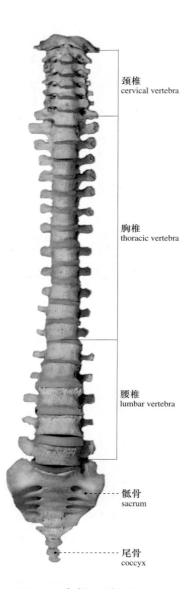

颈椎
cervical vertebra

胸椎
thoracic vertebra

腰椎
lumbar vertebra

骶骨
sacrum

尾骨
coccyx

图 11　脊柱（前面观）
Vertebral column (anterior aspect)

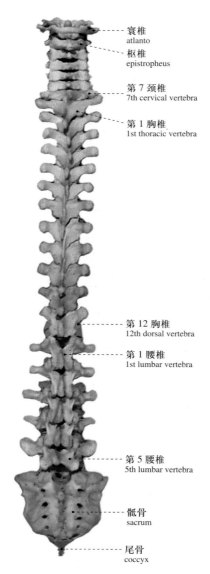

寰椎
atlanto

枢椎
epistropheus

第 7 颈椎
7th cervical vertebra

第 1 胸椎
1st thoracic vertebra

第 12 胸椎
12th dorsal vertebra

第 1 腰椎
1st lumbar vertebra

第 5 腰椎
5th lumbar vertebra

骶骨
sacrum

尾骨
coccyx

图 12　脊柱（后面观）
Vertebral column (posterior aspect)

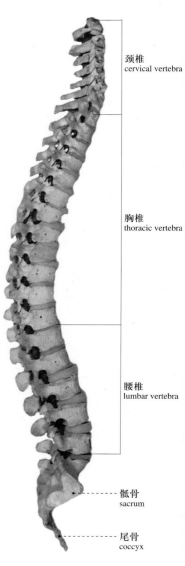

颈椎
cervical vertebra

胸椎
thoracic vertebra

腰椎
lumbar vertebra

骶骨
sacrum

尾骨
coccyx

图 13　脊柱（侧面观）
Vertebral column (lateral aspect)

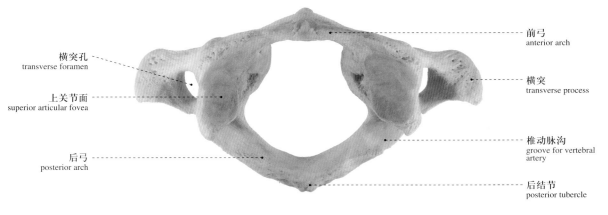

横突孔
transverse foramen

上关节面
superior articular fovea

后弓
posterior arch

前弓
anterior arch

横突
transverse process

椎动脉沟
groove for vertebral artery

后结节
posterior tubercle

图 14　寰椎（上面观）
Atlas (superior aspect)

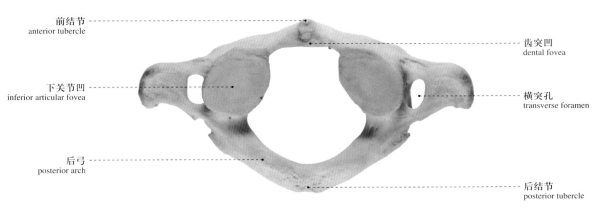

前结节
anterior tubercle

下关节凹
inferior articular fovea

后弓
posterior arch

齿突凹
dental fovea

横突孔
transverse foramen

后结节
posterior tubercle

图 15　寰椎（下面观）
Atlas (inferior aspect)

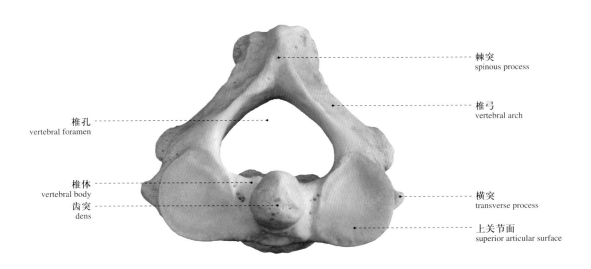

椎孔
vertebral foramen

椎体
vertebral body

齿突
dens

棘突
spinous process

椎弓
vertebral arch

横突
transverse process

上关节面
superior articular surface

图 16　枢椎（上面观）
Axis (superior aspect)

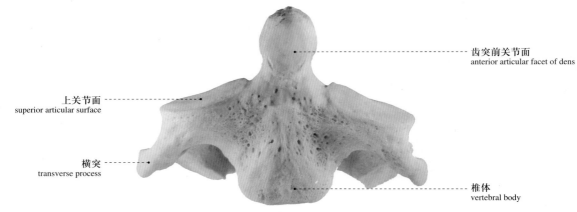

齿突前关节面
anterior articular facet of dens

上关节面
superior articular surface

横突
transverse process

椎体
vertebral body

图 17　枢椎（前面观）
Axis (anterior aspect)

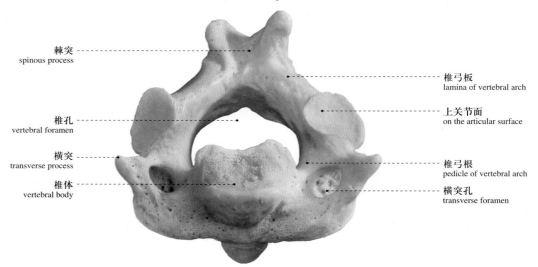

棘突
spinous process

椎孔
vertebral foramen

横突
transverse process

椎体
vertebral body

椎弓板
lamina of vertebral arch

上关节面
on the articular surface

椎弓根
pedicle of vertebral arch

横突孔
transverse foramen

图 18　枢椎（下面观）
Axis (inferior aspect)

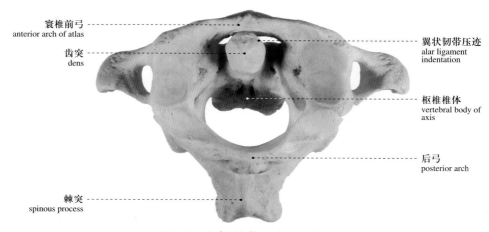

寰椎前弓
anterior arch of atlas

齿突
dens

翼状韧带压迹
alar ligament
indentation

枢椎椎体
vertebral body of
axis

后弓
posterior arch

棘突
spinous process

图 19　寰枢关节（上面观）
Atlanto-axial joint (superior aspect)

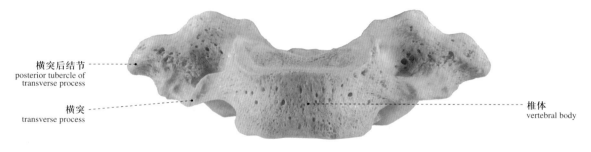

横突后结节
posterior tubercle of
transverse process

横突
transverse process

椎体
vertebral body

图 20　隆椎（前面观）
Vertebra prominens (anterior aspect)

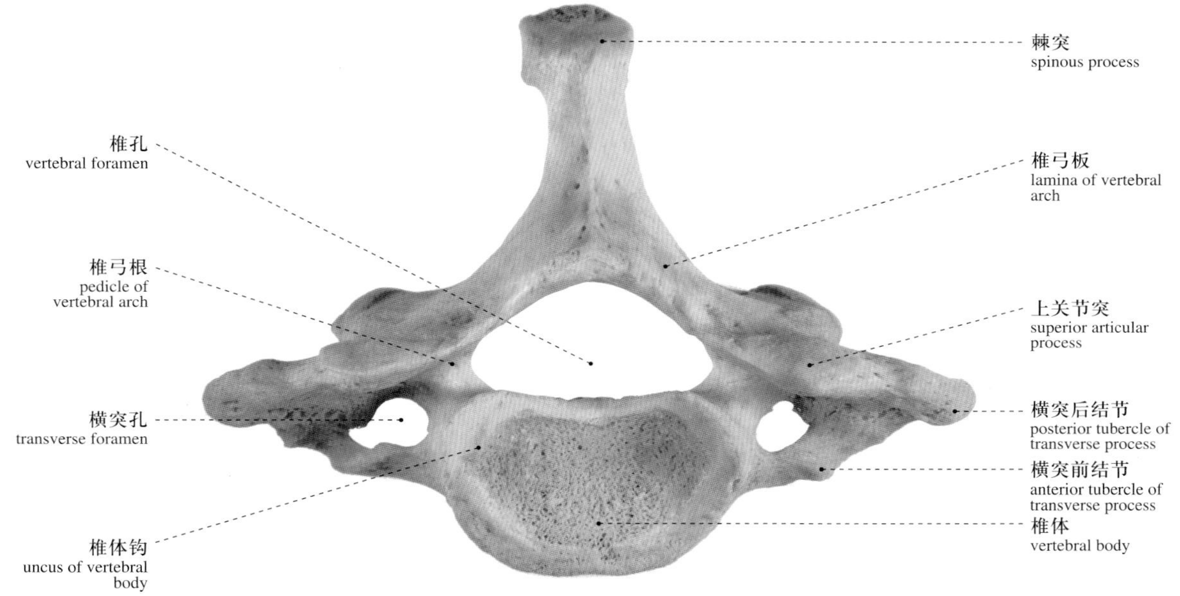

棘突
spinous process

椎孔
vertebral foramen

椎弓板
lamina of vertebral
arch

椎弓根
pedicle of
vertebral arch

上关节突
superior articular
process

横突孔
transverse foramen

横突后结节
posterior tubercle of
transverse process

椎体钩
uncus of vertebral
body

横突前结节
anterior tubercle of
transverse process

椎体
vertebral body

图 21　隆椎（上面观）
Vertebra prominens (superior aspect)

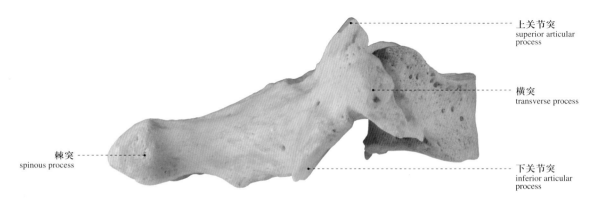

上关节突
superior articular
process

横突
transverse process

棘突
spinous process

下关节突
inferior articular
process

图 22　隆椎（侧面观）
Vertebra prominens (lateral aspect)

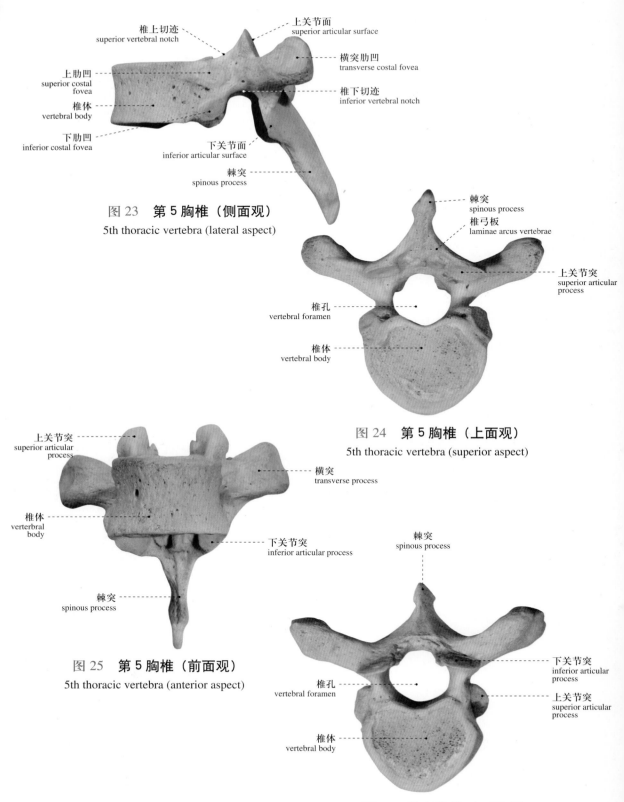

椎上切迹
superior vertebral notch

上关节面
superior articular surface

横突肋凹
transverse costal fovea

上肋凹
superior costal fovea

椎下切迹
inferior vertebral notch

椎体
vertebral body

下肋凹
inferior costal fovea

下关节面
inferior articular surface

棘突
spinous process

图 23　第 5 胸椎（侧面观）
5th thoracic vertebra (lateral aspect)

棘突
spinous process

椎弓板
laminae arcus vertebrae

上关节突
superior articular process

椎孔
vertebral foramen

椎体
vertebral body

图 24　第 5 胸椎（上面观）
5th thoracic vertebra (superior aspect)

上关节突
superior articular process

横突
transverse process

椎体
verterbral body

下关节突
inferior articular process

棘突
spinous process

图 25　第 5 胸椎（前面观）
5th thoracic vertebra (anterior aspect)

棘突
spinous process

下关节突
inferior articular process

椎孔
vertebral foramen

上关节突
superior articular process

椎体
vertebral body

图 26　第 5 胸椎（下面观）
5th thoracic vertebra (inferior aspect)

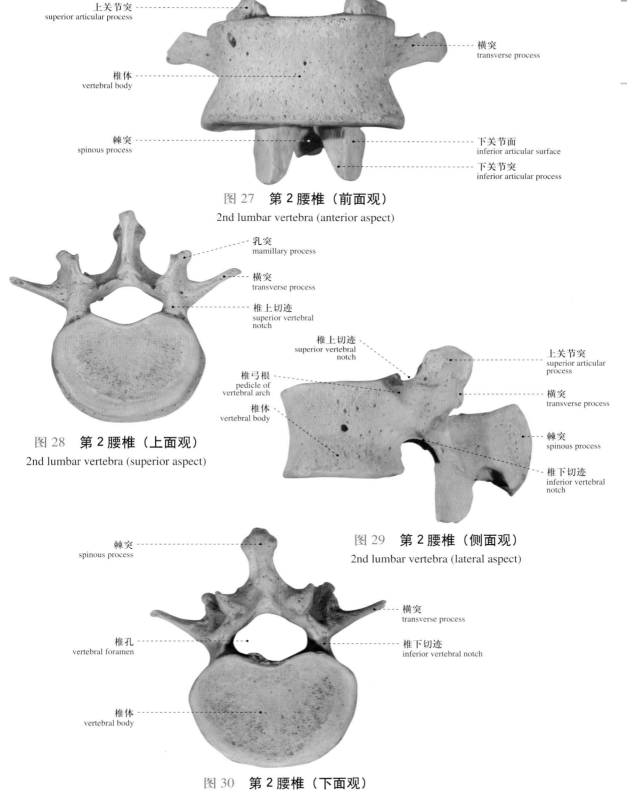

上关节突
superior articular process

横突
transverse process

椎体
vertebral body

棘突
spinous process

下关节面
inferior articular surface

下关节突
inferior articular process

图 27 第 2 腰椎（前面观）
2nd lumbar vertebra (anterior aspect)

乳突
mamillary process

横突
transverse process

椎上切迹
superior vertebral notch

图 28 第 2 腰椎（上面观）
2nd lumbar vertebra (superior aspect)

椎上切迹
superior vertebral notch

椎弓根
pedicle of vertebral arch

椎体
vertebral body

上关节突
superior articular process

横突
transverse process

棘突
spinous process

椎下切迹
inferior vertebral notch

图 29 第 2 腰椎（侧面观）
2nd lumbar vertebra (lateral aspect)

棘突
spinous process

椎孔
vertebral foramen

椎体
vertebral body

横突
transverse process

椎下切迹
inferior vertebral notch

图 30 第 2 腰椎（下面观）
2nd lumbar vertebra (inferior aspect)

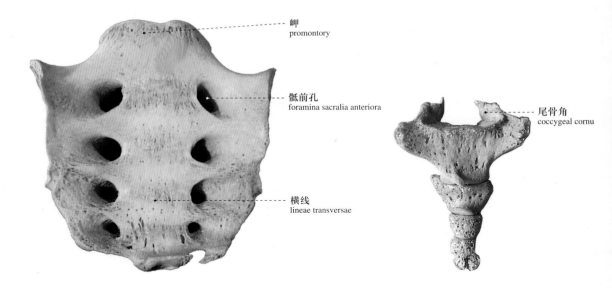

岬
promontory

骶前孔
foramina sacralia anteriora

横线
lineae transversae

尾骨角
coccygeal cornu

图 31　骶骨和尾骨（前面观）
Sacrum and coccyx (anterior aspect)

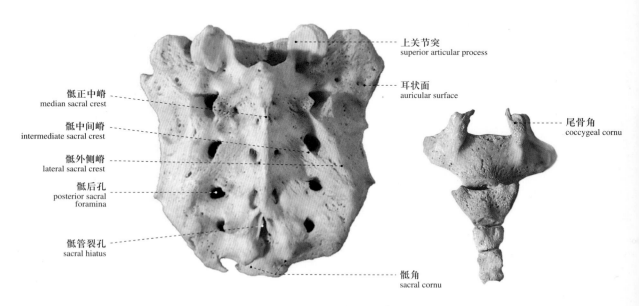

上关节突
superior articular process

耳状面
auricular surface

骶正中嵴
median sacral crest

骶中间嵴
intermediate sacral crest

骶外侧嵴
lateral sacral crest

骶后孔
posterior sacral foramina

骶管裂孔
sacral hiatus

尾骨角
coccygeal cornu

骶角
sacral cornu

图 32　骶骨和尾骨（后面观）
Sacrum and coccyx (posterior aspect)

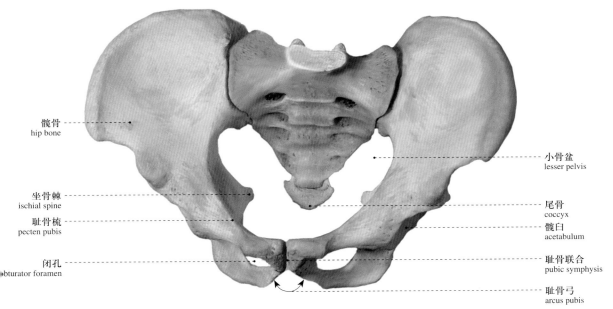

髋骨
hip bone

坐骨棘
ischial spine

耻骨梳
pecten pubis

闭孔
obturator foramen

小骨盆
lesser pelvis

尾骨
coccyx

髋臼
acetabulum

耻骨联合
pubic symphysis

耻骨弓
arcus pubis

图 33　**男性骨盆（前面观）**
Male pelvis (anterior aspect)

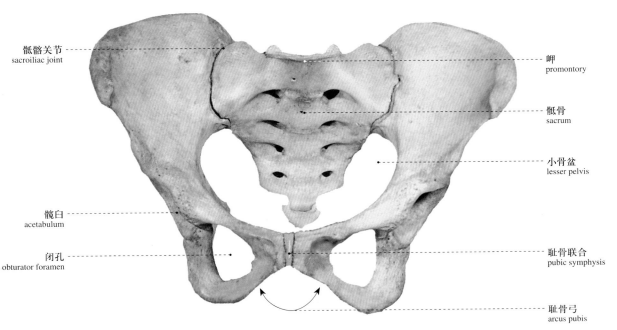

骶髂关节
sacroiliac joint

髋臼
acetabulum

闭孔
obturator foramen

岬
promontory

骶骨
sacrum

小骨盆
lesser pelvis

耻骨联合
pubic symphysis

耻骨弓
arcus pubis

图 34　**女性骨盆（前面观）**
Female pelvis (anterior aspect)

15

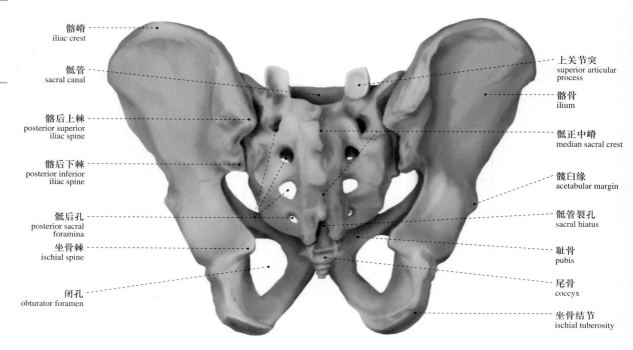

髂嵴
iliac crest

骶管
sacral canal

髂后上棘
posterior superior
iliac spine

髂后下棘
posterior inferior
iliac spine

骶后孔
posterior sacral
foramina

坐骨棘
ischial spine

闭孔
obturator foramen

上关节突
superior articular
process

髂骨
ilium

骶正中嵴
median sacral crest

髋臼缘
acetabular margin

骶管裂孔
sacral hiatus

耻骨
pubis

尾骨
coccyx

坐骨结节
ischial tuberosity

图 35　骨盆（后面观）
Pelvis (posterior aspect)

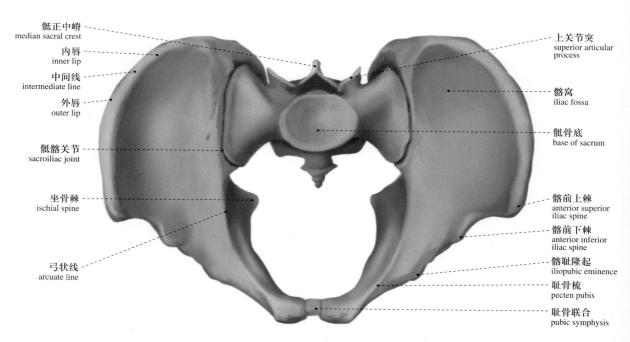

骶正中嵴
median sacral crest

内唇
inner lip

中间线
intermediate line

外唇
outer lip

骶髂关节
sacroiliac joint

坐骨棘
ischial spine

弓状线
arcuate line

上关节突
superior articular
process

髂窝
iliac fossa

骶骨底
base of sacrum

髂前上棘
anterior superior
iliac spine

髂前下棘
anterior inferior
iliac spine

髂耻隆起
iliopubic eminence

耻骨梳
pecten pubis

耻骨联合
pubic symphysis

图 36　男性骨盆（上面观）
Male pelvis (superior aspect)

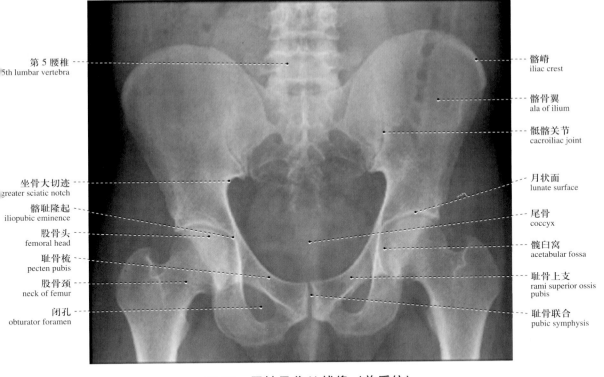

第 5 腰椎
5th lumbar vertebra

坐骨大切迹
greater sciatic notch

髂耻隆起
iliopubic eminence

股骨头
femoral head

耻骨梳
pecten pubis

股骨颈
neck of femur

闭孔
obturator foramen

髂嵴
iliac crest

髂骨翼
ala of ilium

骶髂关节
cacroiliac joint

月状面
lunate surface

尾骨
coccyx

髋臼窝
acetabular fossa

耻骨上支
rami superior ossis pubis

耻骨联合
pubic symphysis

图 37　男性骨盆 X 线像（前后位）
Radiograph of the male pelvis (anteroposterior view)

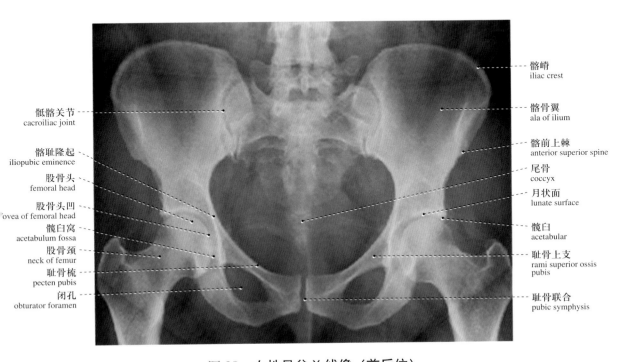

骶髂关节
cacroiliac joint

髂耻隆起
iliopubic eminence

股骨头
femoral head

股骨头凹
fovea of femoral head

髋臼窝
acetabulum fossa

股骨颈
neck of femur

耻骨梳
pecten pubis

闭孔
obturator foramen

髂嵴
iliac crest

髂骨翼
ala of ilium

髂前上棘
anterior superior spine

尾骨
coccyx

月状面
lunate surface

髋臼
acetabular

耻骨上支
rami superior ossis pubis

耻骨联合
pubic symphysis

图 38　女性骨盆 X 线像（前后位）
Radiograph of the female pelvis (anteroposterior view)

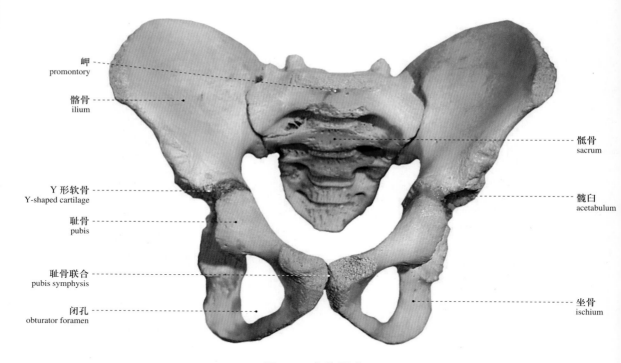

岬
promontory

髂骨
ilium

Y 形软骨
Y-shaped cartilage

耻骨
pubis

耻骨联合
pubis symphysis

闭孔
obturator foramen

骶骨
sacrum

髋臼
acetabulum

坐骨
ischium

图 39　小儿骨盆
Pelvis of an infant

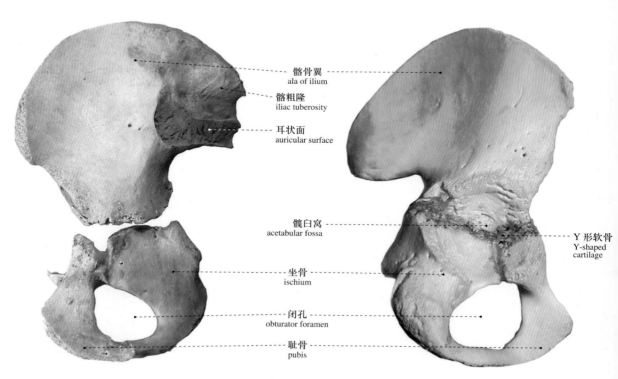

髂骨翼
ala of ilium

髂粗隆
iliac tuberosity

耳状面
auricular surface

髋臼窝
acetabular fossa

Y 形软骨
Y-shaped cartilage

坐骨
ischium

闭孔
obturator foramen

耻骨
pubis

图 40　小儿髋骨（内面观）
Hip bone of an infant (internal aspect)

图 41　小儿髋骨（外面观）
Hip bone of an infant (external aspect)

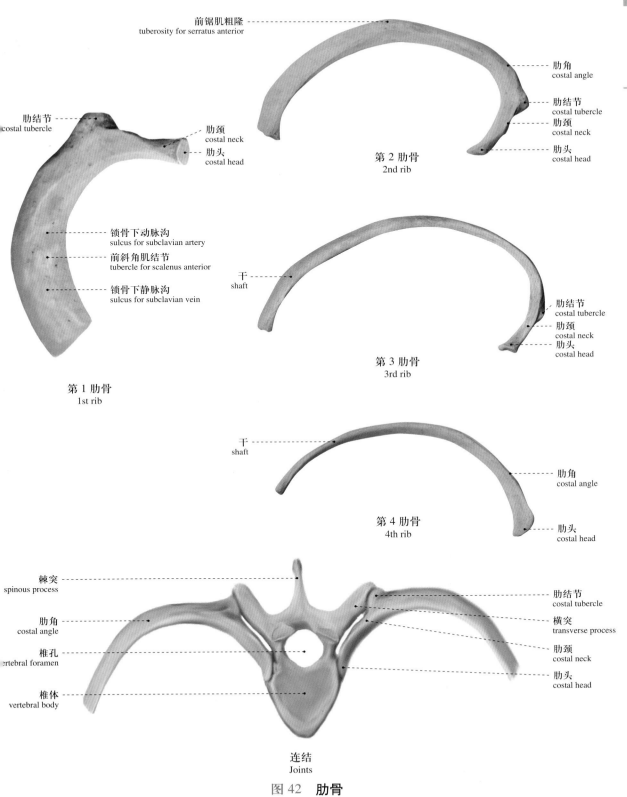

前锯肌粗隆
tuberosity for serratus anterior

肋角
costal angle

肋结节
costal tubercle

肋颈
costal neck

肋头
costal head

第 2 肋骨
2nd rib

肋结节
costal tubercle

肋颈
costal neck

肋头
costal head

锁骨下动脉沟
sulcus for subclavian artery

前斜角肌结节
tubercle for scalenus anterior

锁骨下静脉沟
sulcus for subclavian vein

干
shaft

肋结节
costal tubercle

肋颈
costal neck

肋头
costal head

第 3 肋骨
3rd rib

第 1 肋骨
1st rib

干
shaft

肋角
costal angle

肋头
costal head

第 4 肋骨
4th rib

棘突
spinous process

肋角
costal angle

椎孔
vertebral foramen

椎体
vertebral body

肋结节
costal tubercle

横突
transverse process

肋颈
costal neck

肋头
costal head

连结
Joints

图 42　肋骨
Ribs

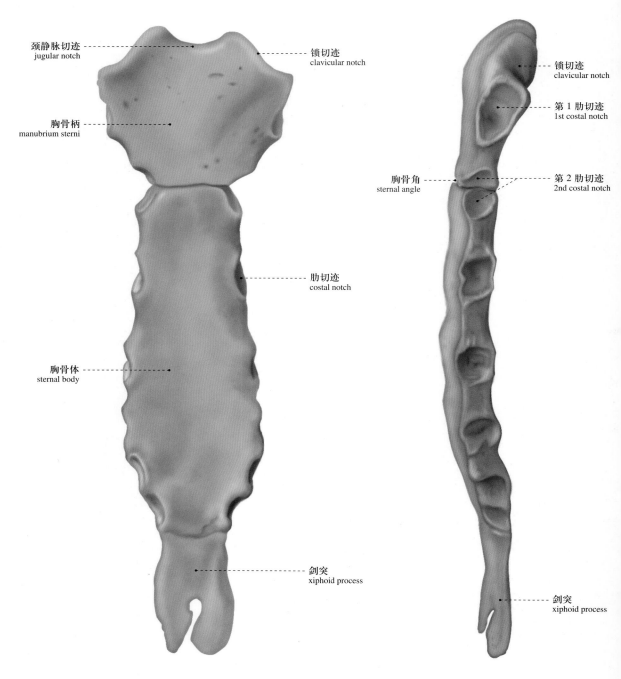

颈静脉切迹
jugular notch

锁切迹
clavicular notch

胸骨柄
manubrium sterni

肋切迹
costal notch

胸骨体
sternal body

剑突
xiphoid process

锁切迹
clavicular notch

第 1 肋切迹
1st costal notch

胸骨角
sternal angle

第 2 肋切迹
2nd costal notch

剑突
xiphoid process

图 43　胸骨（前面观）
Sternum (anterior aspect)

图 44　胸骨（侧面观）
Sternum (lateral aspect)

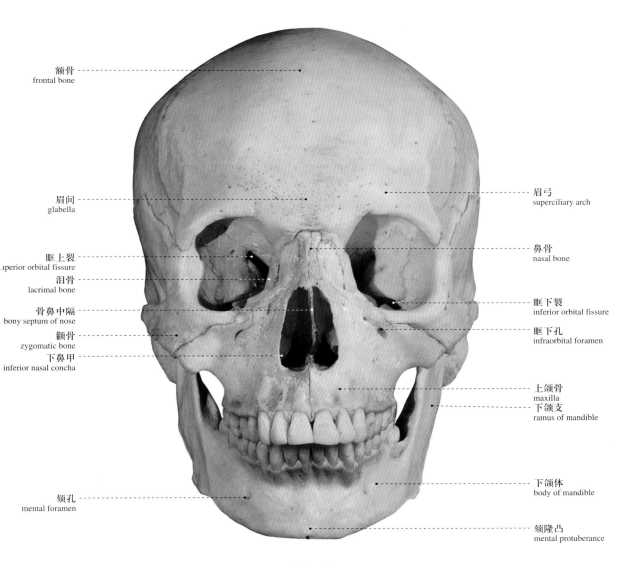

额骨
frontal bone

眉间
glabella

眶上裂
superior orbital fissure

泪骨
lacrimal bone

骨鼻中隔
bony septum of nose

颧骨
zygomatic bone

下鼻甲
inferior nasal concha

颏孔
mental foramen

眉弓
superciliary arch

鼻骨
nasal bone

眶下裂
inferior orbital fissure

眶下孔
infraorbital foramen

上颌骨
maxilla

下颌支
ramus of mandible

下颌体
body of mandible

颏隆凸
mental protuberance

图 45　颅（前面观）

Skull (anterior aspect)

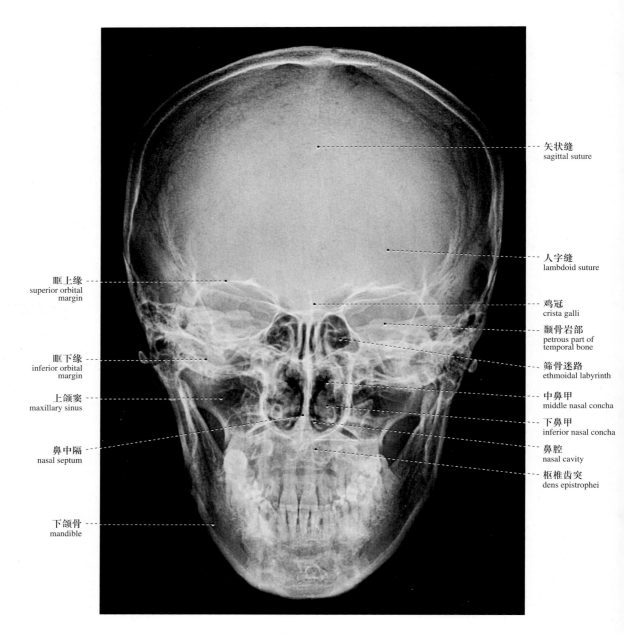

矢状缝
sagittal suture

人字缝
lambdoid suture

鸡冠
crista galli

颞骨岩部
petrous part of
temporal bone

筛骨迷路
ethmoidal labyrinth

中鼻甲
middle nasal concha

下鼻甲
inferior nasal concha

鼻腔
nasal cavity

枢椎齿突
dens epistrophei

眶上缘
superior orbital
margin

眶下缘
inferior orbital
margin

上颌窦
maxillary sinus

鼻中隔
nasal septum

下颌骨
mandible

图 46　颅 X 线像（前后位）
Radiograph of the skull (anteroposterior view)

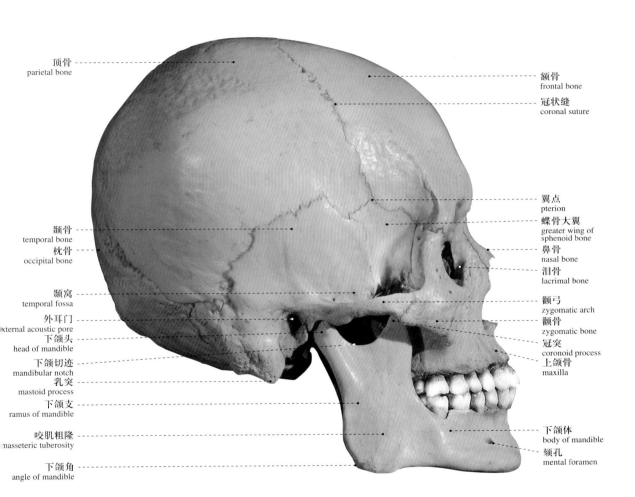

顶骨
parietal bone

额骨
frontal bone

冠状缝
coronal suture

颞骨
temporal bone

枕骨
occipital bone

翼点
pterion

蝶骨大翼
greater wing of
sphenoid bone

鼻骨
nasal bone

泪骨
lacrimal bone

颞窝
temporal fossa

外耳门
external acoustic pore

下颌头
head of mandible

颧弓
zygomatic arch

颧骨
zygomatic bone

冠突
coronoid process

上颌骨
maxilla

下颌切迹
mandibular notch

乳突
mastoid process

下颌支
ramus of mandible

咬肌粗隆
masseteric tuberosity

下颌体
body of mandible

颏孔
mental foramen

下颌角
angle of mandible

图 47　颅（侧面观）
Skull (lateral aspect)

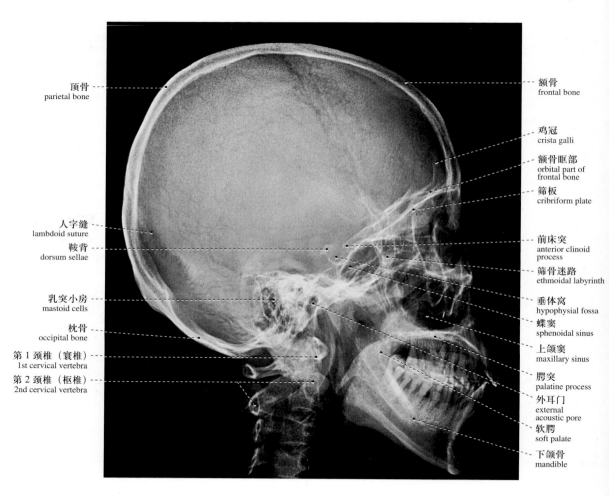

顶骨
parietal bone

额骨
frontal bone

鸡冠
crista galli

额骨眶部
orbital part of
frontal bone

筛板
cribriform plate

人字缝
lambdoid suture

鞍背
dorsum sellae

前床突
anterior clinoid
process

筛骨迷路
ethmoidal labyrinth

乳突小房
mastoid cells

垂体窝
hypophysial fossa

蝶窦
sphenoidal sinus

枕骨
occipital bone

上颌窦
maxillary sinus

第 1 颈椎（寰椎）
1st cervical vertebra

腭突
palatine process

第 2 颈椎（枢椎）
2nd cervical vertebra

外耳门
external
acoustic pore

软腭
soft palate

下颌骨
mandible

图 48　颅 X 线像（侧位）

Radiograph of the skull (lateral view)

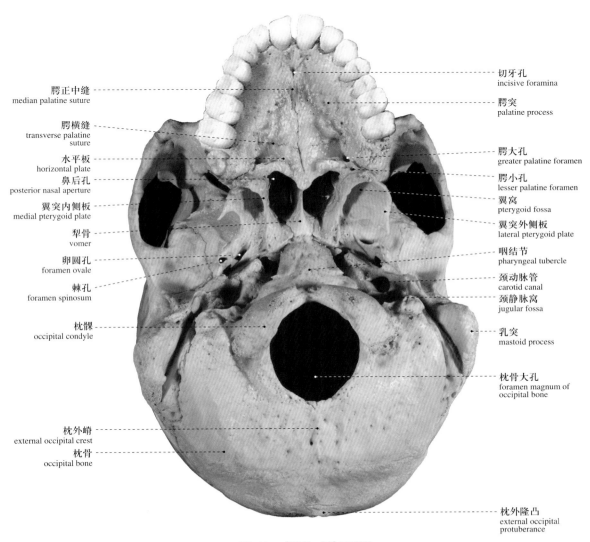

膊正中缝
median palatine suture

膊横缝
transverse palatine suture

水平板
horizontal plate

鼻后孔
posterior nasal aperture

翼突内侧板
medial pterygoid plate

犁骨
vomer

卵圆孔
foramen ovale

棘孔
foramen spinosum

枕髁
occipital condyle

枕外嵴
external occipital crest

枕骨
occipital bone

切牙孔
incisive foramina

膊突
palatine process

膊大孔
greater palatine foramen

膊小孔
lesser palatine foramen

翼窝
pterygoid fossa

翼突外侧板
lateral pterygoid plate

咽结节
pharyngeal tubercle

颈动脉管
carotid canal

颈静脉窝
jugular fossa

乳突
mastoid process

枕骨大孔
foramen magnum of occipital bone

枕外隆凸
external occipital protuberance

图 49　颅底（外面观）
Base of the skull (external aspect)

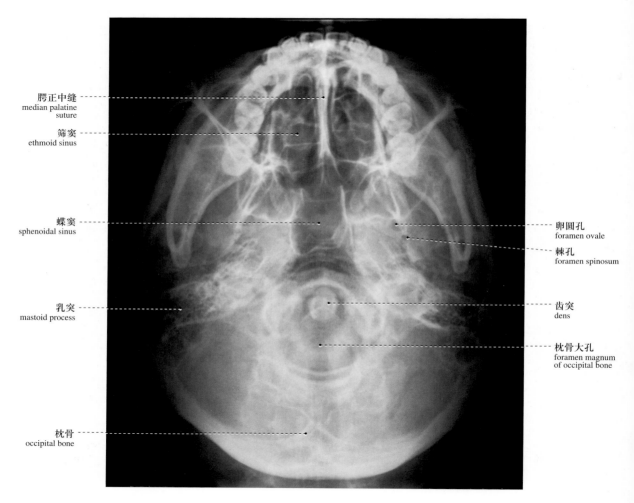

腭正中缝
median palatine
suture

筛窦
ethmoid sinus

蝶窦
sphenoidal sinus

卵圆孔
foramen ovale

棘孔
foramen spinosum

乳突
mastoid process

齿突
dens

枕骨大孔
foramen magnum
of occipital bone

枕骨
occipital bone

图 50　颅 X 线像（下颌顶位）

Radiograph of the base of the skull (SMV)

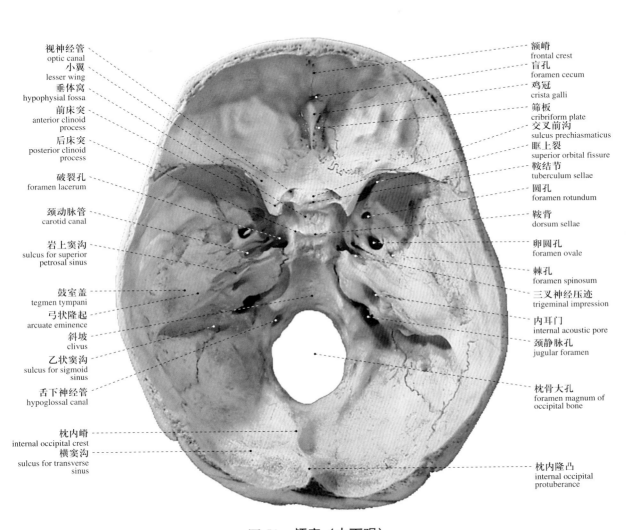

视神经管
optic canal

小翼
lesser wing

垂体窝
hypophysial fossa

前床突
anterior clinoid
process

后床突
posterior clinoid
process

破裂孔
foramen lacerum

颈动脉管
carotid canal

岩上窦沟
sulcus for superior
petrosal sinus

鼓室盖
tegmen tympani

弓状隆起
arcuate eminence

斜坡
clivus

乙状窦沟
sulcus for sigmoid
sinus

舌下神经管
hypoglossal canal

枕内嵴
internal occipital crest

横窦沟
sulcus for transverse
sinus

额嵴
frontal crest

盲孔
foramen cecum

鸡冠
crista galli

筛板
cribriform plate

交叉前沟
sulcus prechiasmaticus

眶上裂
superior orbital fissure

鞍结节
tuberculum sellae

圆孔
foramen rotundum

鞍背
dorsum sellae

卵圆孔
foramen ovale

棘孔
foramen spinosum

三叉神经压迹
trigeminal impression

内耳门
internal acoustic pore

颈静脉孔
jugular foramen

枕骨大孔
foramen magnum of
occipital bone

枕内隆凸
internal occipital
protuberance

图 51 颅底（内面观）
Base of the skull (internal aspect)

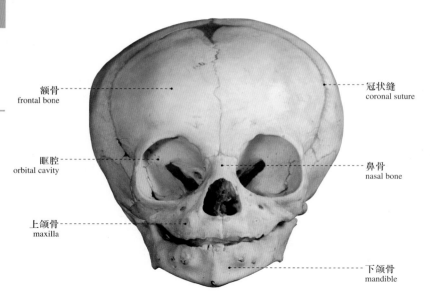

额骨
frontal bone

眶腔
orbital cavity

上颌骨
maxilla

冠状缝
coronal suture

鼻骨
nasal bone

下颌骨
mandible

图 52　婴儿颅（前面观）
Skull of an infant (anterior aspect)

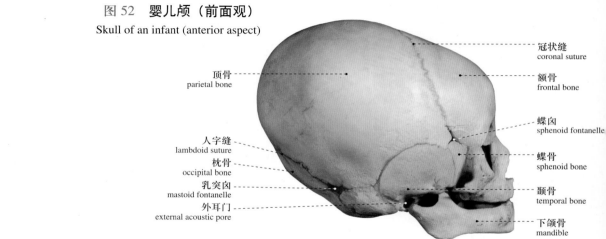

顶骨
parietal bone

人字缝
lambdoid suture

枕骨
occipital bone

乳突囟
mastoid fontanelle

外耳门
external acoustic pore

冠状缝
coronal suture

额骨
frontal bone

蝶囟
sphenoid fontanelle

蝶骨
sphenoid bone

颞骨
temporal bone

下颌骨
mandible

图 53　婴儿颅（侧面观）
Skull of an infant (lateral aspect)

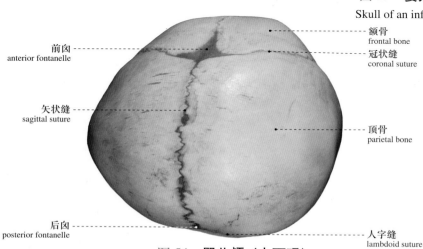

前囟
anterior fontanelle

矢状缝
sagittal suture

后囟
posterior fontanelle

额骨
frontal bone

冠状缝
coronal suture

顶骨
parietal bone

人字缝
lambdoid suture

图 54　婴儿颅（上面观）
Skull of an infant (superior aspect)

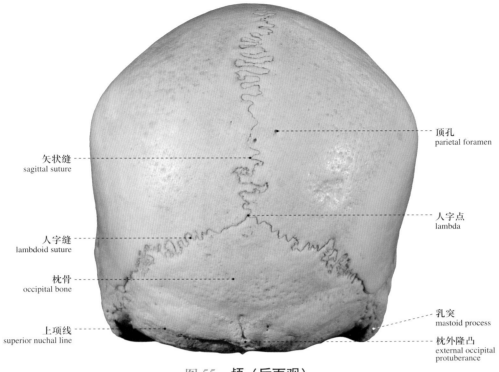

矢状缝
sagittal suture

人字缝
lambdoid suture

枕骨
occipital bone

上项线
superior nuchal line

顶孔
parietal foramen

人字点
lambda

乳突
mastoid process

枕外隆凸
external occipital protuberance

图 55　颅（后面观）
Skull (posterior aspect)

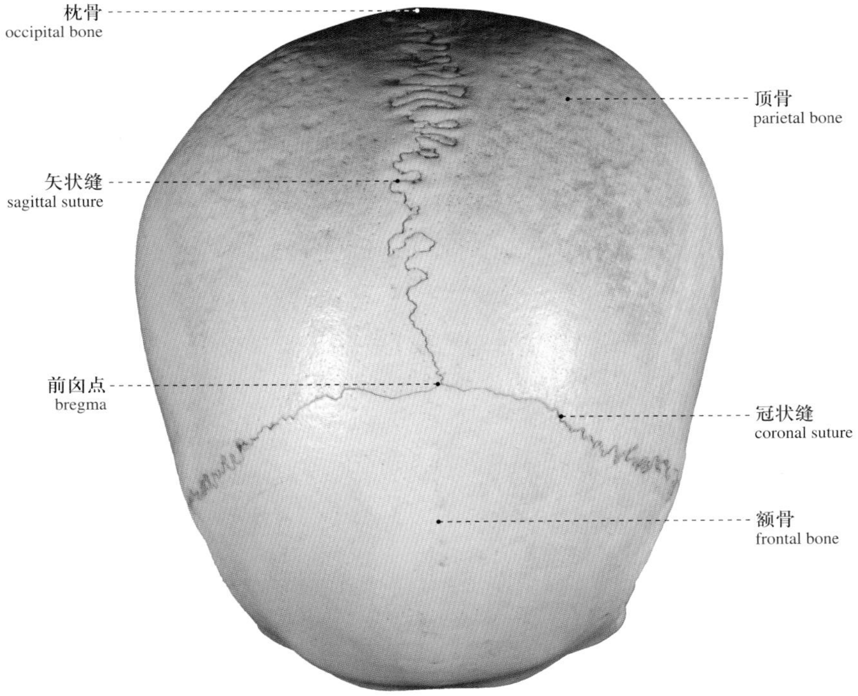

枕骨
occipital bone

矢状缝
sagittal suture

前囟点
bregma

顶骨
parietal bone

冠状缝
coronal suture

额骨
frontal bone

图 56　颅（上面观）
Skull (superior aspect)

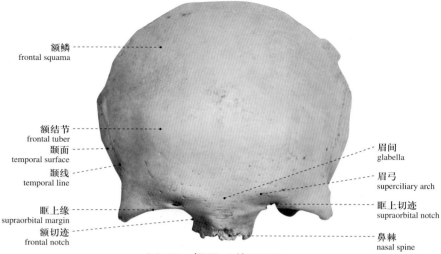

额鳞
frontal squama

额结节
frontal tuber

颞面
temporal surface

颞线
temporal line

眶上缘
supraorbital margin

额切迹
frontal notch

眉间
glabella

眉弓
superciliary arch

眶上切迹
supraorbital notch

鼻棘
nasal spine

图 57　额骨（前面观）

Frontal bone (anterior aspect)

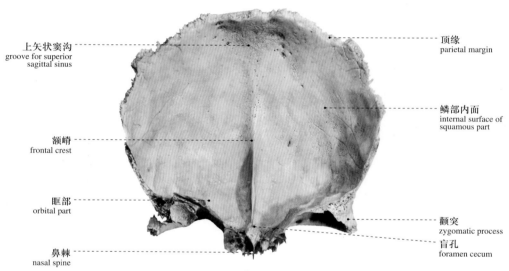

上矢状窦沟
groove for superior
sagittal sinus

额嵴
frontal crest

眶部
orbital part

鼻棘
nasal spine

顶缘
parietal margin

鳞部内面
internal surface of
squamous part

颧突
zygomatic process

盲孔
foramen cecum

图 58　额骨（内面观）

Frontal bone (internal aspect)

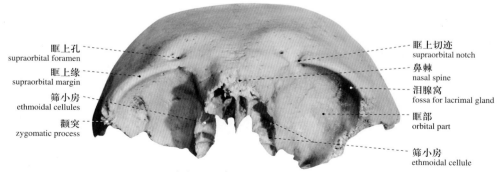

眶上孔
supraorbital foramen

眶上缘
supraorbital margin

筛小房
ethmoidal cellules

颧突
zygomatic process

眶上切迹
supraorbital notch

鼻棘
nasal spine

泪腺窝
fossa for lacrimal gland

眶部
orbital part

筛小房
ethmoidal cellule

图 59　额骨（下面观）

Frontal bone (inferior aspect)

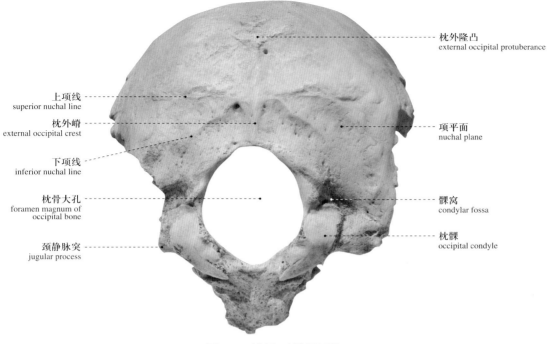

枕外隆凸
external occipital protuberance

上项线
superior nuchal line

枕外嵴
external occipital crest

下项线
inferior nuchal line

枕骨大孔
foramen magnum of occipital bone

颈静脉突
jugular process

项平面
nuchal plane

髁窝
condylar fossa

枕髁
occipital condyle

图 60　**枕骨（外面观）**
Occipital bone (external aspect)

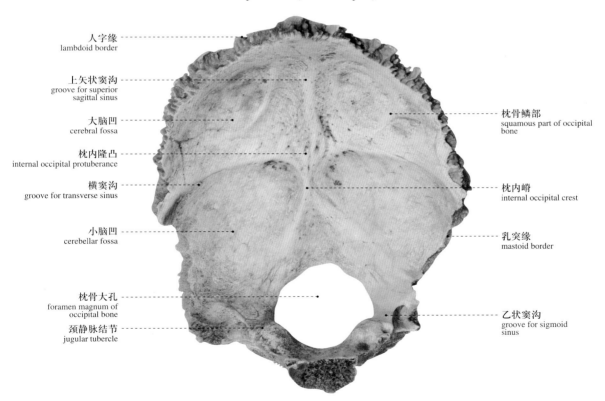

人字缘
lambdoid border

上矢状窦沟
groove for superior sagittal sinus

大脑凹
cerebral fossa

枕内隆凸
internal occipital protuberance

横窦沟
groove for transverse sinus

小脑凹
cerebellar fossa

枕骨大孔
foramen magnum of occipital bone

颈静脉结节
jugular tubercle

枕骨鳞部
squamous part of occipital bone

枕内嵴
internal occipital crest

乳突缘
mastoid border

乙状窦沟
groove for sigmoid sinus

图 61　**枕骨（内面观）**
Occipital bone (internal aspect)

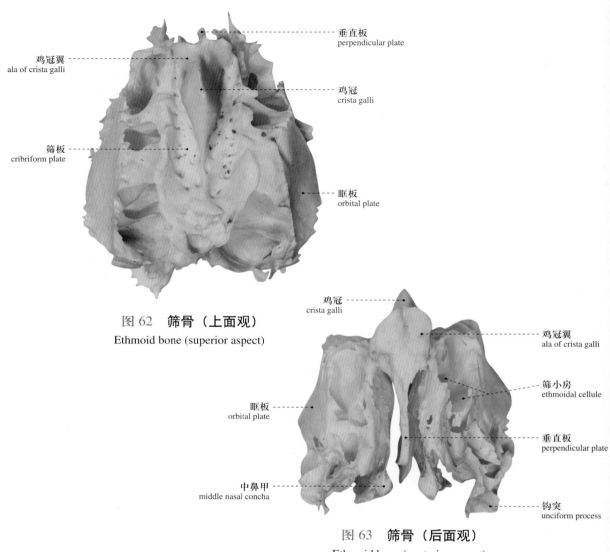

垂直板
perpendicular plate

鸡冠翼
ala of crista galli

鸡冠
crista galli

筛板
cribriform plate

眶板
orbital plate

图 62　筛骨（上面观）
Ethmoid bone (superior aspect)

鸡冠
crista galli

鸡冠翼
ala of crista galli

筛小房
ethmoidal cellule

眶板
orbital plate

垂直板
perpendicular plate

中鼻甲
middle nasal concha

钩突
unciform process

图 63　筛骨（后面观）
Ethmoid bone (posterior aspect)

眶板
orbital plate

鸡冠
crista galli

鸡冠翼
ala of crista galli

筛小房
ethmoidal cellules

图 64　筛骨（侧面观）
Ethmoid bone (lateral aspect)

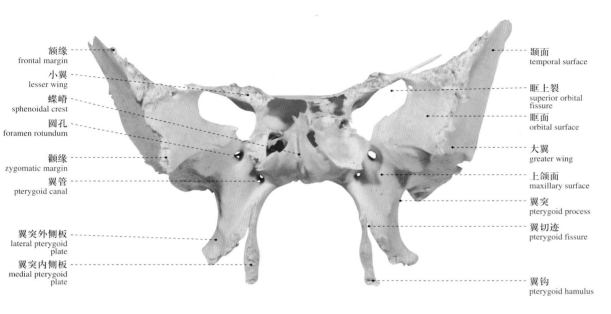

额缘
frontal margin

小翼
lesser wing

蝶嵴
sphenoidal crest

圆孔
foramen rotundum

颧缘
zygomatic margin

翼管
pterygoid canal

翼突外侧板
lateral pterygoid plate

翼突内侧板
medial pterygoid plate

颞面
temporal surface

眶上裂
superior orbital fissure

眶面
orbital surface

大翼
greater wing

上颌面
maxillary surface

翼突
pterygoid process

翼切迹
pterygoid fissure

翼钩
pterygoid hamulus

图 65　蝶骨（前面观）

Sphenoid bone (anterior aspect)

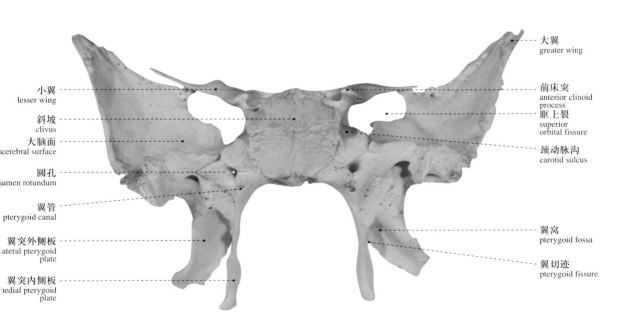

小翼
lesser wing

斜坡
clivus

大脑面
cerebral surface

圆孔
foramen rotundum

翼管
pterygoid canal

翼突外侧板
lateral pterygoid plate

翼突内侧板
medial pterygoid plate

大翼
greater wing

前床突
anterior clinoid process

眶上裂
superior orbital fissure

颈动脉沟
carotid sulcus

翼窝
pterygoid fossa

翼切迹
pterygoid fissure

图 66　蝶骨（后面观）

Sphenoid bone (posterior aspect)

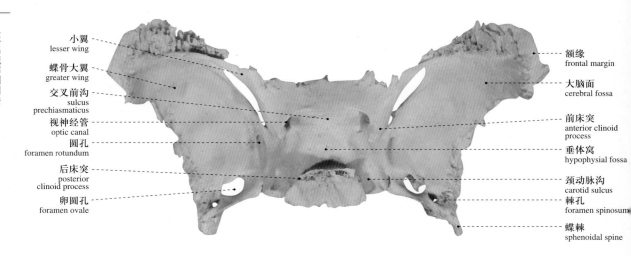

小翼
lesser wing

蝶骨大翼
greater wing

交叉前沟
sulcus
prechiasmaticus

视神经管
optic canal

圆孔
foramen rotundum

后床突
posterior
clinoid process

卵圆孔
foramen ovale

额缘
frontal margin

大脑面
cerebral fossa

前床突
anterior clinoid
process

垂体窝
hypophysial fossa

颈动脉沟
carotid sulcus

棘孔
foramen spinosum

蝶棘
sphenoidal spine

图 67　蝶骨（上面观）
Sphenoid bone (superior aspect)

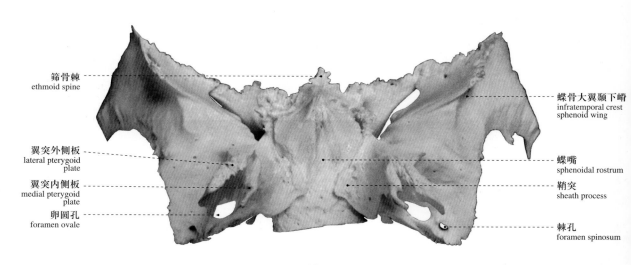

筛骨棘
ethmoid spine

翼突外侧板
lateral pterygoid
plate

翼突内侧板
medial pterygoid
plate

卵圆孔
foramen ovale

蝶骨大翼颞下嵴
infratemporal crest
sphenoid wing

蝶嘴
sphenoidal rostrum

鞘突
sheath process

棘孔
foramen spinosum

图 68　蝶骨（下面观）
Sphenoid (inferior aspect)

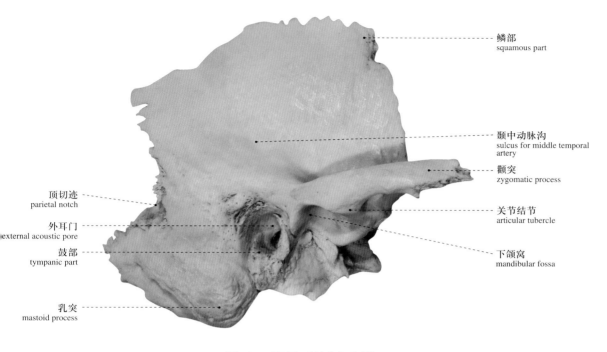

鳞部
squamous part

颞中动脉沟
sulcus for middle temporal
artery

颧突
zygomatic process

顶切迹
parietal notch

外耳门
external acoustic pore

鼓部
tympanic part

乳突
mastoid process

关节结节
articular tubercle

下颌窝
mandibular fossa

图 69　颞骨（外侧面观）
Temporal bone (lateral aspect)

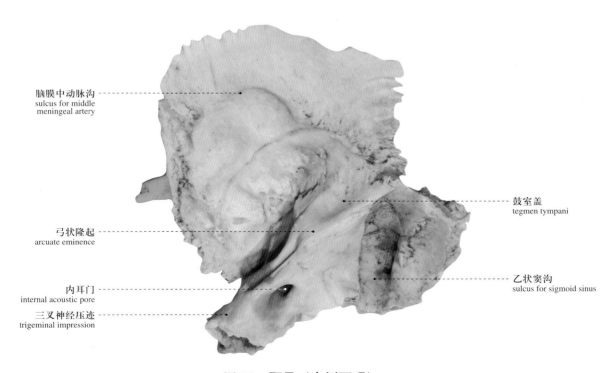

脑膜中动脉沟
sulcus for middle
meningeal artery

弓状隆起
arcuate eminence

内耳门
internal acoustic pore

三叉神经压迹
trigeminal impression

鼓室盖
tegmen tympani

乙状窦沟
sulcus for sigmoid sinus

图 70　颞骨（内侧面观）
Temporal bone (medial aspect)

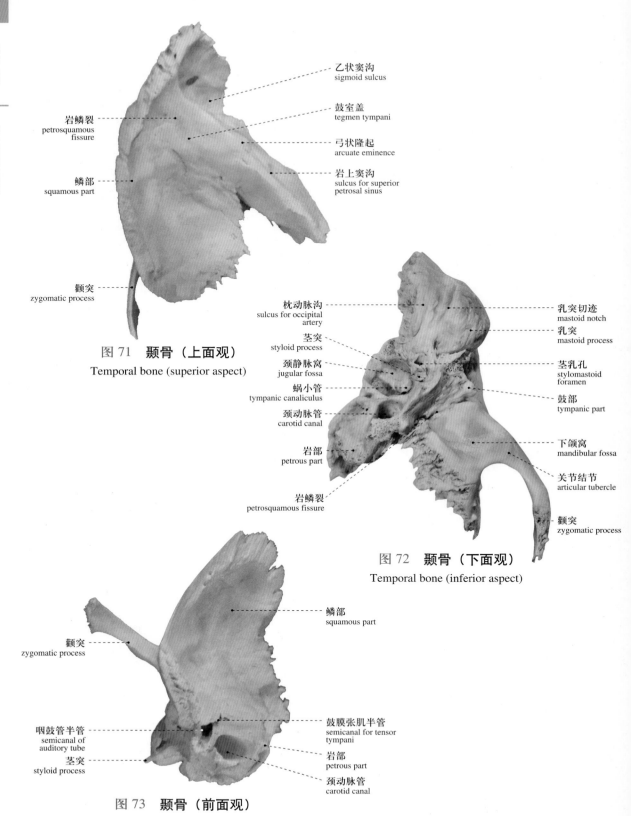

乙状窦沟
sigmoid sulcus

鼓室盖
tegmen tympani

弓状隆起
arcuate eminence

岩上窦沟
sulcus for superior
petrosal sinus

岩鳞裂
petrosquamous
fissure

鳞部
squamous part

颧突
zygomatic process

图 71　颞骨（上面观）
Temporal bone (superior aspect)

枕动脉沟
sulcus for occipital
artery

茎突
styloid process

颈静脉窝
jugular fossa

蜗小管
tympanic canaliculus

颈动脉管
carotid canal

岩部
petrous part

岩鳞裂
petrosquamous fissure

乳突切迹
mastoid notch

乳突
mastoid process

茎乳孔
stylomastoid
foramen

鼓部
tympanic part

下颌窝
mandibular fossa

关节结节
articular tubercle

颧突
zygomatic process

图 72　颞骨（下面观）
Temporal bone (inferior aspect)

鳞部
squamous part

颧突
zygomatic process

咽鼓管半管
semicanal of
auditory tube

茎突
styloid process

鼓膜张肌半管
semicanal for tensor
tympani

岩部
petrous part

颈动脉管
carotid canal

图 73　颞骨（前面观）
Temporal bone (anterior aspect)

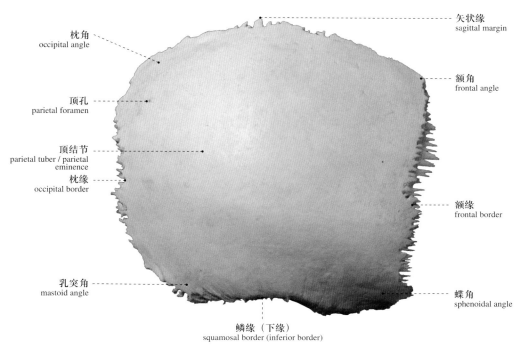

枕角
occipital angle

顶孔
parietal foramen

顶结节
parietal tuber / parietal
eminence

枕缘
occipital border

乳突角
mastoid angle

矢状缘
sagittal margin

额角
frontal angle

额缘
frontal border

蝶角
sphenoidal angle

鳞缘（下缘）
squamosal border (inferior border)

图 74　右侧顶骨（外侧面观）
Right parietal bone (lateral aspect)

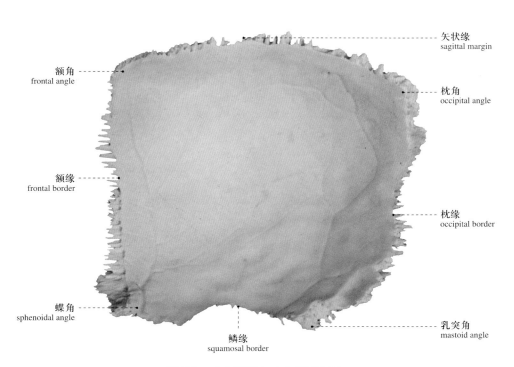

额角
frontal angle

额缘
frontal border

蝶角
sphenoidal angle

矢状缘
sagittal margin

枕角
occipital angle

枕缘
occipital border

乳突角
mastoid angle

鳞缘
squamosal border

图 75　右侧顶骨（内侧面观）
Right parietal bone (medial aspect)

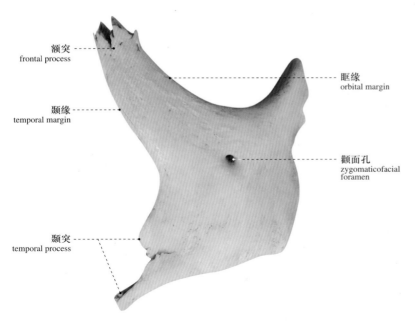

额突
frontal process

眶缘
orbital margin

颞缘
temporal margin

颧面孔
zygomaticofacial
foramen

颞突
temporal process

图 76　**右侧颧骨（外侧面观）**
Right zygomatic bone (lateral aspect)

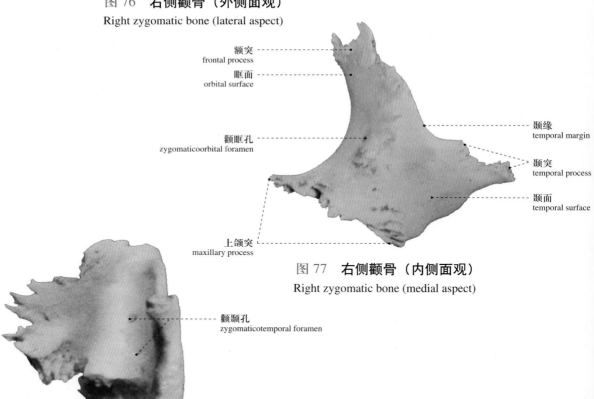

额突
frontal process

眶面
orbital surface

颞缘
temporal margin

颧眶孔
zygomaticoorbital foramen

颞突
temporal process

颞面
temporal surface

上颌突
maxillary process

图 77　**右侧颧骨（内侧面观）**
Right zygomatic bone (medial aspect)

颧颞孔
zygomaticotemporal foramen

图 78　**右侧颧骨（后面观）**
Right zygomatic bone (posterior aspect)

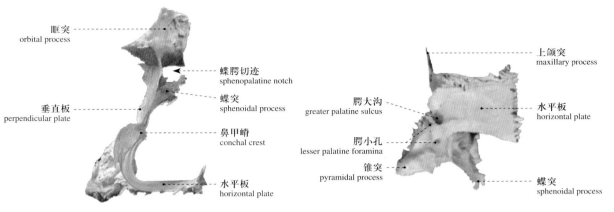

眶突
orbital process

蝶腭切迹
sphenopalatine notch

蝶突
sphenoidal process

鼻甲嵴
conchal crest

水平板
horizontal plate

垂直板
perpendicular plate

图 79 右侧腭骨（前面观）
Right palatine bone (anterior aspect)

上颌突
maxillary process

腭大沟
greater palatine sulcus

水平板
horizontal plate

腭小孔
lesser palatine foramina

锥突
pyramidal process

蝶突
sphenoidal process

图 80 右侧腭骨（下面观）
Right palatine bone (inferior aspect)

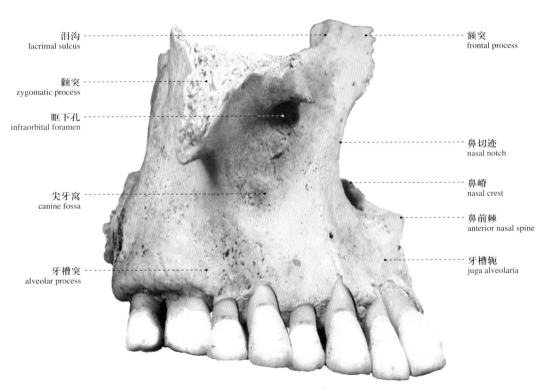

泪沟
lacrimal sulcus

颧突
zygomatic process

眶下孔
infraorbital foramen

尖牙窝
canine fossa

牙槽突
alveolar process

额突
frontal process

鼻切迹
nasal notch

鼻嵴
nasal crest

鼻前棘
anterior nasal spine

牙槽轭
juga alveolaria

图 81 右侧上颌骨（前面观）
Right maxillary bone (anterior aspect)

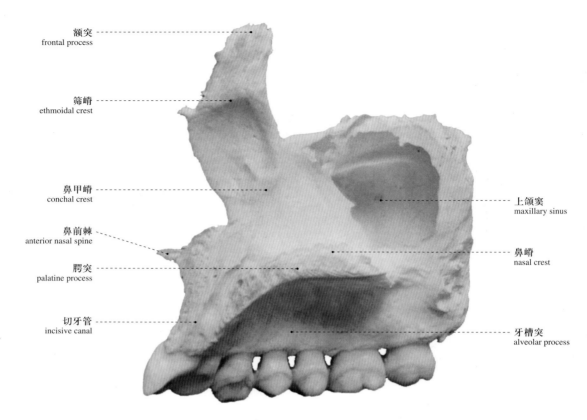

额突
frontal process

筛嵴
ethmoidal crest

鼻甲嵴
conchal crest

鼻前棘
anterior nasal spine

腭突
palatine process

切牙管
incisive canal

上颌窦
maxillary sinus

鼻嵴
nasal crest

牙槽突
alveolar process

图 82　右侧上颌骨（内侧面观）
Right maxillary (medial aspect)

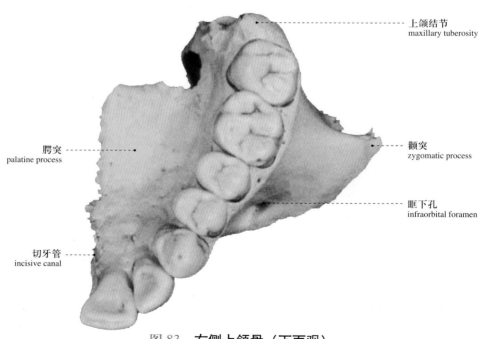

上颌结节
maxillary tuberosity

腭突
palatine process

颧突
zygomatic process

眶下孔
infraorbital foramen

切牙管
incisive canal

图 83　右侧上颌骨（下面观）
Right maxillary (inferior aspect)

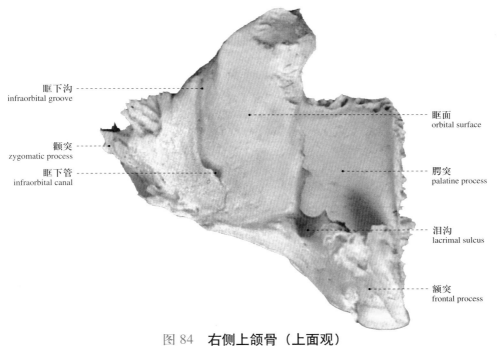

眶下沟
infraorbital groove

颧突
zygomatic process

眶下管
infraorbital canal

眶面
orbital surface

腭突
palatine process

泪沟
lacrimal sulcus

额突
frontal process

图 84　右侧上颌骨（上面观）
Right maxillary (superior aspect)

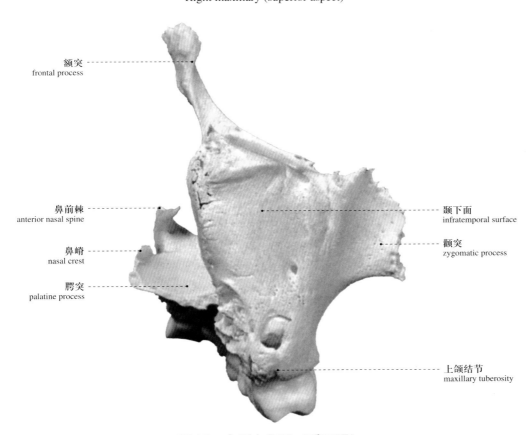

额突
frontal process

鼻前棘
anterior nasal spine

鼻嵴
nasal crest

腭突
palatine process

颞下面
infratemporal surface

颧突
zygomatic process

上颌结节
maxillary tuberosity

图 85　右侧上颌骨（后面观）
Right maxillary (posterior aspect)

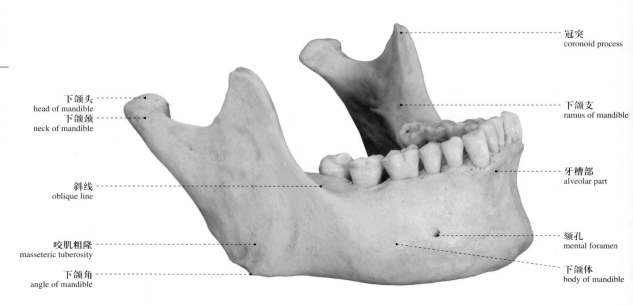

冠突
coronoid process

下颌头
head of mandible

下颌颈
neck of mandible

下颌支
ramus of mandible

斜线
oblique line

牙槽部
alveolar part

咬肌粗隆
masseteric tuberosity

颏孔
mental foramen

下颌角
angle of mandible

下颌体
body of mandible

图 86　下颌骨（外侧面观）
Mandible (lateral aspect)

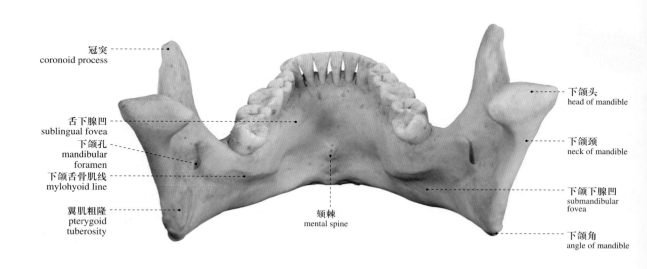

冠突
coronoid process

舌下腺凹
sublingual fovea

下颌孔
mandibular foramen

下颌舌骨肌线
mylohyoid line

翼肌粗隆
pterygoid tuberosity

颏棘
mental spine

下颌头
head of mandible

下颌颈
neck of mandible

下颌下腺凹
submandibular fovea

下颌角
angle of mandible

图 87　下颌骨（后面观）
Mandible (posterior aspect)

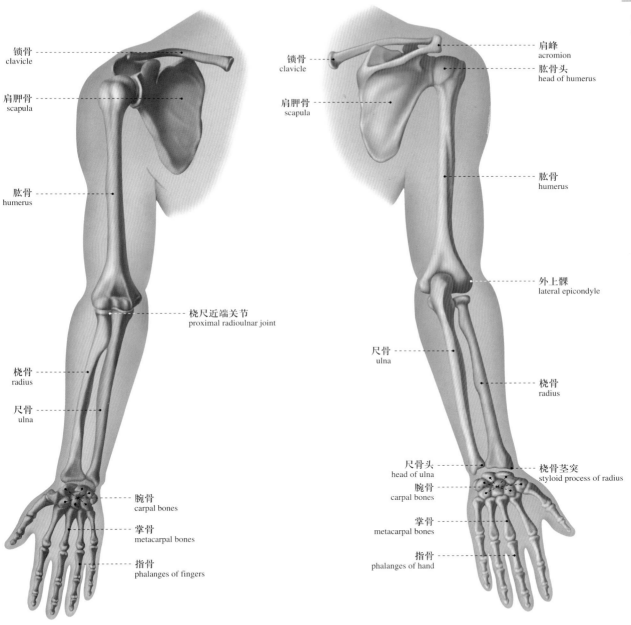

锁骨
clavicle

肩胛骨
scapula

肱骨
humerus

桡尺近端关节
proximal radioulnar joint

桡骨
radius

尺骨
ulna

腕骨
carpal bones

掌骨
metacarpal bones

指骨
phalanges of fingers

锁骨
clavicle

肩胛骨
scapula

肩峰
acromion

肱骨头
head of humerus

肱骨
humerus

外上髁
lateral epicondyle

尺骨
ulna

桡骨
radius

尺骨头
head of ulna

桡骨茎突
styloid process of radius

腕骨
carpal bones

掌骨
metacarpal bones

指骨
phalanges of hand

图 88　上肢骨（前面观）
Bones of the upper limb (anterior aspect)

图 89　上肢骨（后面观）
Bones of the upper limb (posterior aspect)

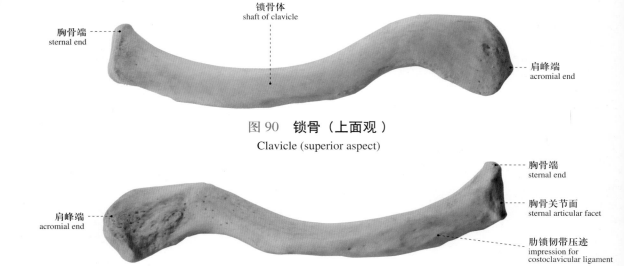

图 90　锁骨（上面观）
Clavicle (superior aspect)

胸骨端
sternal end

锁骨体
shaft of clavicle

肩峰端
acromial end

肩峰端
acromial end

胸骨端
sternal end

胸骨关节面
sternal articular facet

肋锁韧带压迹
impression for
costoclavicular ligament

图 91　锁骨（下面观）
Clavicle (inferior aspect)

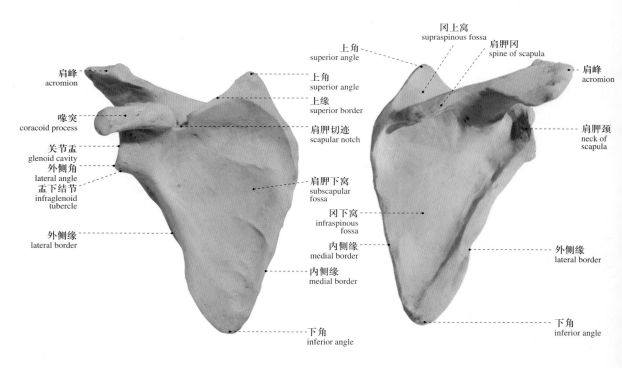

肩峰
acromion

喙突
coracoid process

关节盂
glenoid cavity

外侧角
lateral angle

盂下结节
infraglenoid
tubercle

外侧缘
lateral border

上角
superior angle

上角
superior angle

上缘
superior border

肩胛切迹
scapular notch

肩胛下窝
subscapular
fossa

内侧缘
medial border

内侧缘
medial border

下角
inferior angle

图 92　肩胛骨（前面观）
Scapula (anterior aspect)

冈上窝
supraspinous fossa

肩胛冈
spine of scapula

肩峰
acromion

肩胛颈
neck of
scapula

冈下窝
infraspinous fossa

外侧缘
lateral border

下角
inferior angle

图 93　肩胛骨（后面观）
Scapula (posterior aspect)

44

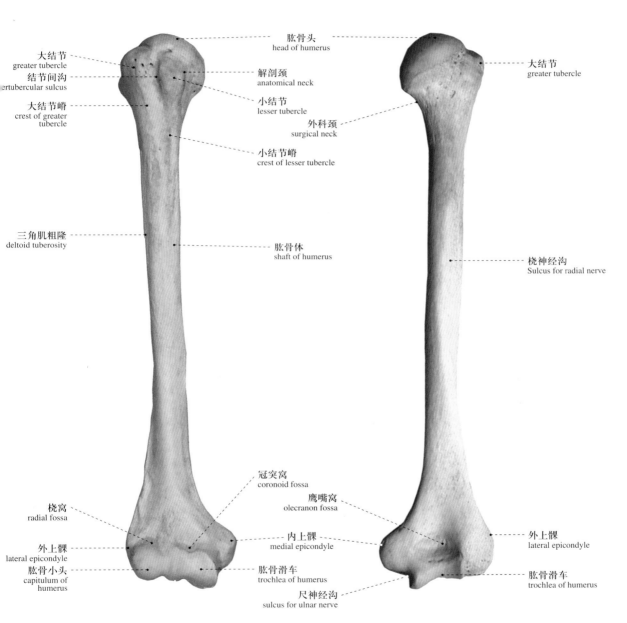

肱骨头
head of humerus

大结节
greater tubercle

大结节
greater tubercle

结节间沟
ertubercular sulcus

解剖颈
anatomical neck

大结节嵴
crest of greater
tubercle

小结节
lesser tubercle

外科颈
surgical neck

小结节嵴
crest of lesser tubercle

三角肌粗隆
deltoid tuberosity

肱骨体
shaft of humerus

桡神经沟
Sulcus for radial nerve

冠突窝
coronoid fossa

鹰嘴窝
olecranon fossa

桡窝
radial fossa

外上髁
lateral epicondyle

肱骨小头
capitulum of
humerus

内上髁
medial epicondyle

肱骨滑车
trochlea of humerus

尺神经沟
sulcus for ulnar nerve

外上髁
lateral epicondyle

肱骨滑车
trochlea of humerus

图 94　肱骨（前面观）
Humerus (anterior aspect)

图 95　肱骨（后面观）
Humerus (posterior aspect)

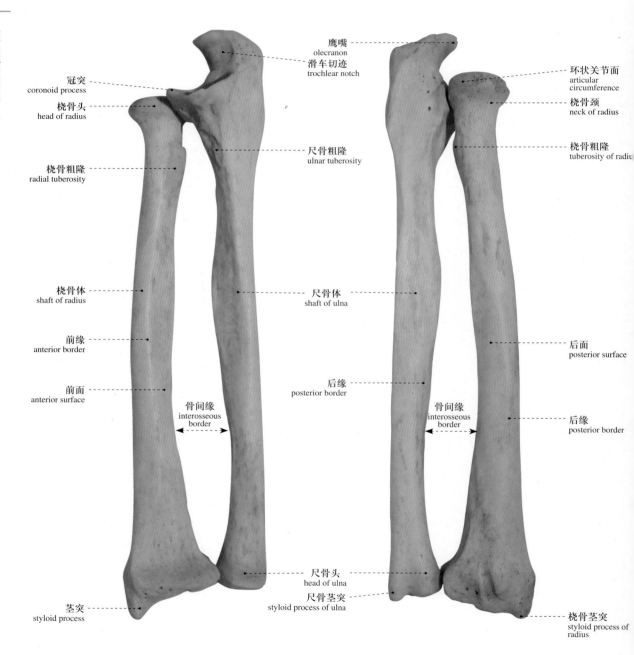

鹰嘴
olecranon

滑车切迹
trochlear notch

冠突
coronoid process

桡骨头
head of radius

环状关节面
articular circumference

桡骨颈
neck of radius

尺骨粗隆
ulnar tuberosity

桡骨粗隆
tuberosity of radius

桡骨粗隆
radial tuberosity

桡骨体
shaft of radius

尺骨体
shaft of ulna

前缘
anterior border

后面
posterior surface

前面
anterior surface

后缘
posterior border

后缘
posterior border

骨间缘
interosseous border

骨间缘
interosseous border

尺骨头
head of ulna

尺骨茎突
styloid process of ulna

茎突
styloid process

桡骨茎突
styloid process of radius

图 96　桡骨和尺骨（前面观）
Radius and the ulna (anterior aspect)

图 97　桡骨和尺骨（后面观）
Radius and the ulna (posterior aspect)

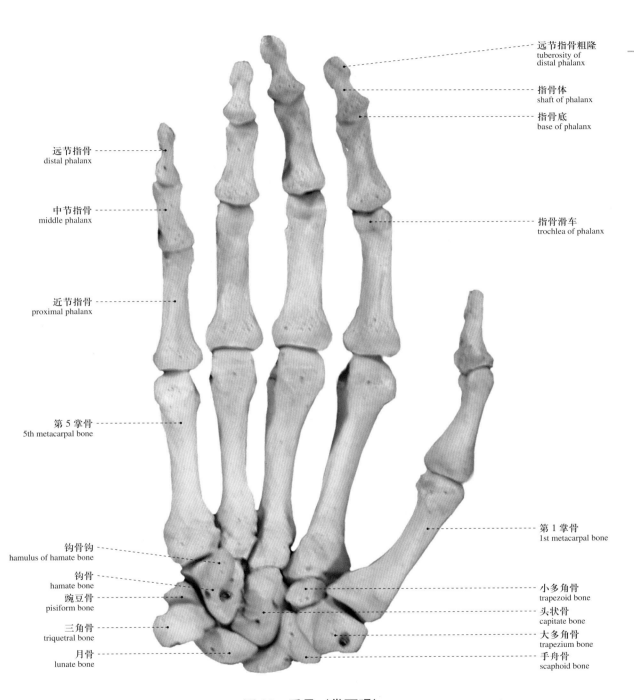

远节指骨粗隆
tuberosity of
distal phalanx

指骨体
shaft of phalanx

指骨底
base of phalanx

远节指骨
distal phalanx

中节指骨
middle phalanx

指骨滑车
trochlea of phalanx

近节指骨
proximal phalanx

第 5 掌骨
5th metacarpal bone

第 1 掌骨
1st metacarpal bone

钩骨钩
hamulus of hamate bone

钩骨
hamate bone

豌豆骨
pisiform bone

小多角骨
trapezoid bone

头状骨
capitate bone

三角骨
triquetral bone

大多角骨
trapezium bone

月骨
lunate bone

手舟骨
scaphoid bone

图 98　手骨（掌面观）
Bones of the hand (palmar aspect)

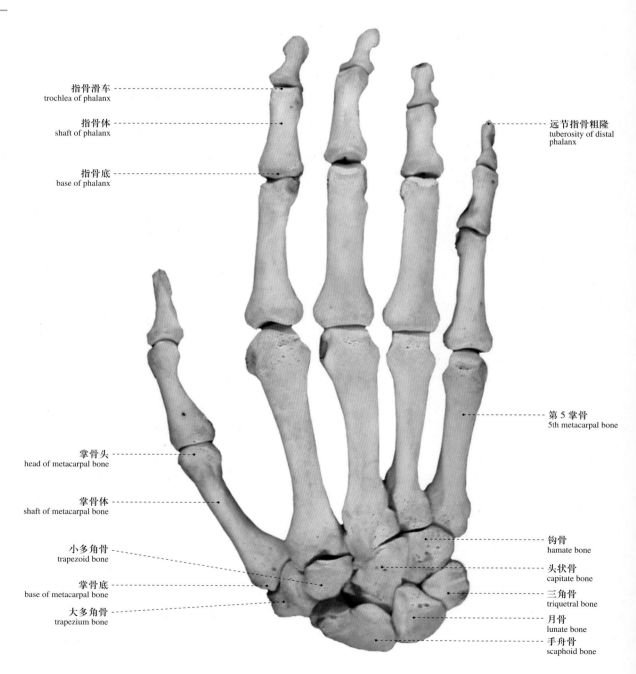

指骨滑车
trochlea of phalanx

指骨体
shaft of phalanx

指骨底
base of phalanx

远节指骨粗隆
tuberosity of distal phalanx

第 5 掌骨
5th metacarpal bone

掌骨头
head of metacarpal bone

掌骨体
shaft of metacarpal bone

小多角骨
trapezoid bone

掌骨底
base of metacarpal bone

大多角骨
trapezium bone

钩骨
hamate bone

头状骨
capitate bone

三角骨
triquetral bone

月骨
lunate bone

手舟骨
scaphoid bone

图 99　手骨（背面观）
Bones of the hand (dorsal aspect)

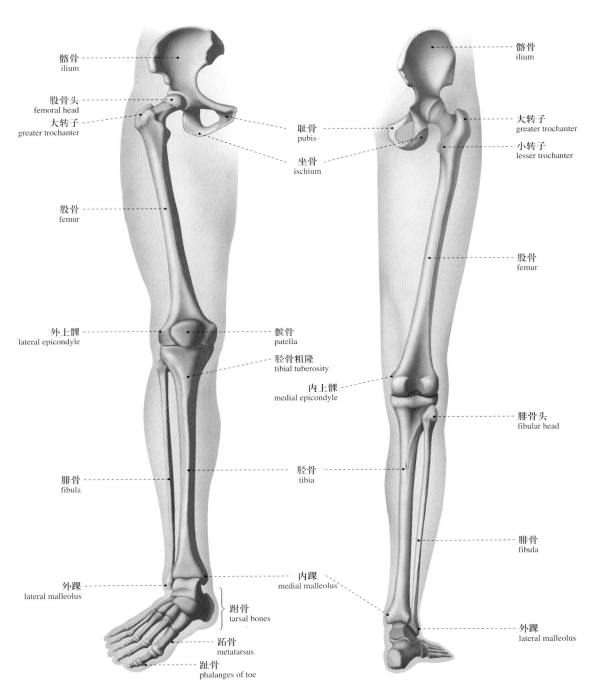

髂骨
ilium

股骨头
femoral head

大转子
greater trochanter

股骨
femur

外上髁
lateral epicondyle

腓骨
fibula

外踝
lateral malleolus

髂骨
ilium

大转子
greater trochanter

小转子
lesser trochanter

股骨
femur

耻骨
pubis

坐骨
ischium

髌骨
patella

胫骨粗隆
tibial tuberosity

内上髁
medial epicondyle

腓骨头
fibular head

胫骨
tibia

腓骨
fibula

内踝
medial malleolus

外踝
lateral malleolus

跗骨
tarsal bones

跖骨
metatarsus

趾骨
phalanges of toe

图 100　下肢骨（前面观）
Bones of the lower limb (anterior aspect)

图 101　下肢骨（后面观）
Bones of the lower limb (posterior aspect)

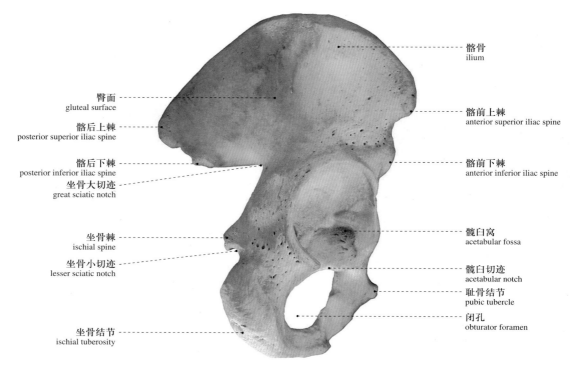

臀面
gluteal surface

髂后上棘
posterior superior iliac spine

髂后下棘
posterior inferior iliac spine

坐骨大切迹
great sciatic notch

坐骨棘
ischial spine

坐骨小切迹
lesser sciatic notch

坐骨结节
ischial tuberosity

髂骨
ilium

髂前上棘
anterior superior iliac spine

髂前下棘
anterior inferior iliac spine

髋臼窝
acetabular fossa

髋臼切迹
acetabular notch

耻骨结节
pubic tubercle

闭孔
obturator foramen

图 102　右髋骨（外侧面观）
Right hip bone (lateral aspect)

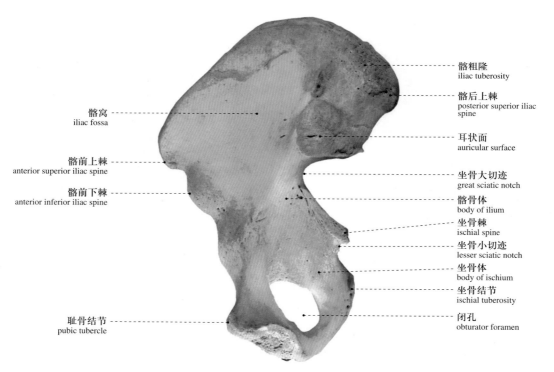

髂窝
iliac fossa

髂前上棘
anterior superior iliac spine

髂前下棘
anterior inferior iliac spine

耻骨结节
pubic tubercle

髂粗隆
iliac tuberosity

髂后上棘
posterior superior iliac spine

耳状面
auricular surface

坐骨大切迹
great sciatic notch

髂骨体
body of ilium

坐骨棘
ischial spine

坐骨小切迹
lesser sciatic notch

坐骨体
body of ischium

坐骨结节
ischial tuberosity

闭孔
obturator foramen

图 103　右髋骨（内侧面观）
Right hip bone (medial aspect)

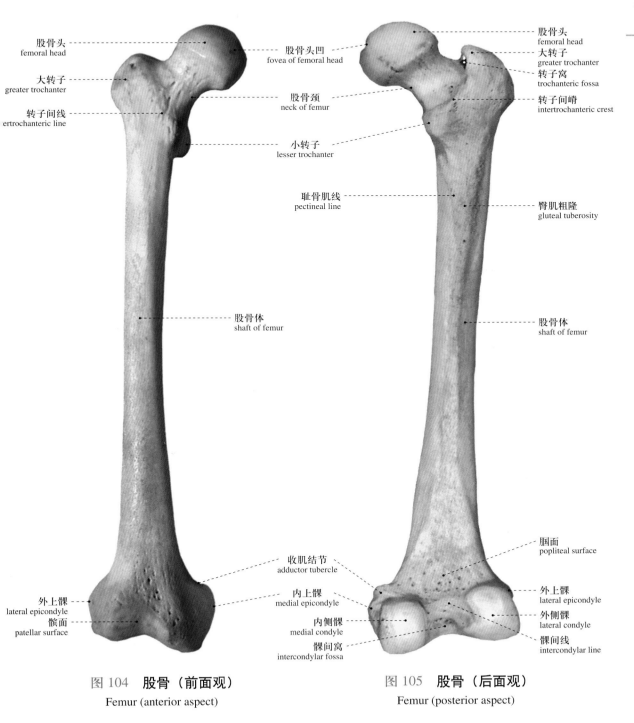

股骨头
femoral head

股骨头凹
fovea of femoral head

大转子
greater trochanter

转子间线
ertrochanteric line

股骨颈
neck of femur

小转子
lesser trochanter

耻骨肌线
pectineal line

股骨体
shaft of femur

收肌结节
adductor tubercle

内上髁
medial epicondyle

内侧髁
medial condyle

髁间窝
intercondylar fossa

外上髁
lateral epicondyle

髌面
patellar surface

图 104　股骨（前面观）
Femur (anterior aspect)

股骨头
femoral head

大转子
greater trochanter

转子窝
trochanteric fossa

转子间嵴
intertrochanteric crest

臀肌粗隆
gluteal tuberosity

股骨体
shaft of femur

腘面
popliteal surface

外上髁
lateral epicondyle

外侧髁
lateral condyle

髁间线
intercondylar line

图 105　股骨（后面观）
Femur (posterior aspect)

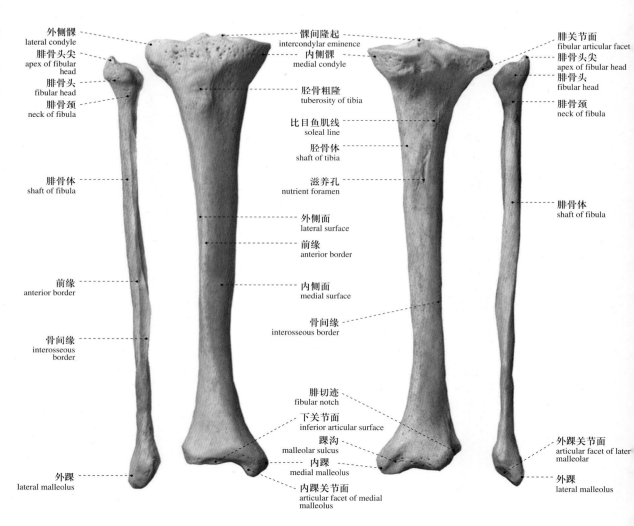

外侧髁
lateral condyle

腓骨头尖
apex of fibular head

腓骨头
fibular head

腓骨颈
neck of fibula

腓骨体
shaft of fibula

前缘
anterior border

骨间缘
interosseous border

外踝
lateral malleolus

髁间隆起
intercondylar eminence

内侧髁
medial condyle

胫骨粗隆
tuberosity of tibia

比目鱼肌线
soleal line

胫骨体
shaft of tibia

滋养孔
nutrient foramen

外侧面
lateral surface

前缘
anterior border

内侧面
medial surface

骨间缘
interosseous border

腓切迹
fibular notch

下关节面
inferior articular surface

踝沟
malleolar sulcus

内踝
medial malleolus

内踝关节面
articular facet of medial malleolus

腓关节面
fibular articular facet

腓骨头尖
apex of fibular head

腓骨头
fibular head

腓骨颈
neck of fibula

腓骨体
shaft of fibula

外踝关节面
articular facet of later malleolar

外踝
lateral malleolus

图 106　胫、腓骨（前面观）
Tibia and the fibula (anterior aspect)

图 107　胫、腓骨（后面观）
Tibia and the fibula (posterior aspect)

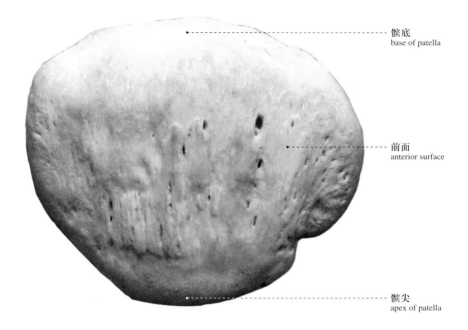

髌底
base of patella

前面
anterior surface

髌尖
apex of patella

图 108　髌骨（前面观）
Patella (anterior aspect)

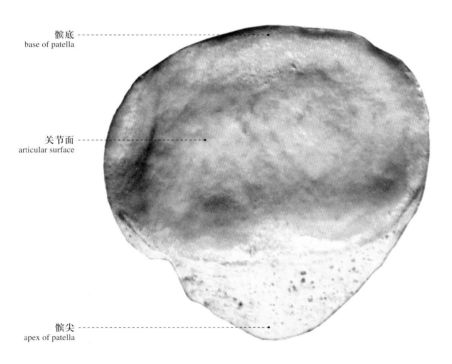

髌底
base of patella

关节面
articular surface

髌尖
apex of patella

图 109　髌骨（后面观）
Patella (posterior aspect)

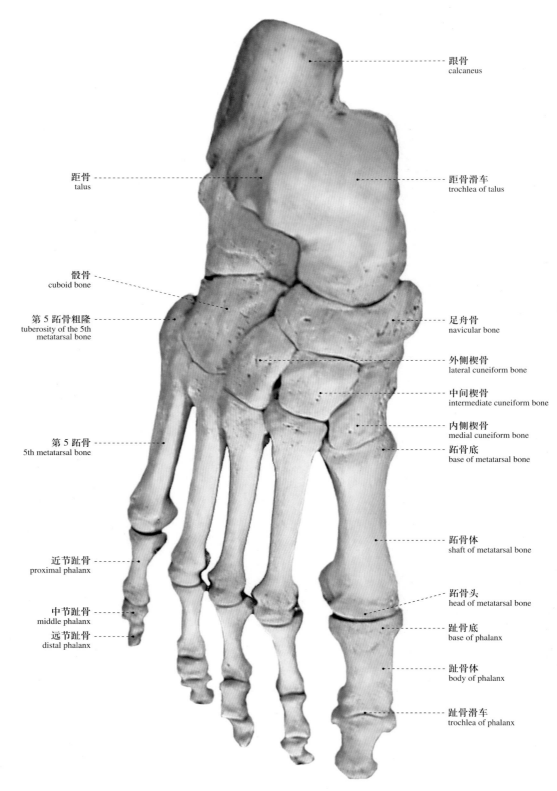

跟骨
calcaneus

距骨
talus

距骨滑车
trochlea of talus

骰骨
cuboid bone

足舟骨
navicular bone

第 5 跖骨粗隆
tuberosity of the 5th metatarsal bone

外侧楔骨
lateral cuneiform bone

中间楔骨
intermediate cuneiform bone

内侧楔骨
medial cuneiform bone

第 5 跖骨
5th metatarsal bone

跖骨底
base of metatarsal bone

跖骨体
shaft of metatarsal bone

近节趾骨
proximal phalanx

跖骨头
head of metatarsal bone

趾骨底
base of phalanx

中节趾骨
middle phalanx

远节趾骨
distal phalanx

趾骨体
body of phalanx

趾骨滑车
trochlea of phalanx

图 110 足骨（背面观）
Bones of the foot (dorsal aspect)

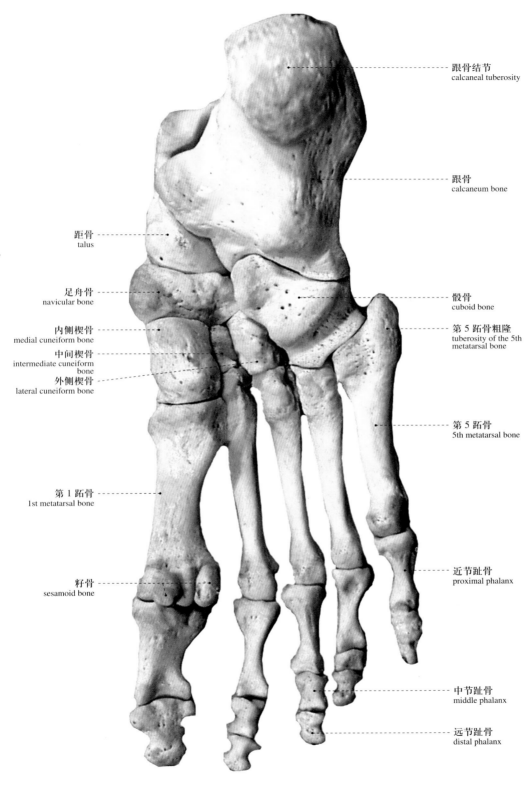

跟骨结节
calcaneal tuberosity

跟骨
calcaneum bone

距骨
talus

足舟骨
navicular bone

骰骨
cuboid bone

内侧楔骨
medial cuneiform bone

第 5 跖骨粗隆
tuberosity of the 5th
metatarsal bone

中间楔骨
intermediate cuneiform
bone

外侧楔骨
lateral cuneiform bone

第 5 跖骨
5th metatarsal bone

第 1 跖骨
1st metatarsal bone

近节趾骨
proximal phalanx

籽骨
sesamoid bone

中节趾骨
middle phalanx

远节趾骨
distal phalanx

图 111　足骨（跖面观）
Bones of the foot (plantar aspect)

第一节

骨连结的方式

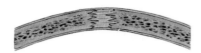

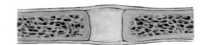

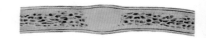

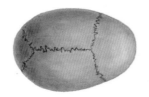

图 112　纤维连结（颅的缝）
Fibrous joint (suture)

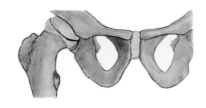

图 113　软骨连结（耻骨联合）
Cartilaginous joint (pubic symphysis)

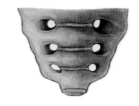

图 114　骨性结合（融合骶骨）
Synostoses (fused sacrum)

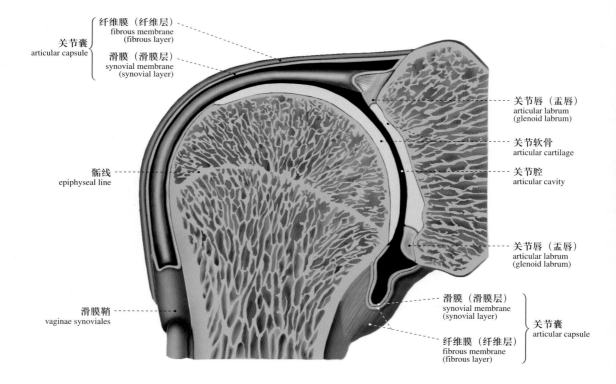

关节囊 { 纤维膜（纤维层）fibrous membrane (fibrous layer)
articular capsule { 滑膜（滑膜层）synovial membrane (synovial layer)

关节唇（盂唇）articular labrum (glenoid labrum)

关节软骨 articular cartilage

骺线 epiphyseal line

关节腔 articular cavity

关节唇（盂唇）articular labrum (glenoid labrum)

滑膜鞘 vaginae synoviales

滑膜（滑膜层）synovial membrane (synovial layer)

纤维膜（纤维层）fibrous membrane (fibrous layer)

关节囊 articular capsule

图 115　滑膜关节
Synovial joint

第二节

中轴骨的连结

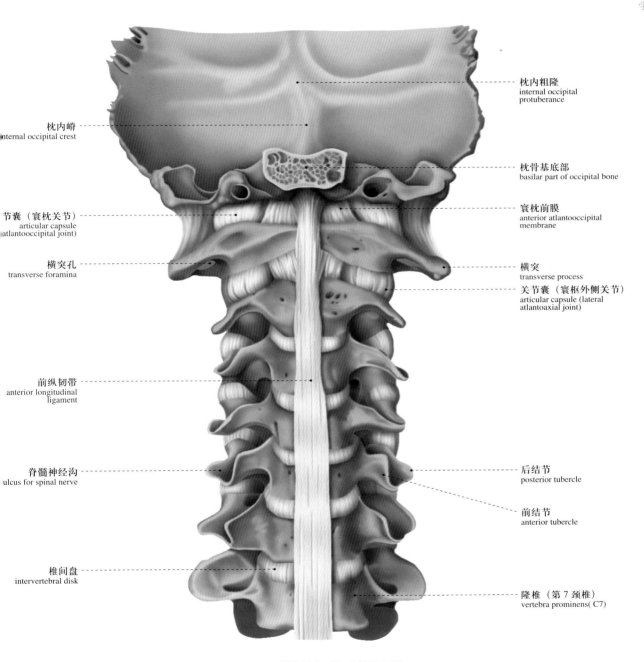

枕内粗隆
internal occipital protuberance

枕内嵴
internal occipital crest

枕骨基底部
basilar part of occipital bone

节囊（寰枕关节）
articular capsule (atlantooccipital joint)

寰枕前膜
anterior atlantooccipital membrane

横突孔
transverse foramina

横突
transverse process

关节囊（寰枢外侧关节）
articular capsule (lateral atlantoaxial joint)

前纵韧带
anterior longitudinal ligament

脊髓神经沟
sulcus for spinal nerve

后结节
posterior tubercle

前结节
anterior tubercle

椎间盘
intervertebral disk

隆椎（第7颈椎）
vertebra prominens(C7)

图 116　颈椎的韧带（前面观）
Ligaments of the cervical vertebrae (anterior aspect)

57

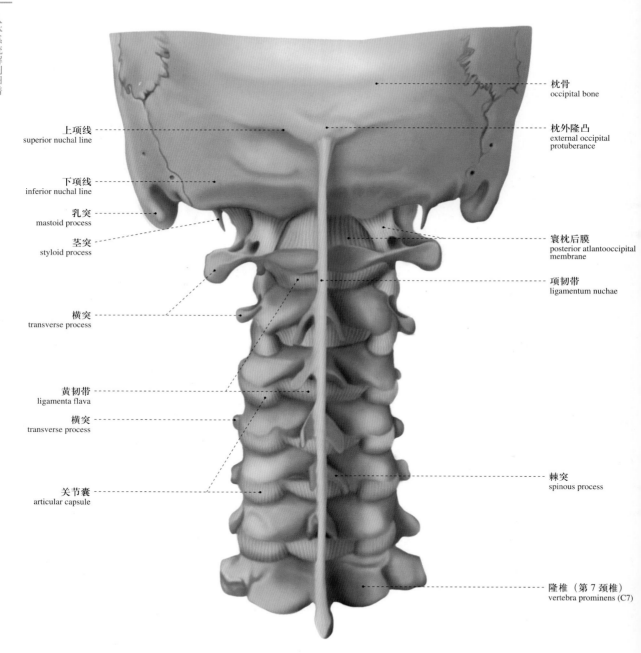

枕骨
occipital bone

上项线
superior nuchal line

枕外隆凸
external occipital protuberance

下项线
inferior nuchal line

乳突
mastoid process

茎突
styloid process

寰枕后膜
posterior atlantooccipital membrane

项韧带
ligamentum nuchae

横突
transverse process

黄韧带
ligamenta flava

横突
transverse process

棘突
spinous process

关节囊
articular capsule

隆椎（第 7 颈椎）
vertebra prominens (C7)

图 117　颈椎的韧带（后面观）
Ligaments of the cervical vertebrae (posterior aspect)

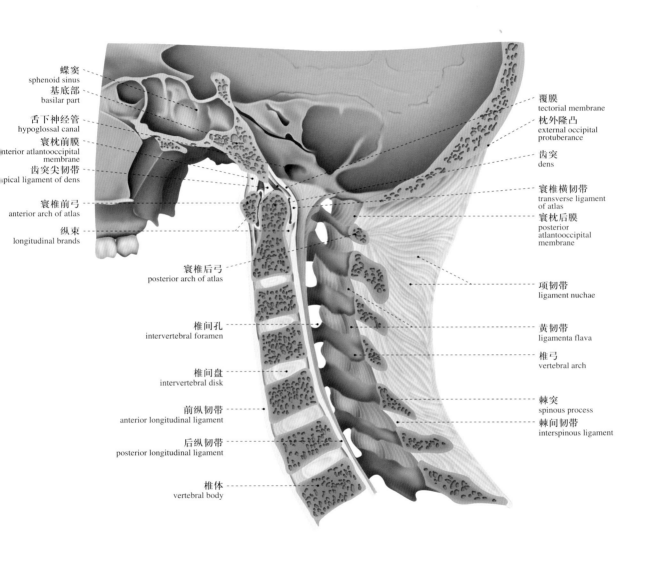

蝶窦
sphenoid sinus

基底部
basilar part

舌下神经管
hypoglossal canal

寰枕前膜
anterior atlantooccipital membrane

齿突尖韧带
apical ligament of dens

寰椎前弓
anterior arch of atlas

纵束
longitudinal brands

寰椎后弓
posterior arch of atlas

椎间孔
intervertebral foramen

椎间盘
intervertebral disk

前纵韧带
anterior longitudinal ligament

后纵韧带
posterior longitudinal ligament

椎体
vertebral body

覆膜
tectorial membrane

枕外隆凸
external occipital protuberance

齿突
dens

寰椎横韧带
transverse ligament of atlas

寰枕后膜
posterior atlantooccipital membrane

项韧带
ligament nuchae

黄韧带
ligamenta flava

椎弓
vertebral arch

棘突
spinous process

棘间韧带
interspinous ligament

图 118　颈椎的韧带（侧面观）

Ligaments of the cervical vertebrae (lateral aspect)

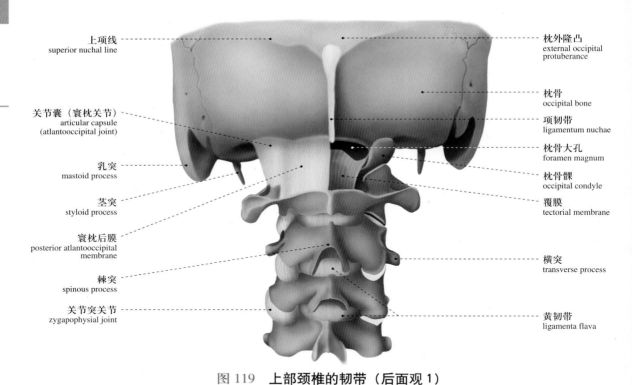

上项线
superior nuchal line

枕外隆凸
external occipital
protuberance

关节囊（寰枕关节）
articular capsule
(atlantooccipital joint)

枕骨
occipital bone

项韧带
ligamentum nuchae

乳突
mastoid process

枕骨大孔
foramen magnum

茎突
styloid process

枕骨髁
occipital condyle

寰枕后膜
posterior atlantooccipital
membrane

覆膜
tectorial membrane

棘突
spinous process

横突
transverse process

关节突关节
zygapophysial joint

黄韧带
ligamenta flava

图 119　上部颈椎的韧带（后面观 1）
Ligaments of the upper cervical spine (posterior aspect 1)

颞骨
temporal bone

枕外隆凸
external occipital
protuberance

枕外嵴
external occipital crest

寰枕后膜
posterior atlantooccipital
membrane

乳突
mastoid process

寰枕关节
atlantooccipital joint

茎突
styloid process

关节囊（寰枕关节）
articular capsule
(atlantooccipital joint)

覆膜
tectorial membrane

后纵韧带
posterior longitudinal
ligament

椎弓
vertebral arch

图 120　上部颈椎的韧带（后面观 2）
Ligaments of the upper cervical spine (posterior aspect 2)

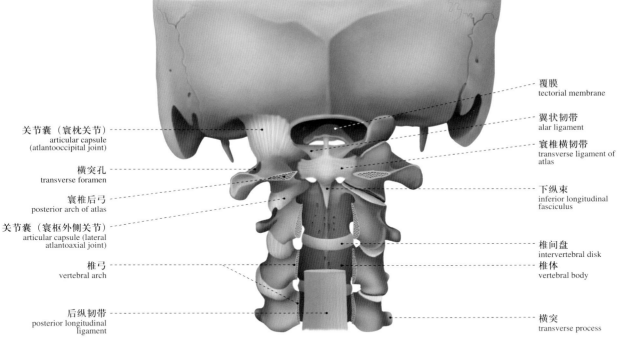

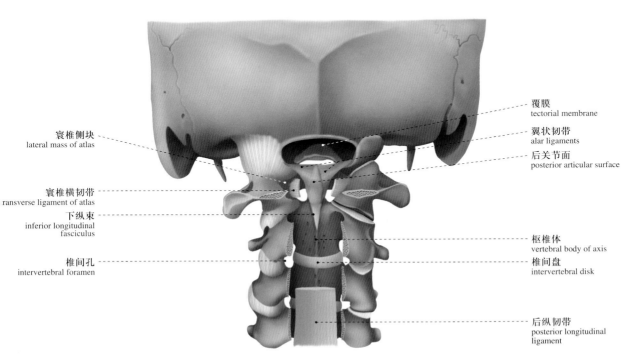

图 121　上部颈椎的韧带（后面观 3）

Ligaments of the upper cervical spine (posterior aspect 3)

关节囊（寰枕关节）
articular capsule
(atlantooccipital joint)

横突孔
transverse foramen

寰椎后弓
posterior arch of atlas

关节囊（寰枢外侧关节）
articular capsule (lateral
atlantoaxial joint)

椎弓
vertebral arch

后纵韧带
posterior longitudinal
ligament

覆膜
tectorial membrane

翼状韧带
alar ligament

寰椎横韧带
transverse ligament of
atlas

下纵束
inferior longitudinal
fasciculus

椎间盘
intervertebral disk

椎体
vertebral body

横突
transverse process

寰椎侧块
lateral mass of atlas

寰椎横韧带
 transverse ligament of atlas

下纵束
inferior longitudinal
fasciculus

椎间孔
intervertebral foramen

覆膜
tectorial membrane

翼状韧带
alar ligaments

后关节面
posterior articular surface

枢椎体
vertebral body of axis

椎间盘
intervertebral disk

后纵韧带
posterior longitudinal
ligament

图 122　上部颈椎的韧带（后面观 4）

Ligaments of the upper cervical spine (posterior aspect 4)

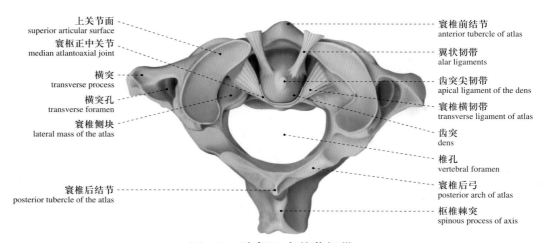

上关节面
superior articular surface
寰枢正中关节
median atlantoaxial joint
横突
transverse process
横突孔
transverse foramen
寰椎侧块
lateral mass of the atlas
寰椎后结节
posterior tubercle of the atlas

寰椎前结节
anterior tubercle of atlas
翼状韧带
alar ligaments
齿突尖韧带
apical ligament of the dens
寰椎横韧带
transverse ligament of atlas
齿突
dens
椎孔
vertebral foramen
寰椎后弓
posterior arch of atlas
枢椎棘突
spinous process of axis

图 123 寰枢正中关节韧带

Ligaments of the median atlanto-axial joint

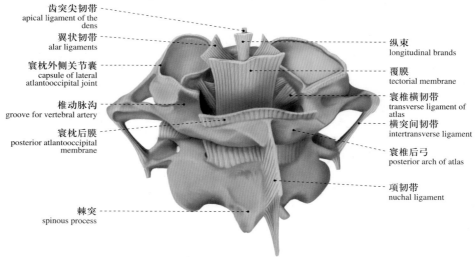

齿突尖韧带
apical ligament of the dens
翼状韧带
alar ligaments
寰枕外侧关节囊
capsule of lateral atlantooccipital joint
椎动脉沟
groove for vertebral artery
寰枕后膜
posterior atlantooccipital membrane
棘突
spinous process

纵束
longitudinal brands
覆膜
tectorial membrane
寰椎横韧带
transverse ligament of atlas
横突间韧带
intertransverse ligament
寰椎后弓
posterior arch of atlas
项韧带
nuchal ligament

图 124 颅颈关节韧带（后上面观）

Ligaments of the craniovertebral joints (posterosuperior aspect)

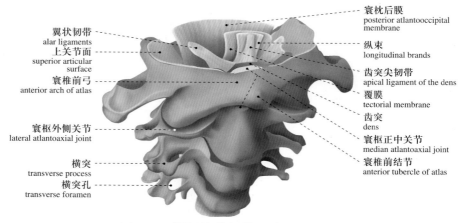

翼状韧带
alar ligaments
上关节面
superior articular surface
寰椎前弓
anterior arch of atlas
寰枢外侧关节
lateral atlantoaxial joint
横突
transverse process
横突孔
transverse foramen

寰枕后膜
posterior atlantooccipital membrane
纵束
longitudinal brands
齿突尖韧带
apical ligament of the dens
覆膜
tectorial membrane
齿突
dens
寰枢正中关节
median atlantaxial joint
寰椎前结节
anterior tubercle of atlas

图 125 颅颈关节韧带（前上面观）

Ligaments of the craniovertebral joints (antersuperior aspect)

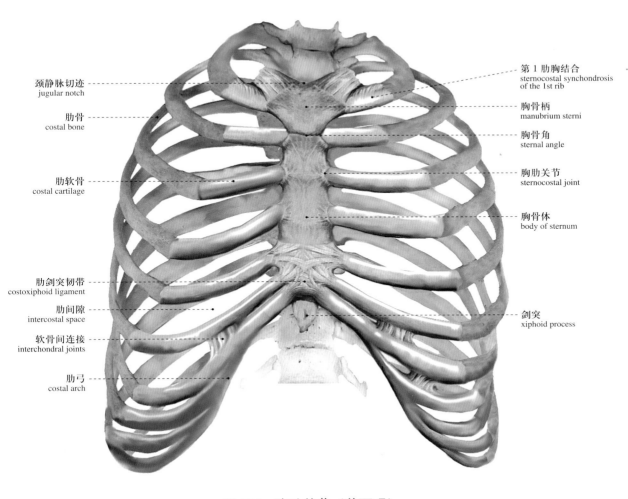

颈静脉切迹
jugular notch

肋骨
costal bone

肋软骨
costal cartilage

肋剑突韧带
costoxiphoid ligament

肋间隙
intercostal space

软骨间连接
interchondral joints

肋弓
costal arch

第 1 肋胸结合
sternocostal synchondrosis
of the 1st rib

胸骨柄
manubrium sterni

胸骨角
sternal angle

胸肋关节
sternocostal joint

胸骨体
body of sternum

剑突
xiphoid process

图 126　胸肋关节（前面观）
Sternocostal joints (anterior aspect)

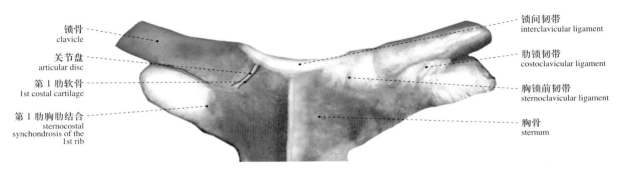

锁骨
clavicle

关节盘
articular disc

第 1 肋软骨
1st costal cartilage

第 1 肋胸肋结合
sternocostal
synchondrosis of the
1st rib

锁间韧带
interclavicular ligament

肋锁韧带
costoclavicular ligament

胸锁前韧带
sternoclavicular ligament

胸骨
sternum

图 127　胸锁关节和第 1 肋胸肋结合（前面观）
Sternoclavicular joint and the sternocostal synchondrosis of the 1st rib (anterior aspect)

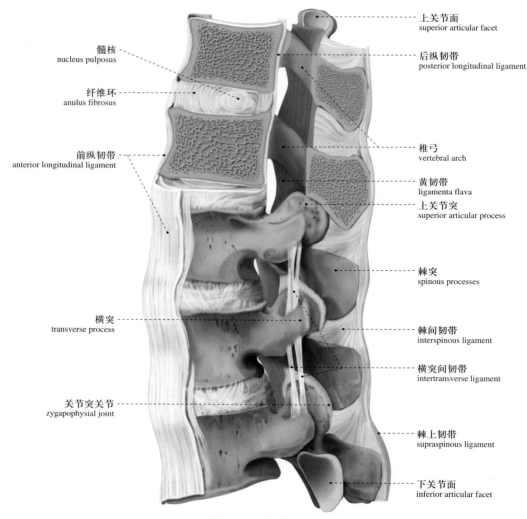

上关节面
superior articular facet

髓核
nucleus pulposus

后纵韧带
posterior longitudinal ligament

纤维环
anulus fibrosus

前纵韧带
anterior longitudinal ligament

椎弓
vertebral arch

黄韧带
ligamenta flava

上关节突
superior articular process

棘突
spinous processes

横突
transverse process

棘间韧带
interspinous ligament

横突间韧带
intertransverse ligament

关节突关节
zygapophysial joint

棘上韧带
supraspinous ligament

下关节面
inferior articular facet

图 128　腰椎周围的韧带（侧面观）
Ligaments surrounding the lumbar spine (lateral aspect)

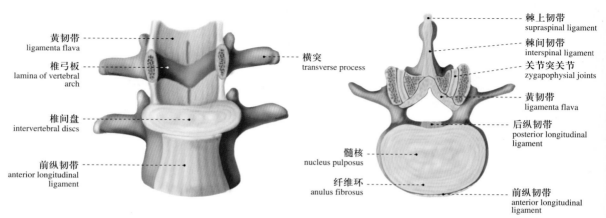

黄韧带
ligamenta flava

椎弓板
lamina of vertebral arch

椎间盘
intervertebral discs

前纵韧带
anterior longitudinal ligament

横突
transverse process

棘上韧带
supraspinal ligament

棘间韧带
interspinal ligament

关节突关节
zygapophysial joints

黄韧带
ligamenta flava

后纵韧带
posterior longitudinal ligament

髓核
nucleus pulposus

纤维环
anulus fibrosus

前纵韧带
anterior longitudinal ligament

图 129　椎骨间的连结（前面观）
Intervertebral joints (anterior aspect)

图 130　椎间盘（上面观）
Intervertebral discs (superior aspect)

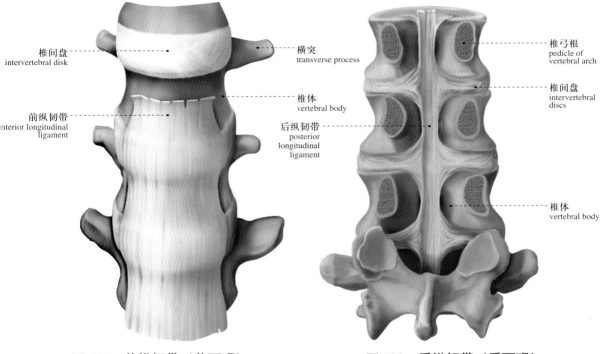

椎间盘
intervertebral disk

横突
transverse process

椎体
vertebral body

前纵韧带
anterior longitudinal
ligament

椎弓根
pedicle of
vertebral arch

椎间盘
intervertebral
discs

后纵韧带
posterior
longitudinal
ligament

椎体
vertebral body

图 131　前纵韧带（前面观）
Anterior longitudinal ligament (anterior aspect)

图 132　后纵韧带（后面观）
Posterior longitudinal ligament (posterior aspect)

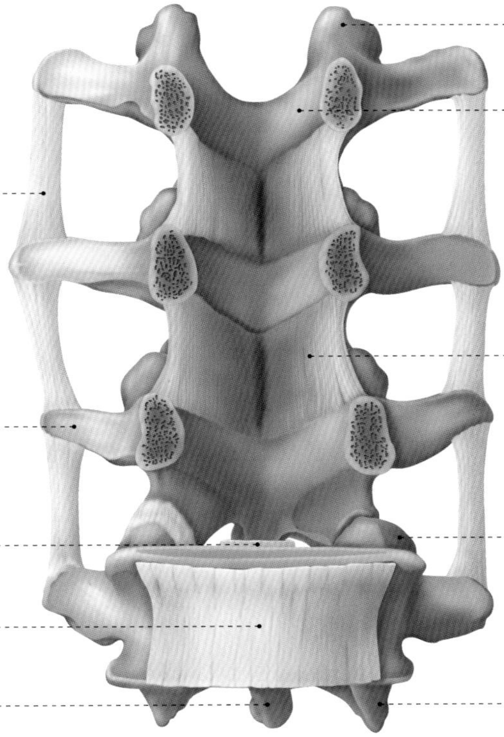

上关节突
superior articular process

椎弓板
lamina of
vertebral arch

横突间韧带
intertransverse
ligament

黄韧带
ligamenta flava

横突
transverse process

后纵韧带
posterior longitudinal ligament

上关节突
superior articular
process

前纵韧带
anterior longitudinal ligament

棘突
spinous process

下关节面
inferior articular
surface

图 133　黄韧带和横突间韧带（前面观）
Ligamenta flava and intertransverse ligaments (anterior aspect)

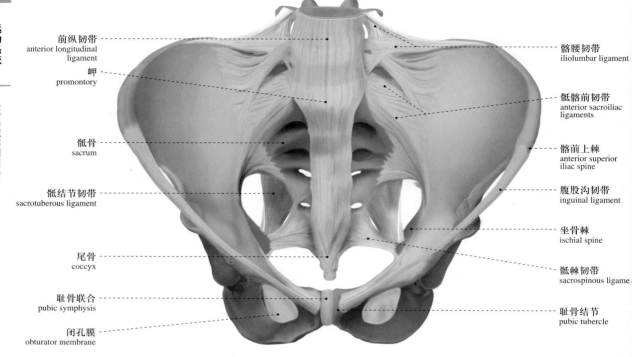

前纵韧带
anterior longitudinal
ligament

岬
promontory

骶骨
sacrum

骶结节韧带
sacrotuberous ligament

尾骨
coccyx

耻骨联合
pubic symphysis

闭孔膜
obturator membrane

髂腰韧带
iliolumbar ligament

骶髂前韧带
anterior sacroiliac
ligaments

髂前上棘
anterior superior
iliac spine

腹股沟韧带
inguinal ligament

坐骨棘
ischial spine

骶棘韧带
sacrospinous ligame

耻骨结节
pubic tubercle

图 134　骨盆韧带（上面观）
Ligaments of the pelvic (superior aspect)

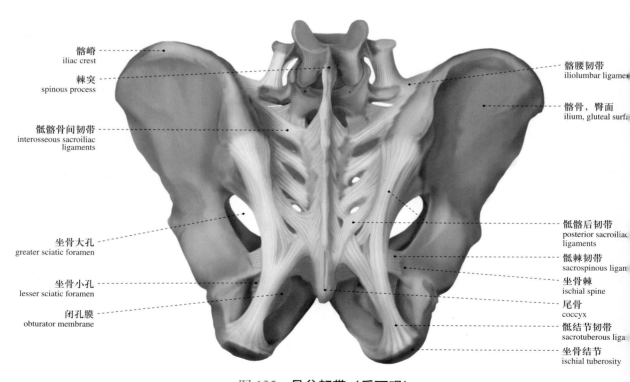

髂嵴
iliac crest

棘突
spinous process

骶髂骨间韧带
interosseous sacroiliac
ligaments

坐骨大孔
greater sciatic foramen

坐骨小孔
lesser sciatic foramen

闭孔膜
obturator membrane

髂腰韧带
iliolumbar ligame

髂骨，臀面
ilium, gluteal surfa

骶髂后韧带
posterior sacroiliac
ligaments

骶棘韧带
sacrospinous ligam

坐骨棘
ischial spine

尾骨
coccyx

骶结节韧带
sacrotuberous liga

坐骨结节
ischial tuberosity

图 135　骨盆韧带（后面观）
Ligaments of the pelvic (posterior aspect)

第三节

附肢骨的连结

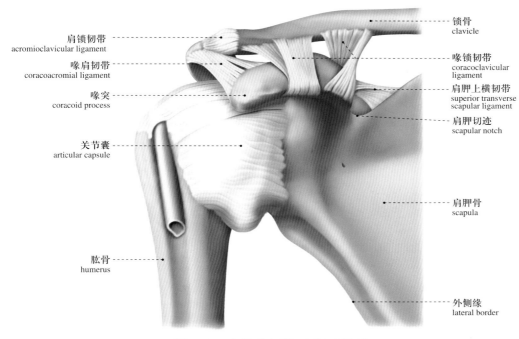

肩锁韧带
acromioclavicular ligament

喙肩韧带
coracoacromial ligament

喙突
coracoid process

关节囊
articular capsule

肱骨
humerus

锁骨
clavicle

喙锁韧带
coracoclavicular ligament

肩胛上横韧带
superior transverse scapular ligament

肩胛切迹
scapular notch

肩胛骨
scapula

外侧缘
lateral border

图 136　肩关节韧带（前面观 1）
Ligaments of the shoulder joint (anterior aspect 1)

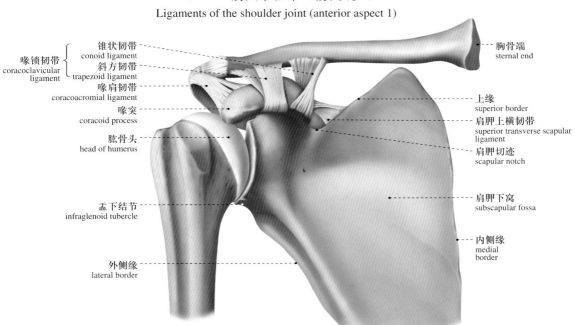

喙锁韧带
coracoclavicular ligament

锥状韧带
conoid ligament

斜方韧带
trapezoid ligament

喙肩韧带
coracoacromial ligament

喙突
coracoid process

肱骨头
head of humerus

盂下结节
infraglenoid tubercle

外侧缘
lateral border

胸骨端
sternal end

上缘
superior border

肩胛上横韧带
superior transverse scapular ligament

肩胛切迹
scapular notch

肩胛下窝
subscapular fossa

内侧缘
medial border

图 137　肩关节韧带（前面观 2）
Ligaments of the shoulder joint (anterior aspect 2)

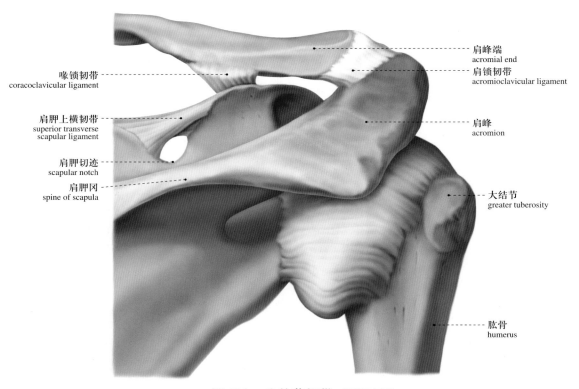

喙锁韧带
coracoclavicular ligament

肩胛上横韧带
superior transverse
scapular ligament

肩胛切迹
scapular notch

肩胛冈
spine of scapula

肩峰端
acromial end

肩锁韧带
acromioclavicular ligament

肩峰
acromion

大结节
greater tuberosity

肱骨
humerus

图 138　肩关节韧带（后面观）

Ligaments of the shoulder joint (posterior aspect)

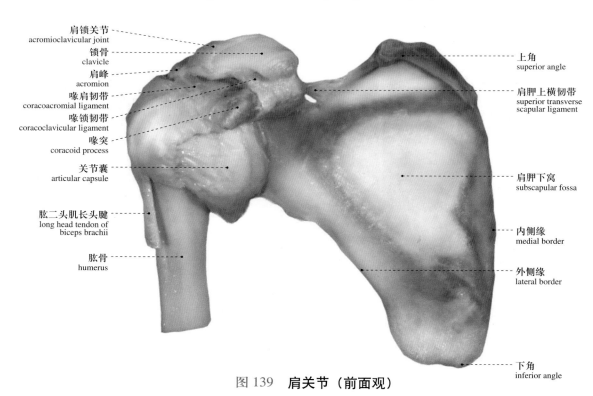

肩锁关节
acromioclavicular joint

锁骨
clavicle

肩峰
acromion

喙肩韧带
coracoacromial ligament

喙锁韧带
coracoclavicular ligament

喙突
coracoid process

关节囊
articular capsule

肱二头肌长头腱
long head tendon of
biceps brachii

肱骨
humerus

上角
superior angle

肩胛上横韧带
superior transverse
scapular ligament

肩胛下窝
subscapular fossa

内侧缘
medial border

外侧缘
lateral border

下角
inferior angle

图 139　肩关节（前面观）

Shoulder joint (anterior aspect)

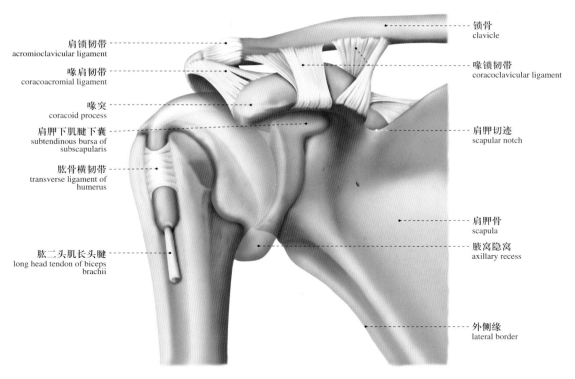

肩锁韧带 acromioclavicular ligament		锁骨 clavicle
喙肩韧带 coracoacromial ligament		喙锁韧带 coracoclavicular ligament
喙突 coracoid process		肩胛切迹 scapular notch
肩胛下肌腱下囊 subtendinous bursa of subscapularis		
肱骨横韧带 transverse ligament of humerus		
		肩胛骨 scapula
肱二头肌长头腱 long head tendon of biceps brachii		腋窝隐窝 axillary recess
		外侧缘 lateral border

图 140　肩关节滑液囊（前面观）

Bursa synovialis of the shoulder joint (anterior aspect)

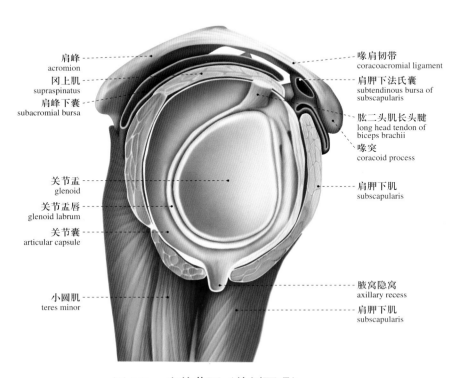

肩峰 acromion		喙肩韧带 coracoacromial ligament
冈上肌 supraspinatus		肩胛下法氏囊 subtendinous bursa of subscapularis
肩峰下囊 subacromial bursa		肱二头肌长头腱 long head tendon of biceps brachii
		喙突 coracoid process
关节盂 glenoid		肩胛下肌 subscapularis
关节盂唇 glenoid labrum		
关节囊 articular capsule		
		腋窝隐窝 axillary recess
小圆肌 teres minor		肩胛下肌 subscapularis

图 141　肩关节面（外侧面观）

Articular surface of the shoulder joint (lateral aspect)

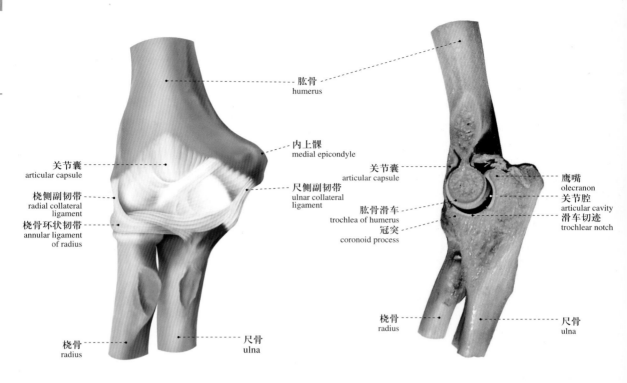

关节囊
articular capsule

桡侧副韧带
radial collateral
ligament

桡骨环状韧带
annular ligament
of radius

桡骨
radius

内上髁
medial epicondyle

尺侧副韧带
ulnar collateral
ligament

尺骨
ulna

肱骨
humerus

图 142　肘关节（前面观）
Elbow joint (anterior aspect)

肱骨
humerus

关节囊
articular capsule

肱骨滑车
trochlea of humerus

冠突
coronoid process

桡骨
radius

鹰嘴
olecranon

关节腔
articular cavity

滑车切迹
trochlear notch

尺骨
ulna

图 143　肘关节（矢状断面）
Elbow joint (sagittal section)

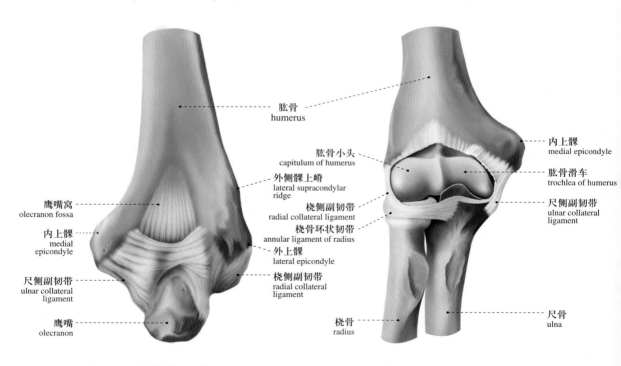

鹰嘴窝
olecranon fossa

内上髁
medial
epicondyle

尺侧副韧带
ulnar collateral
ligament

鹰嘴
olecranon

肱骨
humerus

肱骨小头
capitulum of humerus

外侧髁上嵴
lateral supracondylar
ridge

桡侧副韧带
radial collateral
ligament

桡骨环状韧带
annular ligament of radius

外上髁
lateral epicondyle

桡侧副韧带
radial collateral
ligament

内上髁
medial epicondyle

肱骨滑车
trochlea of humerus

尺侧副韧带
ulnar collateral
ligament

桡骨
radius

尺骨
ulna

图 144　肘关节（后面观 1）
Elbow joint (posterior aspect 1)

图 145　肘关节（后面观 2）
Elbow joint (posterior aspect 2)

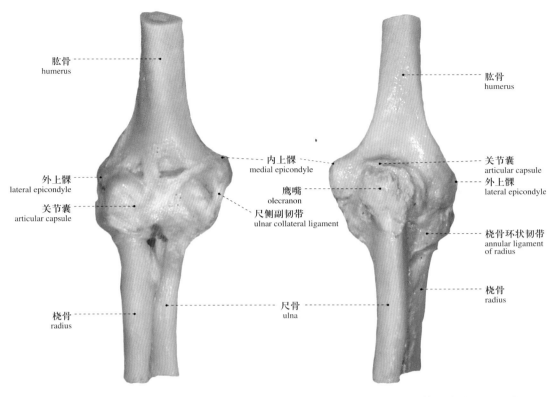

肱骨
humerus

外上髁
lateral epicondyle

关节囊
articular capsule

桡骨
radius

内上髁
medial epicondyle

鹰嘴
olecranon

尺侧副韧带
ulnar collateral ligament

尺骨
ulna

肱骨
humerus

关节囊
articular capsule

外上髁
lateral epicondyle

桡骨环状韧带
annular ligament
of radius

桡骨
radius

图 146　肘关节局部解剖（前面观）
Topography of the elbow joint (anterior aspect)

图 147　肘关节局部解剖（后面观）
Topography of the elbow joint (posterior aspect)

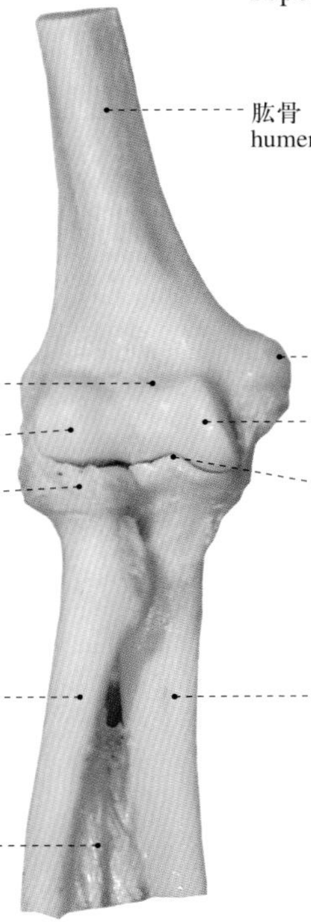

肱骨
humerus

冠突窝
coronoid fossa

肱骨小头
capitulum of humerus

桡骨环状韧带
annular ligament of
radius

桡骨
radius

前臂骨间膜
interosseous
membrane of forearm

内上髁
medial epicondyle

肱骨滑车
trochlea of humerus

冠突
coronoid process

尺骨
ulna

图 148　肘关节局部解剖（囊切开）
Topography of the elbow joint (capsule opened)

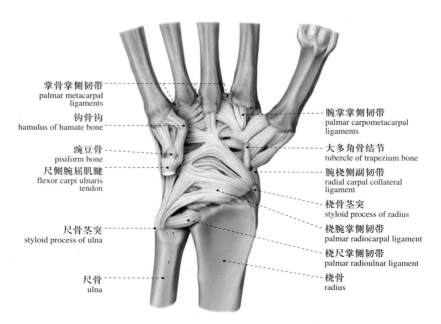

掌骨掌侧韧带
palmar metacarpal
ligaments

钩骨钩
hamulus of hamate bone

豌豆骨
pisiform bone

尺侧腕屈肌腱
flexor carpi ulnaris
tendon

尺骨茎突
styloid process of ulna

尺骨
ulna

腕掌掌侧韧带
palmar carpometacarpal
ligaments

大多角骨结节
tubercle of trapezium bone

腕桡侧副韧带
radial carpal collateral
ligament

桡骨茎突
styloid process of radius

桡腕掌侧韧带
palmar radiocarpal ligament

桡尺掌侧韧带
palmar radioulnar ligament

桡骨
radius

图 149 腕关节韧带（掌面观）
Ligaments of the carpal joint (palmar aspect)

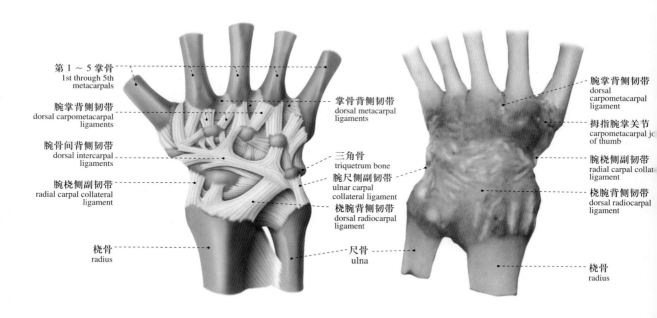

第 1～5 掌骨
1st through 5th
metacarpals

腕掌背侧韧带
dorsal carpometacarpal
ligaments

腕骨间背侧韧带
dorsal intercarpal
ligaments

腕桡侧副韧带
radial carpal collateral
ligament

桡骨
radius

掌骨背侧韧带
dorsal metacarpal
ligaments

三角骨
triquetrum bone

腕尺侧副韧带
ulnar carpal
collateral ligament

桡腕背侧韧带
dorsal radiocarpal
ligament

尺骨
ulna

腕掌背侧韧带
dorsal
carpometacarpal
ligament

拇指腕掌关节
carpometacarpal jo
of thumb

腕桡侧副韧带
radial carpal collat
ligament

桡腕背侧韧带
dorsal radiocarpal
ligament

桡骨
radius

图 150 腕关节韧带（背面观）
Ligaments of the carpal joint (dorsal aspect)

图 151 腕关节韧带局部解剖（背面观）
Topography of the ligaments of the carpal joint
(dorsal aspect)

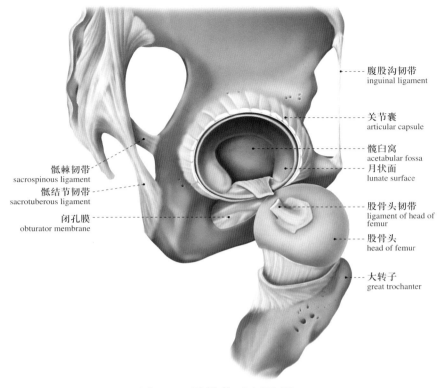

腹股沟韧带
inguinal ligament

关节囊
articular capsule

髋臼窝
acetabular fossa

月状面
lunate surface

股骨头韧带
ligament of head of femur

股骨头
head of femur

大转子
great trochanter

骶棘韧带
sacrospinous ligament

骶结节韧带
sacrotuberous ligament

闭孔膜
obturator membrane

图 152 髋关节（内面观）
Hip joint (internal aspect)

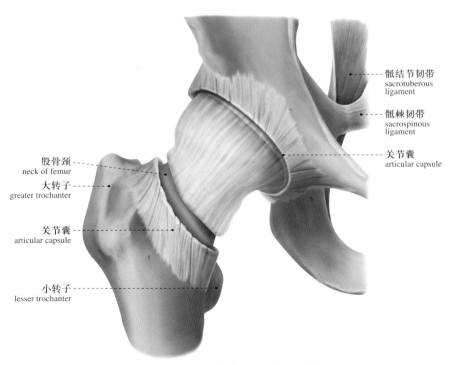

骶结节韧带
sacrotuberous ligament

骶棘韧带
sacrospinous ligament

关节囊
articular capsule

股骨颈
neck of femur

大转子
greater trochanter

关节囊
articular capsule

小转子
lesser trochanter

图 153 髋关节囊（前面观）
Capsule of the hip joint (anterior aspect)

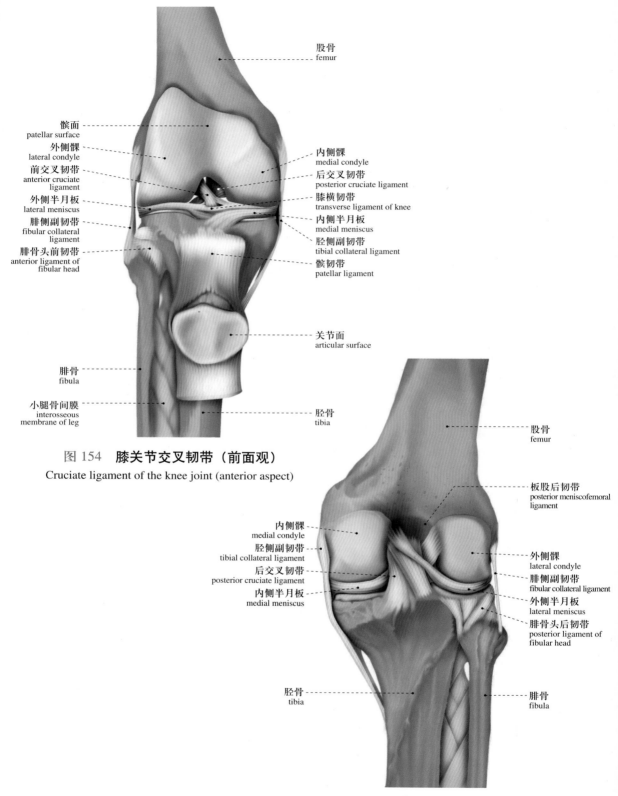

股骨
femur

髌面
patellar surface

外侧髁
lateral condyle

前交叉韧带
anterior cruciate
ligament

外侧半月板
lateral meniscus

腓侧副韧带
fibular collateral
ligament

腓骨头前韧带
anterior ligament of
fibular head

内侧髁
medial condyle

后交叉韧带
posterior cruciate ligament

膝横韧带
transverse ligament of knee

内侧半月板
medial meniscus

胫侧副韧带
tibial collateral ligament

髌韧带
patellar ligament

关节面
articular surface

腓骨
fibula

小腿骨间膜
interosseous
membrane of leg

胫骨
tibia

图 154　膝关节交叉韧带（前面观）
Cruciate ligament of the knee joint (anterior aspect)

股骨
femur

板股后韧带
posterior meniscofemoral
ligament

内侧髁
medial condyle

胫侧副韧带
tibial collateral ligament

后交叉韧带
posterior cruciate ligament

内侧半月板
medial meniscus

外侧髁
lateral condyle

腓侧副韧带
fibular collateral ligament

外侧半月板
lateral meniscus

腓骨头后韧带
posterior ligament of
fibular head

胫骨
tibia

腓骨
fibula

图 155　膝关节交叉韧带（后面观）
Cruciate ligament of the knee joint (posterior aspect)

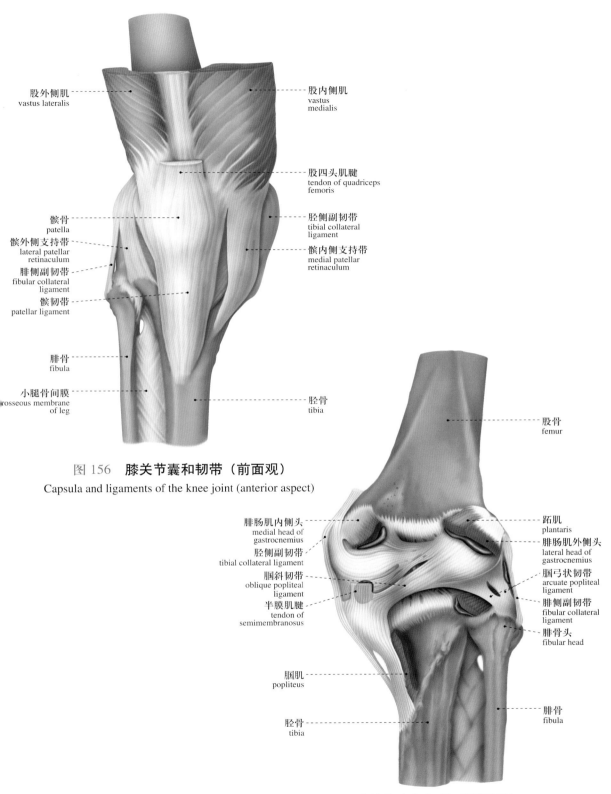

股外侧肌
vastus lateralis

股内侧肌
vastus medialis

股四头肌腱
tendon of quadriceps femoris

髌骨
patella

胫侧副韧带
tibial collateral ligament

髌外侧支持带
lateral patellar retinaculum

髌内侧支持带
medial patellar retinaculum

腓侧副韧带
fibular collateral ligament

髌韧带
patellar ligament

腓骨
fibula

小腿骨间膜
interosseous membrane of leg

胫骨
tibia

图 156　膝关节囊和韧带（前面观）
Capsula and ligaments of the knee joint (anterior aspect)

腓肠肌内侧头
medial head of gastrocnemius

跖肌
plantaris

腓肠肌外侧头
lateral head of gastrocnemius

胫侧副韧带
tibial collateral ligament

腘斜韧带
oblique popliteal ligament

腘弓状韧带
arcuate popliteal ligament

半膜肌腱
tendon of semimembranosus

腓侧副韧带
fibular collateral ligament

腓骨头
fibular head

股骨
femur

腘肌
popliteus

腓骨
fibula

胫骨
tibia

图 157　膝关节囊和韧带（后面观）
Capsula and ligaments of the knee joint (posterior aspect)

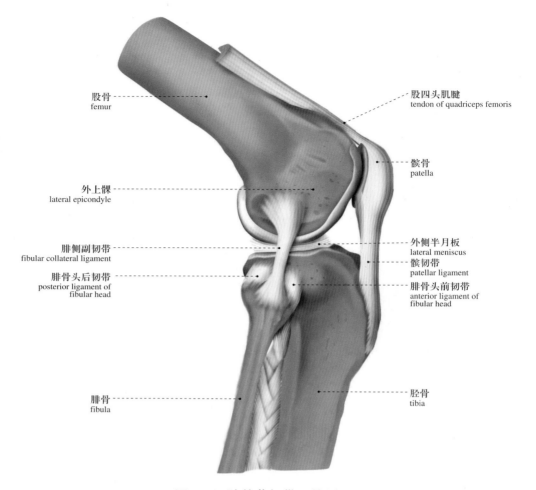

股骨
femur

股四头肌腱
tendon of quadriceps femoris

髌骨
patella

外上髁
lateral epicondyle

外侧半月板
lateral meniscus

腓侧副韧带
fibular collateral ligament

髌韧带
patellar ligament

腓骨头后韧带
posterior ligament of
fibular head

腓骨头前韧带
anterior ligament of
fibular head

腓骨
fibula

胫骨
tibia

图 158　膝关节韧带（外侧面观）
Ligaments of the knee joint (lateral aspect)

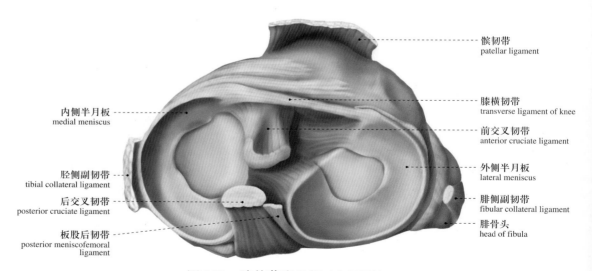

髌韧带
patellar ligament

内侧半月板
medial meniscus

膝横韧带
transverse ligament of knee

前交叉韧带
anterior cruciate ligament

外侧半月板
lateral meniscus

胫侧副韧带
tibial collateral ligament

后交叉韧带
posterior cruciate ligament

腓侧副韧带
fibular collateral ligament

板股后韧带
posterior meniscofemoral
ligament

腓骨头
head of fibula

图 159　膝关节半月板（上面观）
Meniscus of the knee joint (superior aspect)

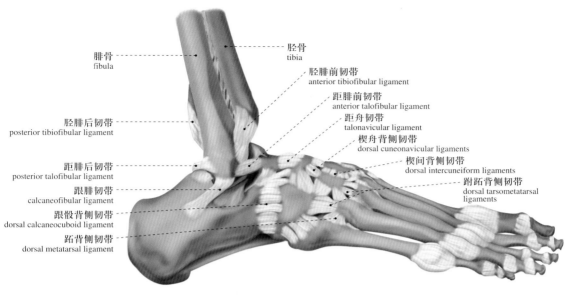

腓骨
fibula

胫骨
tibia

胫腓前韧带
anterior tibiofibular ligament

距腓前韧带
anterior talofibular ligament

距舟韧带
talonavicular ligament

楔舟背侧韧带
dorsal cuneonavicular ligaments

楔间背侧韧带
dorsal intercuneiform ligaments

跗跖背侧韧带
dorsal tarsometatarsal ligaments

胫腓后韧带
posterior tibiofibular ligament

距腓后韧带
posterior talofibular ligament

跟腓韧带
calcaneofibular ligament

跟骰背侧韧带
dorsal calcaneocuboid ligament

跖背侧韧带
dorsal metatarsal ligament

图 160 足的关节和韧带（外侧面观）
Joints and ligaments of the foot (lateral aspect)

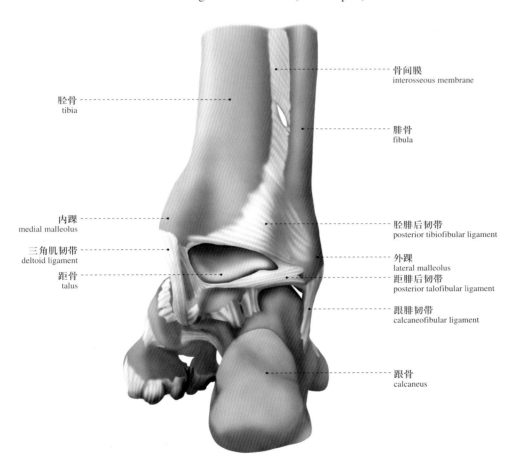

胫骨
tibia

骨间膜
interosseous membrane

腓骨
fibula

内踝
medial malleolus

三角肌韧带
deltoid ligament

距骨
talus

胫腓后韧带
posterior tibiofibular ligament

外踝
lateral malleolus

距腓后韧带
posterior talofibular ligament

跟腓韧带
calcaneofibular ligament

跟骨
calcaneus

图 161 足的关节和韧带（后面观）
Joints and ligaments of the foot (posterior aspect)

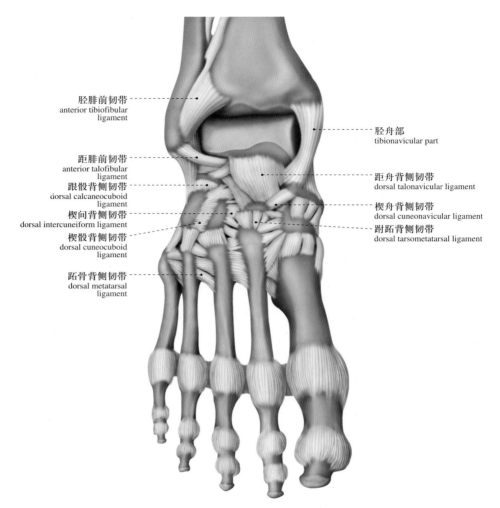

胫腓前韧带
anterior tibiofibular
ligament

距腓前韧带
anterior talofibular
ligament

跟骰背侧韧带
dorsal calcaneocuboid
ligament

楔间背侧韧带
dorsal intercuneiform ligament

楔骰背侧韧带
dorsal cuneocuboid
ligament

跖骨背侧韧带
dorsal metatarsal
ligament

胫舟部
tibionavicular part

距舟背侧韧带
dorsal talonavicular ligament

楔舟背侧韧带
dorsal cuneonavicular ligament

跗跖背侧韧带
dorsal tarsometatarsal ligament

图 162　足的关节和韧带（背面观）

Joints and ligaments of the foot (dorsal aspect)

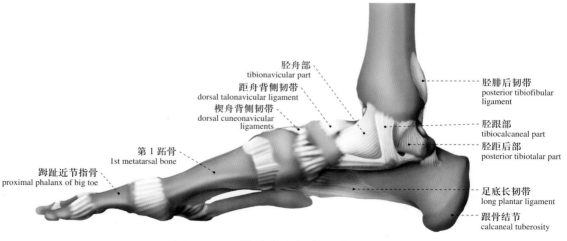

胫舟部
tibionavicular part

距舟背侧韧带
dorsal talonavicular ligament

楔舟背侧韧带
dorsal cuneonavicular
ligaments

第 1 跖骨
1st metatarsal bone

踇趾近节指骨
proximal phalanx of big toe

胫腓后韧带
posterior tibiofibular
ligament

胫跟部
tibiocalcaneal part

胫距后部
posterior tibiotalar part

足底长韧带
long plantar ligament

跟骨结节
calcaneal tuberosity

图 163　足的关节和韧带（内侧面观）

Joints and ligaments of the foot (medial aspect)

全 身 肌 肉

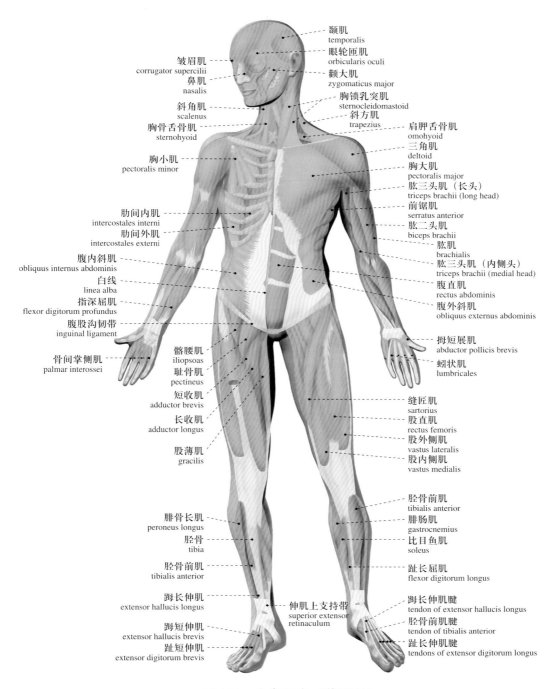

颞肌
temporalis
眼轮匝肌
orbicularis oculi
颧大肌
zygomaticus major
胸锁乳突肌
sternocleidomastoid
斜方肌
trapezius
肩胛舌骨肌
omohyoid
三角肌
deltoid
胸大肌
pectoralis major
肱三头肌（长头）
triceps brachii (long head)
前锯肌
serratus anterior
肱二头肌
biceps brachii
肱肌
brachialis
肱三头肌（内侧头）
triceps brachii (medial head)
腹直肌
rectus abdominis
腹外斜肌
obliquus externus abdominis
拇短展肌
abductor pollicis brevis
蚓状肌
lumbricales
缝匠肌
sartorius
股直肌
rectus femoris
股外侧肌
vastus lateralis
股内侧肌
vastus medialis
胫骨前肌
tibialis anterior
腓肠肌
gastrocnemius
比目鱼肌
soleus
趾长屈肌
flexor digitorum longus
拇长伸肌腱
tendon of extensor hallucis longus
胫骨前肌腱
tendon of tibialis anterior
趾长伸肌腱
tendons of extensor digitorum longus

皱眉肌
corrugator supercilii
鼻肌
nasalis
斜角肌
scalenus
胸骨舌骨肌
sternohyoid
胸小肌
pectoralis minor
肋间内肌
intercostales interni
肋间外肌
intercostales externi
腹内斜肌
obliquus internus abdominis
白线
linea alba
指深屈肌
flexor digitorum profundus
腹股沟韧带
inguinal ligament
骨间掌侧肌
palmar interossei
髂腰肌
iliopsoas
耻骨肌
pectineus
短收肌
adductor brevis
长收肌
adductor longus
股薄肌
gracilis
腓骨长肌
peroneus longus
胫骨
tibia
胫骨前肌
tibialis anterior
拇长伸肌
extensor hallucis longus
拇短伸肌
extensor hallucis brevis
趾短伸肌
extensor digitorum brevis
伸肌上支持带
superior extensor retinaculum

图 164　全身肌肉（前面观）
Muscles of the body (anterior aspect)

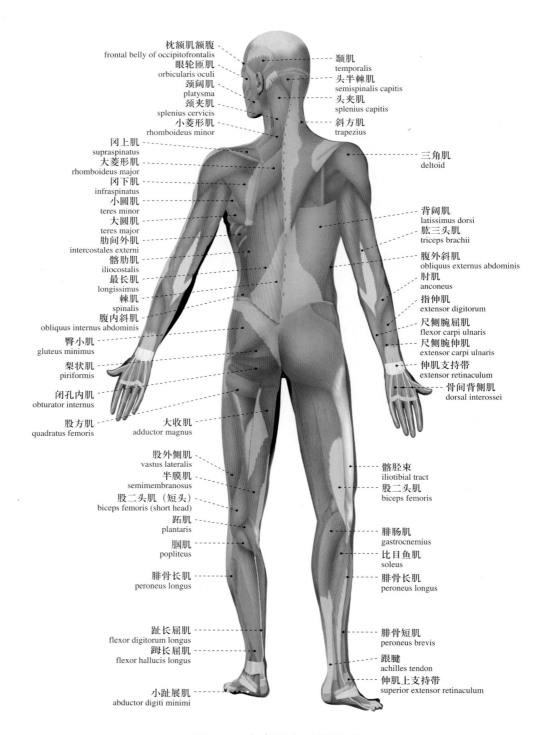

枕额肌额腹
frontal belly of occipitofrontalis
眼轮匝肌
orbicularis oculi
颈阔肌
platysma
颈夹肌
splenius cervicis
小菱形肌
rhomboideus minor
冈上肌
supraspinatus
大菱形肌
rhomboideus major
冈下肌
infraspinatus
小圆肌
teres minor
大圆肌
teres major
肋间外肌
intercostales externi
髂肋肌
iliocostalis
最长肌
longissimus
棘肌
spinalis
腹内斜肌
obliquus internus abdominis
臀小肌
gluteus minimus
梨状肌
piriformis
闭孔内肌
obturator internus
股方肌
quadratus femoris
大收肌
adductor magnus
股外侧肌
vastus lateralis
半膜肌
semimembranosus
股二头肌（短头）
biceps femoris (short head)
跖肌
plantaris
腘肌
popliteus
腓骨长肌
peroneus longus
趾长屈肌
flexor digitorum longus
踇长屈肌
flexor hallucis longus
小趾展肌
abductor digiti minimi

颞肌
temporalis
头半棘肌
semispinalis capitis
头夹肌
splenius capitis
斜方肌
trapezius
三角肌
deltoid
背阔肌
latissimus dorsi
肱三头肌
triceps brachii
腹外斜肌
obliquus externus abdominis
肘肌
anconeus
指伸肌
extensor digitorum
尺侧腕屈肌
flexor carpi ulnaris
尺侧腕伸肌
extensor carpi ulnaris
伸肌支持带
extensor retinaculum
骨间背侧肌
dorsal interossei
髂胫束
iliotibial tract
股二头肌
biceps femoris
腓肠肌
gastrocnemius
比目鱼肌
soleus
腓骨长肌
peroneus longus
腓骨短肌
peroneus brevis
跟腱
achilles tendon
伸肌上支持带
superior extensor retinaculum

图 165　全身肌肉（后面观）
Muscles of the body (posterior aspect)

第二节

肌的各种形态

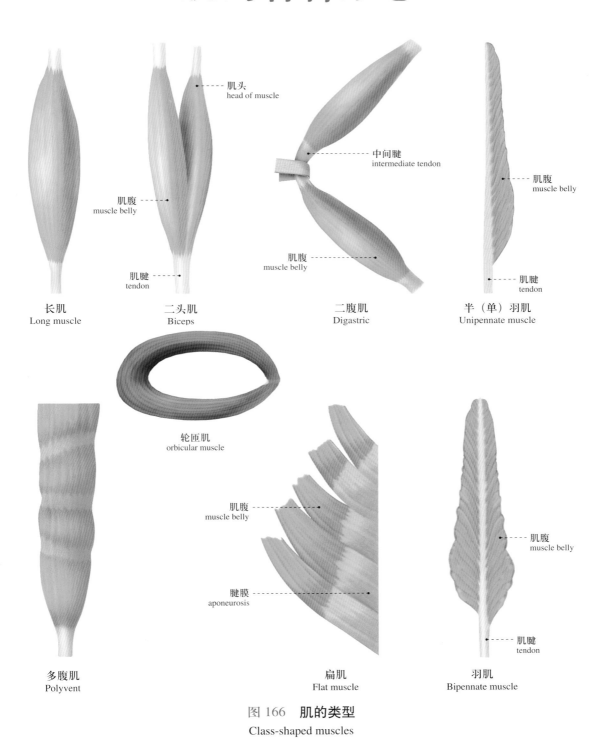

肌头
head of muscle

中间腱
intermediate tendon

肌腹
muscle belly

肌腹
muscle belly

肌腹
muscle belly

肌腱
tendon

肌腹
muscle belly

肌腱
tendon

长肌
Long muscle

二头肌
Biceps

二腹肌
Digastric

半（单）羽肌
Unipennate muscle

轮匝肌
orbicular muscle

肌腹
muscle belly

腱膜
aponeurosis

肌腹
muscle belly

肌腱
tendon

多腹肌
Polyvent

扁肌
Flat muscle

羽肌
Bipennate muscle

图 166 **肌的类型**
Class-shaped muscles

肌肉的构造

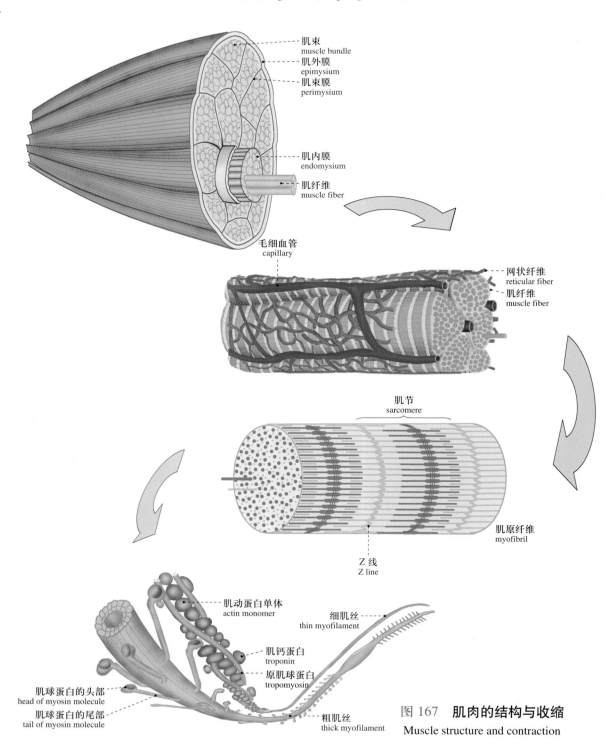

肌束
muscle bundle

肌外膜
epimysium

肌束膜
perimysium

肌内膜
endomysium

肌纤维
muscle fiber

毛细血管
capillary

网状纤维
reticular fiber

肌纤维
muscle fiber

肌节
sarcomere

肌原纤维
myofibril

Z 线
Z line

肌动蛋白单体
actin monomer

细肌丝
thin myofilament

肌钙蛋白
troponin

原肌球蛋白
tropomyosin

肌球蛋白的头部
head of myosin molecule

肌球蛋白的尾部
tail of myosin molecule

粗肌丝
thick myofilament

图 167　肌肉的结构与收缩
Muscle structure and contraction

82

第四节

肌肉的辅助装置

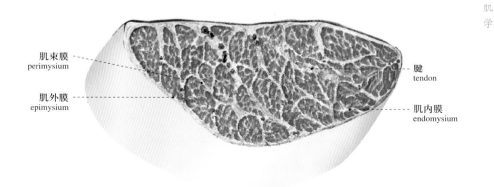

肌束膜 perimysium
肌外膜 epimysium
腱 tendon
肌内膜 endomysium

肌的横断面
Transverse section of muscle

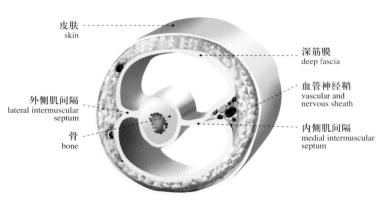

皮肤 skin
深筋膜 deep fascia
血管神经鞘 vascular and nervous sheath
外侧肌间隔 lateral intermuscular septum
内侧肌间隔 medial intermuscular septum
骨 bone

筋膜鞘（模式图）
Fascial sheath (diagram)

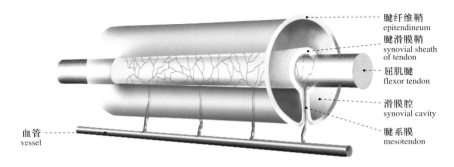

腱纤维鞘 epitendineum
腱滑膜鞘 synovial sheath of tendon
屈肌腱 flexor tendon
滑膜腔 synovial cavity
腱系膜 mesotendon
血管 vessel

腱鞘（模式图）
Tendinous sheath (diagram)

图 168　肌肉的辅助装置
Auxiliary device of the muscle

第五节

头 颈 肌

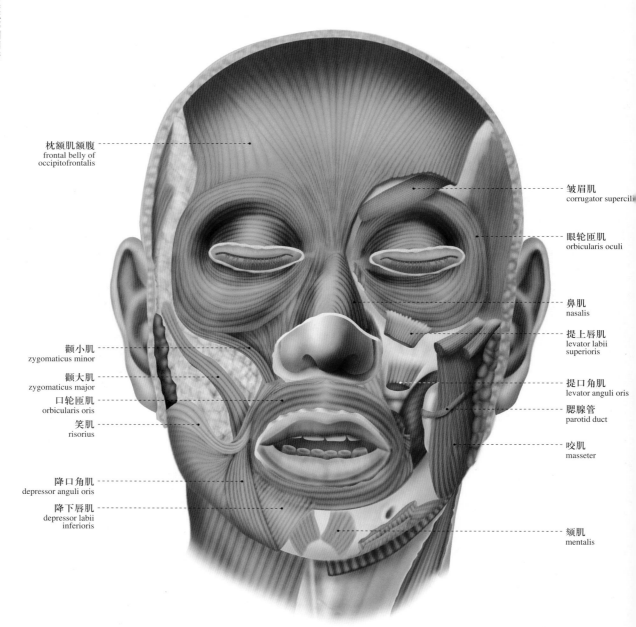

枕额肌额腹
frontal belly of
occipitofrontalis

皱眉肌
corrugator supercil

眼轮匝肌
orbicularis oculi

鼻肌
nasalis

提上唇肌
levator labii
superioris

颧小肌
zygomaticus minor

颧大肌
zygomaticus major

口轮匝肌
orbicularis oris

笑肌
risorius

提口角肌
levator anguli oris

腮腺管
parotid duct

咬肌
masseter

降口角肌
depressor anguli oris

降下唇肌
depressor labii
inferioris

颏肌
mentalis

图 169　面部肌肉（前面观）

Facial muscles (anterior aspect)

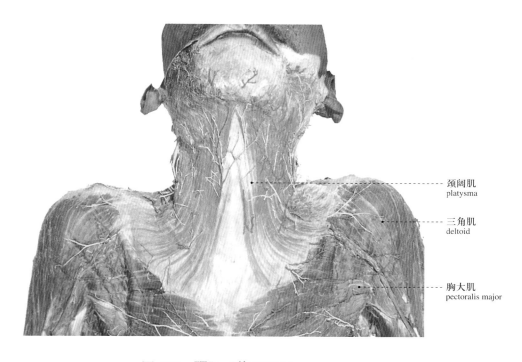

图 170　颈肌（前面观 1）

Lateral cervical muscles (anterior aspect 1)

颈阔肌
platysma

三角肌
deltoid

胸大肌
pectoralis major

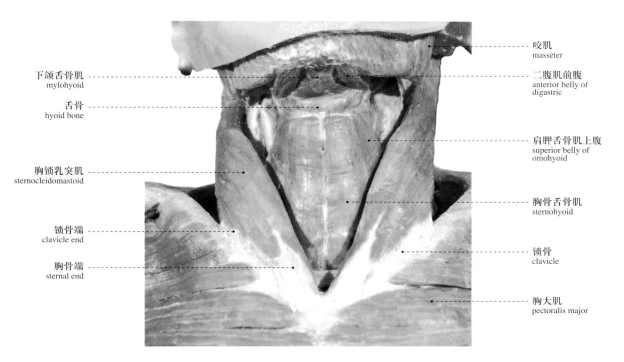

下颌舌骨肌
mylohyoid

舌骨
hyoid bone

胸锁乳突肌
sternocleidomastoid

锁骨端
clavicle end

胸骨端
sternal end

咬肌
masseter

二腹肌前腹
anterior belly of
digastric

肩胛舌骨肌上腹
superior belly of
omohyoid

胸骨舌骨肌
sternohyoid

锁骨
clavicle

胸大肌
pectoralis major

图 171　颈肌（前面观 2）

Cervical muscles (anterior aspect 2)

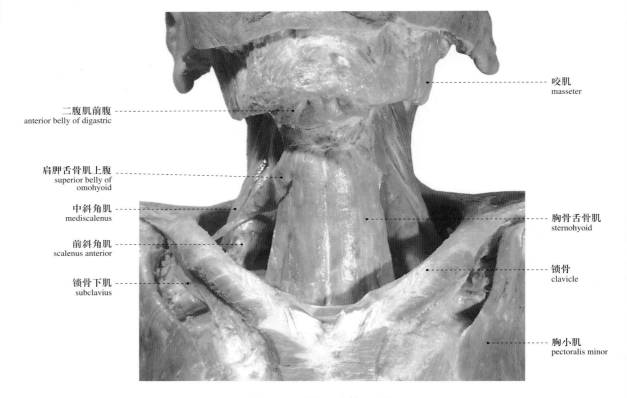

二腹肌前腹
anterior belly of digastric

肩胛舌骨肌上腹
superior belly of
omohyoid

中斜角肌
mediscalenus

前斜角肌
scalenus anterior

锁骨下肌
subclavius

咬肌
masseter

胸骨舌骨肌
sternohyoid

锁骨
clavicle

胸小肌
pectoralis minor

图 172　颈肌（前面观 3）
Cervical muscles (anterior aspect 3)

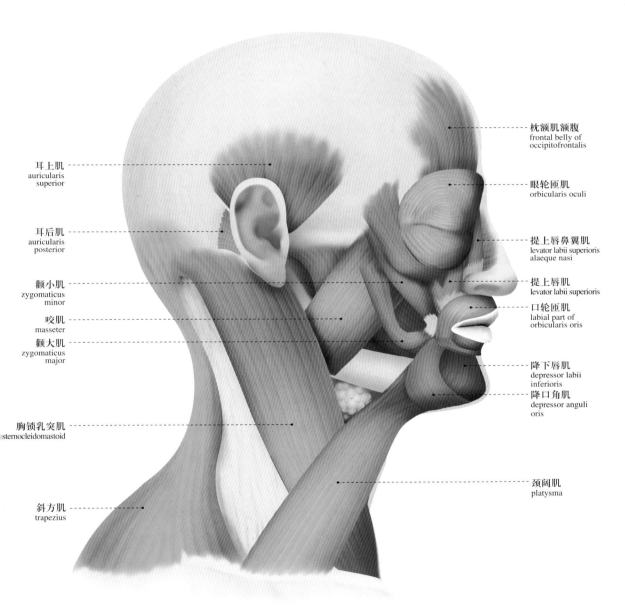

耳上肌
auricularis
superior

耳后肌
auricularis
posterior

颧小肌
zygomaticus
minor

咬肌
masseter

颧大肌
zygomaticus
major

胸锁乳突肌
sternocleidomastoid

斜方肌
trapezius

枕额肌额腹
frontal belly of
occipitofrontalis

眼轮匝肌
orbicularis oculi

提上唇鼻翼肌
levator labii superioris
alaeque nasi

提上唇肌
levator labii superioris

口轮匝肌
labial part of
orbicularis oris

降下唇肌
depressor labii
inferioris

降口角肌
depressor anguli
oris

颈阔肌
platysma

图 173　头颈肌（侧面观 1）
Muscles of the head and neck (lateral aspect 1)

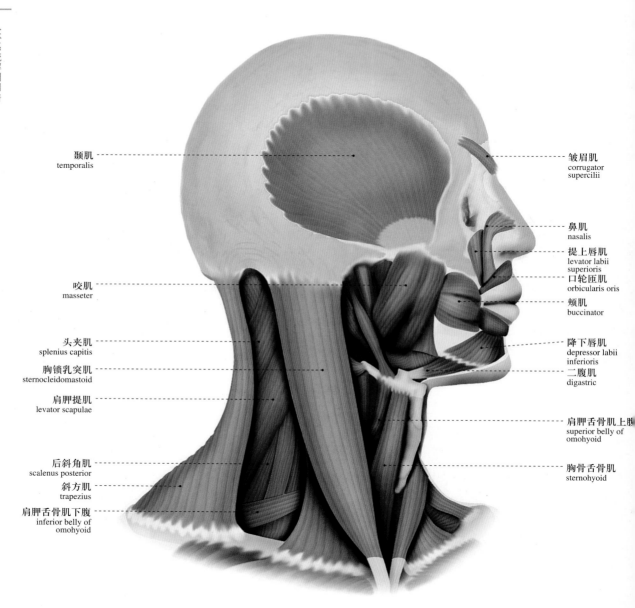

颞肌
temporalis

咬肌
masseter

头夹肌
splenius capitis

胸锁乳突肌
sternocleidomastoid

肩胛提肌
levator scapulae

后斜角肌
scalenus posterior

斜方肌
trapezius

肩胛舌骨肌下腹
inferior belly of
omohyoid

皱眉肌
corrugator
supercilii

鼻肌
nasalis

提上唇肌
levator labii
superioris

口轮匝肌
orbicularis oris

颊肌
buccinator

降下唇肌
depressor labii
inferioris

二腹肌
digastric

肩胛舌骨肌上腹
superior belly of
omohyoid

胸骨舌骨肌
sternohyoid

图 174　头颈肌（侧面观 2）

Muscles of the head and neck (lateral aspect 2)

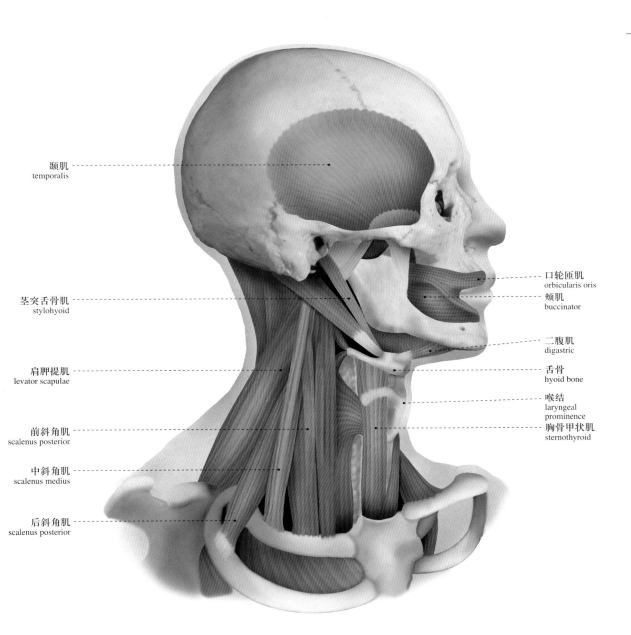

颞肌
temporalis

口轮匝肌
orbicularis oris

颊肌
buccinator

茎突舌骨肌
stylohyoid

二腹肌
digastric

肩胛提肌
levator scapulae

舌骨
hyoid bone

喉结
laryngeal
prominence

前斜角肌
scalenus posterior

胸骨甲状肌
sternothyroid

中斜角肌
scalenus medius

后斜角肌
scalenus posterior

图 175　头颈肌（侧面观 3）

Muscles of the head and neck (lateral aspect 3)

第六节

躯 干 肌

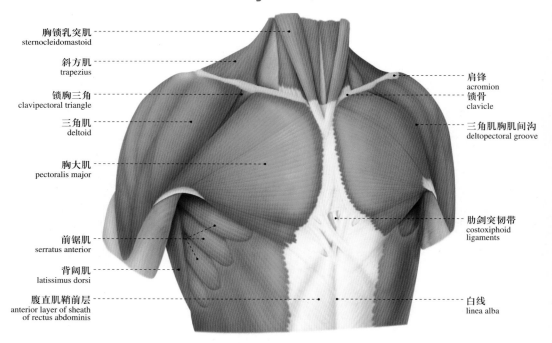

胸锁乳突肌
sternocleidomastoid

斜方肌
trapezius

锁胸三角
clavipectoral triangle

三角肌
deltoid

胸大肌
pectoralis major

前锯肌
serratus anterior

背阔肌
latissimus dorsi

腹直肌鞘前层
anterior layer of sheath
of rectus abdominis

肩锋
acromion

锁骨
clavicle

三角肌胸肌间沟
deltopectoral groove

肋剑突韧带
costoxiphoid
ligaments

白线
linea alba

图 176　胸部肌肉（浅层）
Chest muscles (superficial layer)

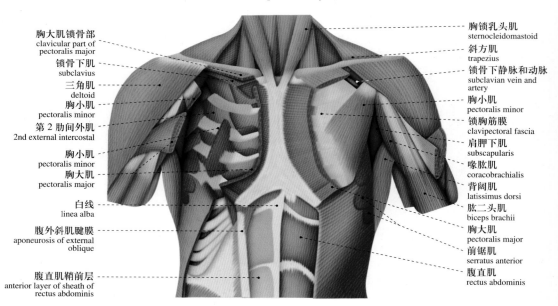

胸大肌锁骨部
clavicular part of
pectoralis major

锁骨下肌
subclavius

三角肌
deltoid

胸小肌
pectoralis minor

第 2 肋间外肌
2nd external intercostal

胸小肌
pectoralis minor

胸大肌
pectoralis major

白线
linea alba

腹外斜肌腱膜
aponeurosis of external
oblique

腹直肌鞘前层
anterior layer of sheath of
rectus abdominis

胸锁乳头肌
sternocleidomastoid

斜方肌
trapezius

锁骨下静脉和动脉
subclavian vein and
artery

胸小肌
pectoralis minor

锁胸筋膜
clavipectoral fascia

肩胛下肌
subscapularis

喙肱肌
coracobrachialis

背阔肌
latissimus dorsi

肱二头肌
biceps brachii

胸大肌
pectoralis major

前锯肌
serratus anterior

腹直肌
rectus abdominis

图 177　胸部肌肉（深层）
Chest muscles (deep layer)

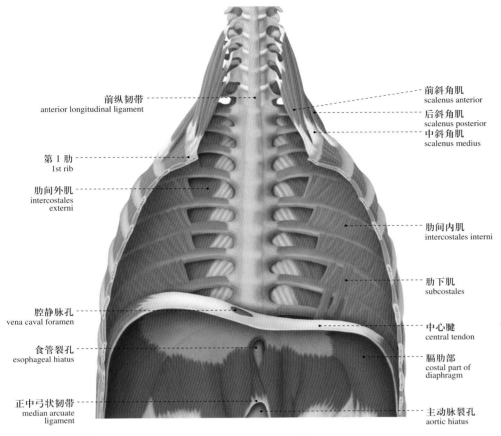

前斜角肌
scalenus anterior

后斜角肌
scalenus posterior

中斜角肌
scalenus medius

前纵韧带
anterior longitudinal ligament

第 1 肋
1st rib

肋间外肌
intercostales
externi

肋间内肌
intercostales interni

肋下肌
subcostales

腔静脉孔
vena caval foramen

中心腱
central tendon

食管裂孔
esophageal hiatus

膈肋部
costal part of
diaphragm

正中弓状韧带
median arcuate
ligament

主动脉裂孔
aortic hiatus

图 178　胸后壁（前面观）
Posterior wall of the chest (anterior aspect)

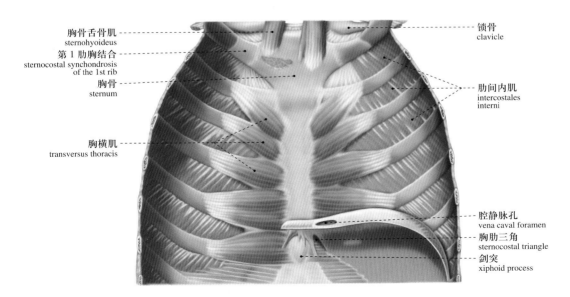

胸骨舌骨肌
sternohyoideus

第 1 肋胸结合
sternocostal synchondrosis
of the 1st rib

胸骨
sternum

胸横肌
transversus thoracis

锁骨
clavicle

肋间内肌
intercostales
interni

腔静脉孔
vena caval foramen

胸肋三角
sternocostal triangle

剑突
xiphoid process

图 179　胸前壁（后面观）
Anterior wall of the chest (posterior aspect)

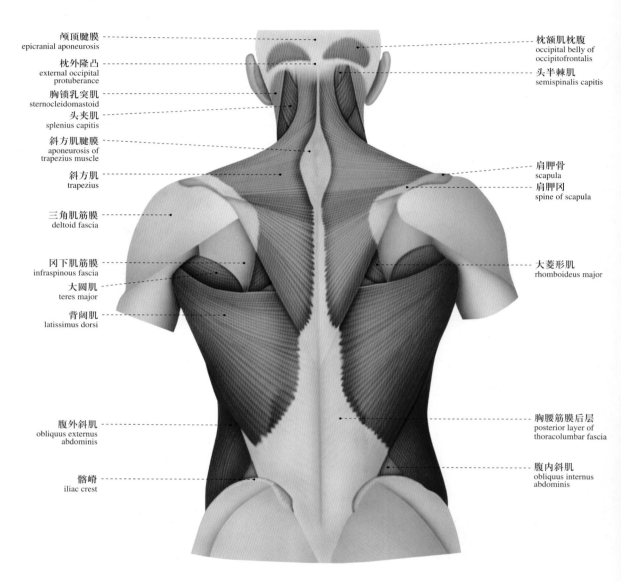

颅顶腱膜
epicranial aponeurosis

枕外隆凸
external occipital
protuberance

胸锁乳突肌
sternocleidomastoid

头夹肌
splenius capitis

斜方肌腱膜
aponeurosis of
trapezius muscle

斜方肌
trapezius

三角肌筋膜
deltoid fascia

冈下肌筋膜
infraspinous fascia

大圆肌
teres major

背阔肌
latissimus dorsi

腹外斜肌
obliquus externus
abdominis

髂嵴
iliac crest

枕额肌枕腹
occipital belly of
occipitofrontalis

头半棘肌
semispinalis capitis

肩胛骨
scapula

肩胛冈
spine of scapula

大菱形肌
rhomboideus major

胸腰筋膜后层
posterior layer of
thoracolumbar fascia

腹内斜肌
obliquus internus
abdominis

图 180　背肌（浅层）

Muscles of the back (superficial layer)

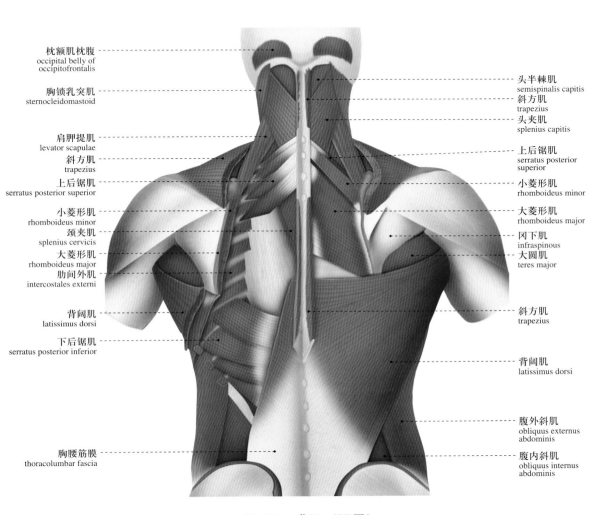

枕额肌枕腹
occipital belly of
occipitofrontalis

胸锁乳突肌
sternocleidomastoid

肩胛提肌
levator scapulae

斜方肌
trapezius

上后锯肌
serratus posterior superior

小菱形肌
rhomboideus minor

颈夹肌
splenius cervicis

大菱形肌
rhomboideus major

肋间外肌
intercostales externi

背阔肌
latissimus dorsi

下后锯肌
serratus posterior inferior

胸腰筋膜
thoracolumbar fascia

头半棘肌
semispinalis capitis

斜方肌
trapezius

头夹肌
splenius capitis

上后锯肌
serratus posterior
superior

小菱形肌
rhomboideus minor

大菱形肌
rhomboideus major

冈下肌
infraspinous

大圆肌
teres major

斜方肌
trapezius

背阔肌
latissimus dorsi

腹外斜肌
obliquus externus
abdominis

腹内斜肌
obliquus internus
abdominis

图 181 背肌（深层）

Muscles of the back (deep layer)

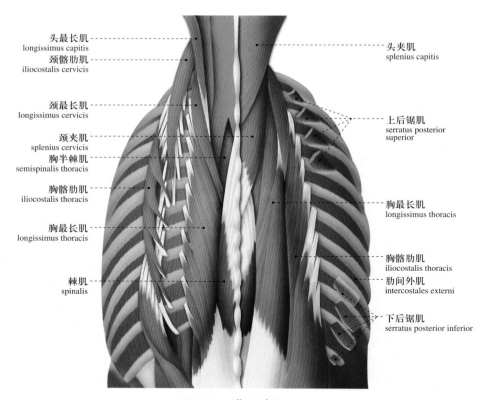

头最长肌
longissimus capitis

颈髂肋肌
iliocostalis cervicis

颈最长肌
longissimus cervicis

颈夹肌
splenius cervicis

胸半棘肌
semispinalis thoracis

胸髂肋肌
iliocostalis thoracis

胸最长肌
longissimus thoracis

棘肌
spinalis

头夹肌
splenius capitis

上后锯肌
serratus posterior superior

胸最长肌
longissimus thoracis

胸髂肋肌
iliocostalis thoracis

肋间外肌
intercostales externi

下后锯肌
serratus posterior inferior

图 182　背固有肌 1
Intrinsic back muscles 1

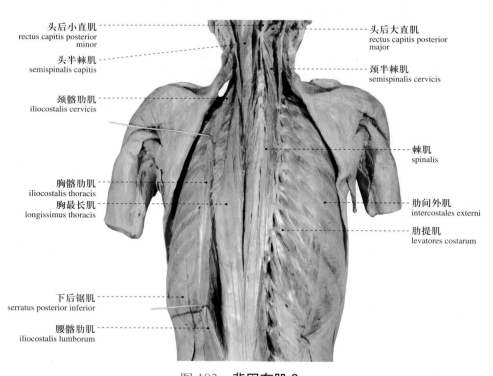

头后小直肌
rectus capitis posterior minor

头半棘肌
semispinalis capitis

颈髂肋肌
iliocostalis cervicis

胸髂肋肌
iliocostalis thoracis

胸最长肌
longissimus thoracis

下后锯肌
serratus posterior inferior

腰髂肋肌
iliocostalis lumborum

头后大直肌
rectus capitis posterior major

颈半棘肌
semispinalis cervicis

棘肌
spinalis

肋间外肌
intercostales externi

肋提肌
levatores costarum

图 183　背固有肌 2
Intrinsic back muscles 2

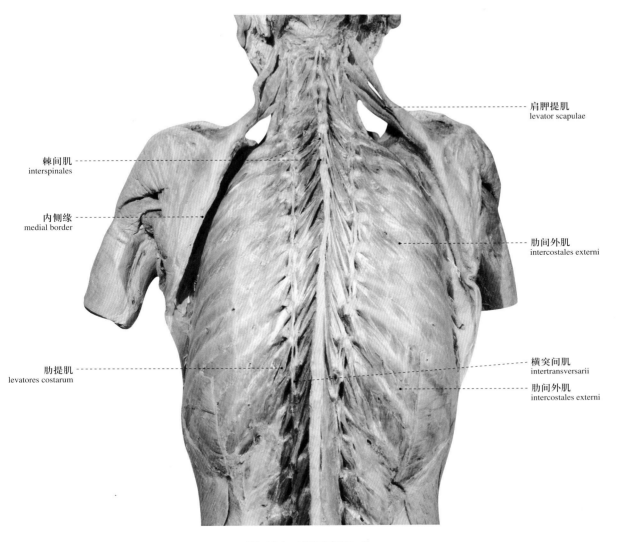

肩胛提肌
levator scapulae

棘间肌
interspinales

内侧缘
medial border

肋间外肌
intercostales externi

肋提肌
levatores costarum

横突间肌
intertransversarii

肋间外肌
intercostales externi

图 184　背固有肌 3

Intrinsic back muscles 3

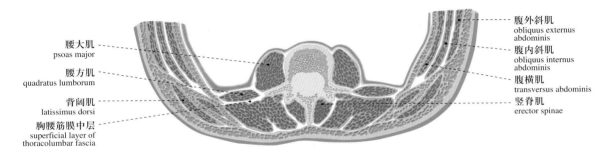

腰大肌
psoas major

腰方肌
quadratus lumborum

背阔肌
latissimus dorsi

胸腰筋膜中层
superficial layer of
thoracolumbar fascia

腹外斜肌
obliquus externus
abdominis

腹内斜肌
obliquus internus
abdominis

腹横肌
transversus abdominis

竖脊肌
erector spinae

图 185　背肌（断面）

Muscles of the back (section)

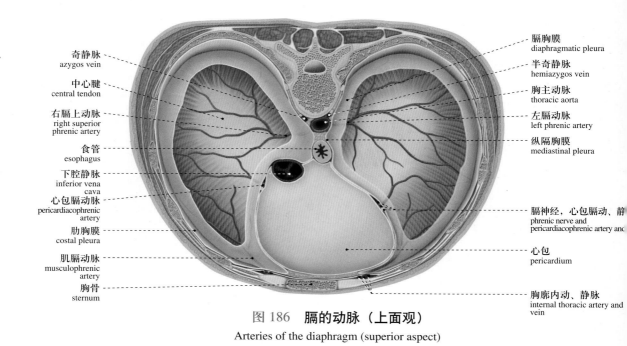

奇静脉
azygos vein

中心腱
central tendon

右膈上动脉
right superior
phrenic artery

食管
esophagus

下腔静脉
inferior vena
cava

心包膈动脉
pericardiacophrenic
artery

肋胸膜
costal pleura

肌膈动脉
musculophrenic
artery

胸骨
sternum

膈胸膜
diaphragmatic pleura

半奇静脉
hemiazygos vein

胸主动脉
thoracic aorta

左膈动脉
left phrenic artery

纵隔胸膜
mediastinal pleura

膈神经，心包膈动、静
phrenic nerve and
pericardiacophrenic artery and

心包
pericardium

胸廓内动、静脉
internal thoracic artery and
vein

图 186　膈的动脉（上面观）
Arteries of the diaphragm (superior aspect)

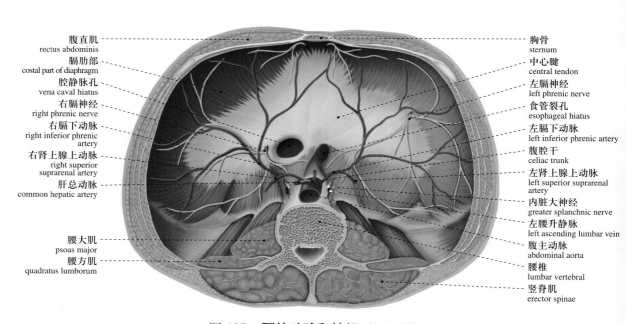

腹直肌
rectus abdominis

膈肋部
costal part of diaphragm

腔静脉孔
vena caval hiatus

右膈神经
right phrenic nerve

右膈下动脉
right inferior phrenic
artery

右肾上腺上动脉
right superior
suprarenal artery

肝总动脉
common hepatic artery

腰大肌
psoas major

腰方肌
quadratus lumborum

胸骨
sternum

中心腱
central tendon

左膈神经
left phrenic nerve

食管裂孔
esophageal hiatus

左膈下动脉
left inferior phrenic artery

腹腔干
celiac trunk

左肾上腺上动脉
left superior suprarenal
artery

内脏大神经
greater splanchnic nerve

左腰升静脉
left ascending lumbar vein

腹主动脉
abdominal aorta

腰椎
lumbar vertebral

竖脊肌
erector spinae

图 187　膈的动脉和神经（下面观）
Arteries and nerves of the diaphragm (inferior aspect)

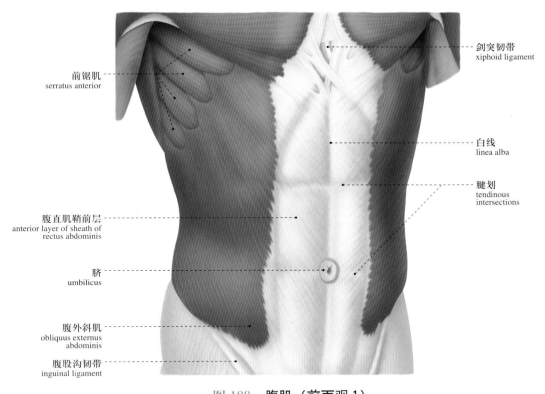

前锯肌
serratus anterior

剑突韧带
xiphoid ligament

白线
linea alba

腱划
tendinous intersections

腹直肌鞘前层
anterior layer of sheath of rectus abdominis

脐
umbilicus

腹外斜肌
obliquus externus abdominis

腹股沟韧带
inguinal ligament

图 188　腹肌（前面观 1）

Muscles of the abdomen (anterior aspect 1)

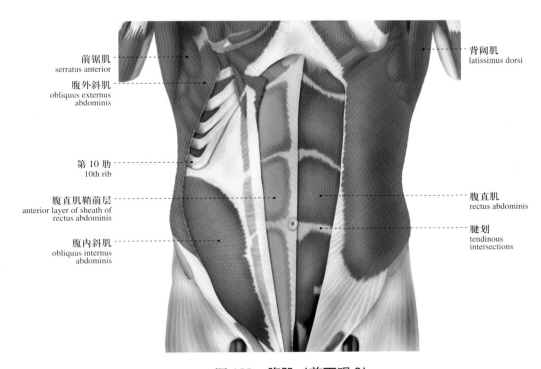

前锯肌
serratus anterior

腹外斜肌
obliquus externus abdominis

背阔肌
latissimus dorsi

第 10 肋
10th rib

腹直肌鞘前层
anterior layer of sheath of rectus abdominis

腹内斜肌
obliquus internus abdominis

腹直肌
rectus abdominis

腱划
tendinous intersections

图 189　腹肌（前面观 2）

Muscles of the abdomen (anterior aspect 2)

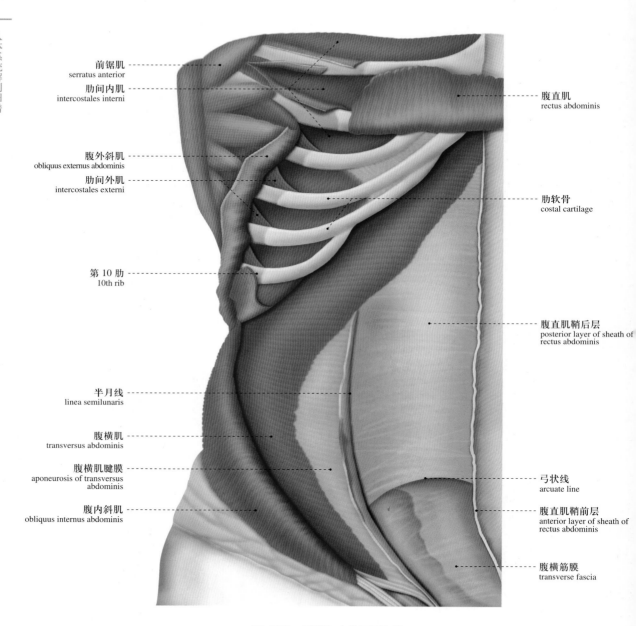

前锯肌
serratus anterior

肋间内肌
intercostales interni

腹外斜肌
obliquus externus abdominis

肋间外肌
intercostales externi

第 10 肋
10th rib

半月线
linea semilunaris

腹横肌
transversus abdominis

腹横肌腱膜
aponeurosis of transversus abdominis

腹内斜肌
obliquus internus abdominis

腹直肌
rectus abdominis

肋软骨
costal cartilage

腹直肌鞘后层
posterior layer of sheath of rectus abdominis

弓状线
arcuate line

腹直肌鞘前层
anterior layer of sheath of rectus abdominis

腹横筋膜
transverse fascia

图 190　腹肌（前面观 3）

Muscles of the abdomen (anterior aspect 3)

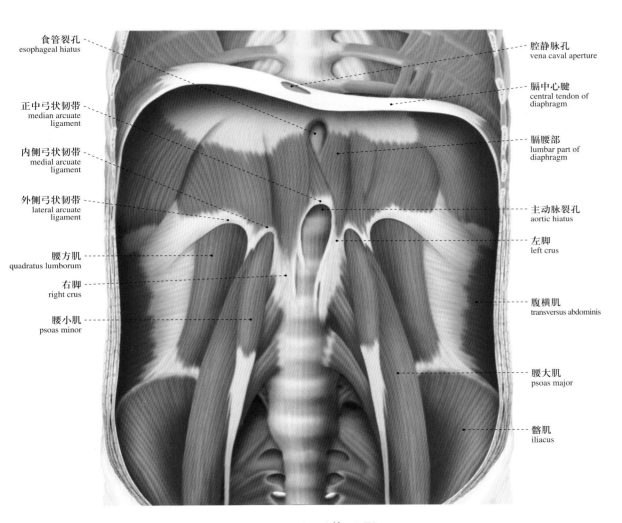

食管裂孔
esophageal hiatus

正中弓状韧带
median arcuate ligament

内侧弓状韧带
medial arcuate ligament

外侧弓状韧带
lateral arcuate ligament

腰方肌
quadratus lumborum

右脚
right crus

腰小肌
psoas minor

腔静脉孔
vena caval aperture

膈中心腱
central tendon of diaphragm

膈腰部
lumbar part of diaphragm

主动脉裂孔
aortic hiatus

左脚
left crus

腹横肌
transversus abdominis

腰大肌
psoas major

髂肌
iliacus

图 191　腰肌（前面观）
Lumbar muscles (anterior aspect)

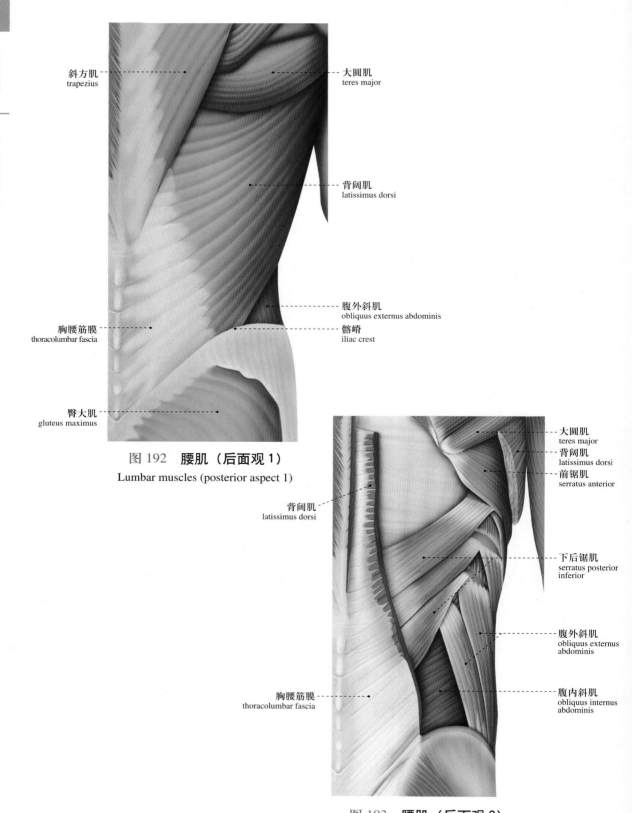

斜方肌
trapezius

大圆肌
teres major

背阔肌
latissimus dorsi

腹外斜肌
obliquus externus abdominis

髂嵴
iliac crest

胸腰筋膜
thoracolumbar fascia

臀大肌
gluteus maximus

图 192　腰肌（后面观 1）
Lumbar muscles (posterior aspect 1)

大圆肌
teres major

背阔肌
latissimus dorsi

前锯肌
serratus anterior

背阔肌
latissimus dorsi

下后锯肌
serratus posterior inferior

腹外斜肌
obliquus externus abdominis

胸腰筋膜
thoracolumbar fascia

腹内斜肌
obliquus internus abdominis

图 193　腰肌（后面观 2）
Lumbar muscles (posterior aspect 2)

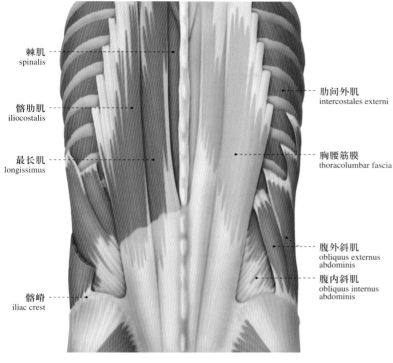

棘肌
spinalis

髂肋肌
iliocostalis

最长肌
longissimus

髂嵴
iliac crest

肋间外肌
intercostales externi

胸腰筋膜
thoracolumbar fascia

腹外斜肌
obliquus externus
abdominis

腹内斜肌
obliquus internus
abdominis

图 194　腰肌（后面观 3）
Lumbar muscles (posterior aspect 3)

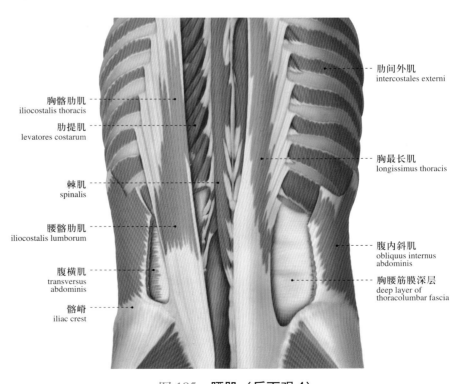

胸髂肋肌
iliocostalis thoracis

肋提肌
levatores costarum

棘肌
spinalis

腰髂肋肌
iliocostalis lumborum

腹横肌
transversus
abdominis

髂嵴
iliac crest

肋间外肌
intercostales externi

胸最长肌
longissimus thoracis

腹内斜肌
obliquus internus
abdominis

胸腰筋膜深层
deep layer of
thoracolumbar fascia

图 195　腰肌（后面观 4）
Lumbar muscles (posterior aspect 4)

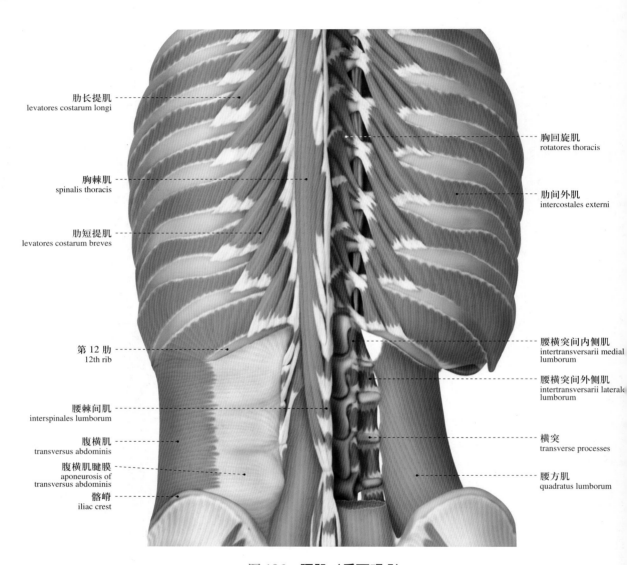

肋长提肌
levatores costarum longi

胸棘肌
spinalis thoracis

肋短提肌
levatores costarum breves

第 12 肋
12th rib

腰棘间肌
interspinales lumborum

腹横肌
transversus abdominis

腹横肌腱膜
aponeurosis of
transversus abdominis

髂嵴
iliac crest

胸回旋肌
rotatores thoracis

肋间外肌
intercostales externi

腰横突间内侧肌
intertransversarii medial
lumborum

腰横突间外侧肌
intertransversarii laterale
lumborum

横突
transverse processes

腰方肌
quadratus lumborum

图 196　腰肌（后面观 5）
Lumbar muscles (posterior aspect 5)

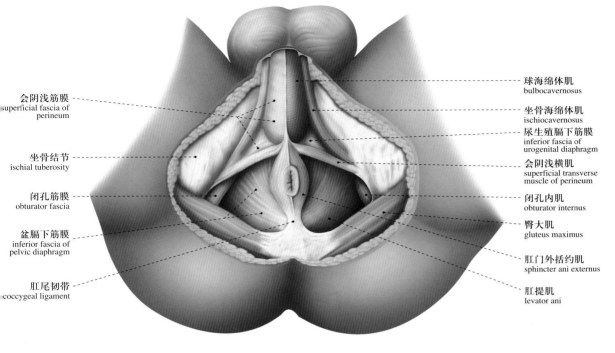

会阴浅筋膜
superficial fascia of
perineum

坐骨结节
ischial tuberosity

闭孔筋膜
obturator fascia

盆膈下筋膜
inferior fascia of
pelvic diaphragm

肛尾韧带
coccygeal ligament

球海绵体肌
bulbocavernosus

坐骨海绵体肌
ischiocavernosus

尿生殖膈下筋膜
inferior fascia of
urogenital diaphragm

会阴浅横肌
superficial transverse
muscle of perineum

闭孔内肌
obturator internus

臀大肌
gluteus maximus

肛门外括约肌
sphincter ani externus

肛提肌
levator ani

图 197　**男性盆底浅层筋膜**

Superficial fasciae of the male pelvic floor

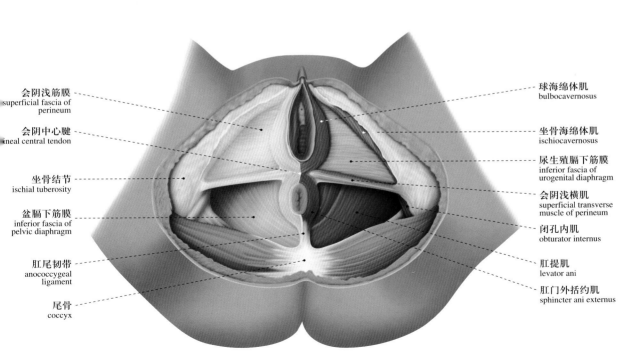

会阴浅筋膜
superficial fascia of
perineum

会阴中心腱
perineal central tendon

坐骨结节
ischial tuberosity

盆膈下筋膜
inferior fascia of
pelvic diaphragm

肛尾韧带
anococcygeal
ligament

尾骨
coccyx

球海绵体肌
bulbocavernosus

坐骨海绵体肌
ischiocavernosus

尿生殖膈下筋膜
inferior fascia of
urogenital diaphragm

会阴浅横肌
superficial transverse
muscle of perineum

闭孔内肌
obturator internus

肛提肌
levator ani

肛门外括约肌
sphincter ani externus

图 198　**女性盆底浅层筋膜**

Superficial fasciae of the female pelvic floor

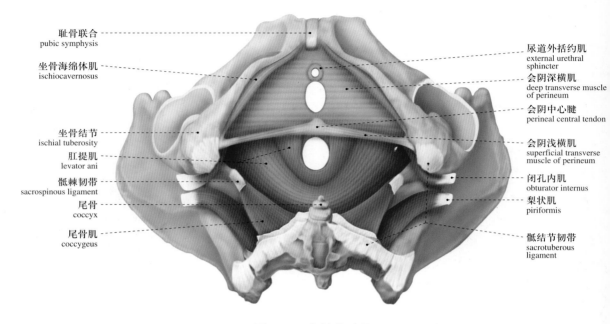

耻骨联合
pubic symphysis

坐骨海绵体肌
ischiocavernosus

坐骨结节
ischial tuberosity

肛提肌
levator ani

骶棘韧带
sacrospinous ligament

尾骨
coccyx

尾骨肌
coccygeus

尿道外括约肌
external urethral sphincter

会阴深横肌
deep transverse muscle of perineum

会阴中心腱
perineal central tendon

会阴浅横肌
superficial transverse muscle of perineum

闭孔内肌
obturator internus

梨状肌
piriformis

骶结节韧带
sacrotuberous ligament

图 199　女性盆底肌 1
Muscles of the female pelvic floor 1

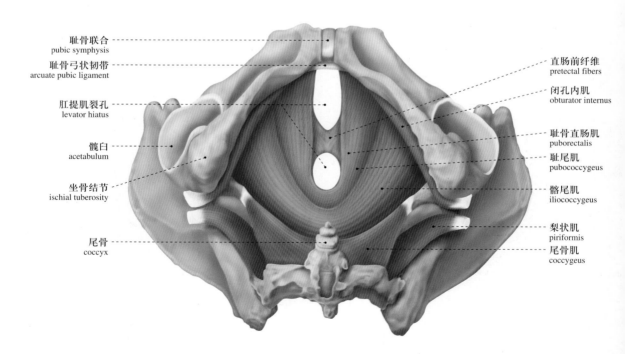

耻骨联合
pubic symphysis

耻骨弓状韧带
arcuate pubic ligament

肛提肌裂孔
levator hiatus

髋臼
acetabulum

坐骨结节
ischial tuberosity

尾骨
coccyx

直肠前纤维
pretectal fibers

闭孔内肌
obturator internus

耻骨直肠肌
puborectalis

耻尾肌
pubococcygeus

髂尾肌
iliococcygeus

梨状肌
piriformis

尾骨肌
coccygeus

图 200　女性盆底肌 2
Muscles of the female pelvic floor 2

第七节

上 肢 肌

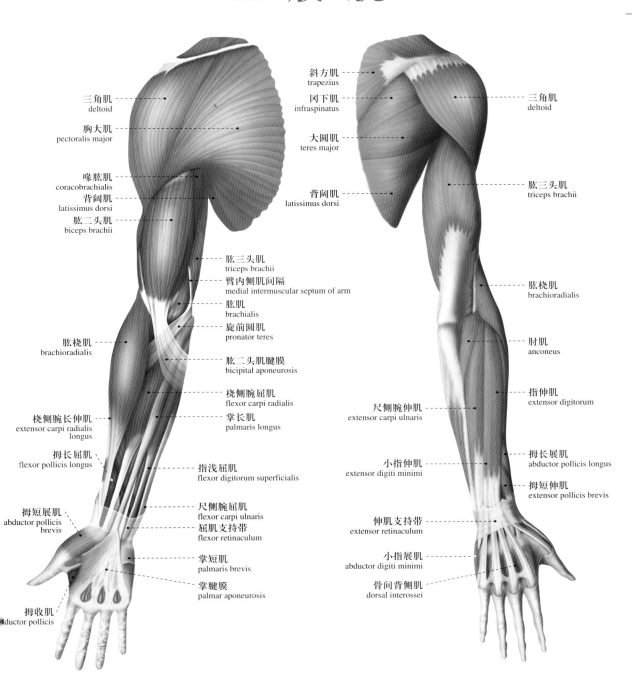

三角肌
deltoid

胸大肌
pectoralis major

喙肱肌
coracobrachialis

背阔肌
latissimus dorsi

肱二头肌
biceps brachii

肱桡肌
brachioradialis

桡侧腕长伸肌
extensor carpi radialis longus

拇长屈肌
flexor pollicis longus

拇短展肌
abductor pollicis brevis

拇收肌
adductor pollicis

斜方肌
trapezius

冈下肌
infraspinatus

大圆肌
teres major

背阔肌
latissimus dorsi

肱三头肌
triceps brachii

臂内侧肌间隔
medial intermuscular septum of arm

肱肌
brachialis

旋前圆肌
pronator teres

肱二头肌腱膜
bicipital aponeurosis

桡侧腕屈肌
flexor carpi radialis

掌长肌
palmaris longus

指浅屈肌
flexor digitorum superficialis

尺侧腕屈肌
flexor carpi ulnaris

屈肌支持带
flexor retinaculum

掌短肌
palmaris brevis

掌腱膜
palmar aponeurosis

三角肌
deltoid

肱三头肌
triceps brachii

肱桡肌
brachioradialis

肘肌
anconeus

指伸肌
extensor digitorum

尺侧腕伸肌
extensor carpi ulnaris

小指伸肌
extensor digiti minimi

拇长展肌
abductor pollicis longus

拇短伸肌
extensor pollicis brevis

伸肌支持带
extensor retinaculum

小指展肌
abductor digiti minimi

骨间背侧肌
dorsal interossei

图 201　上肢肌（前面观）
Muscles of the upper limb (anterior aspect)

图 202　上肢肌（后面观）
Muscles of the upper limb (posterior aspect)

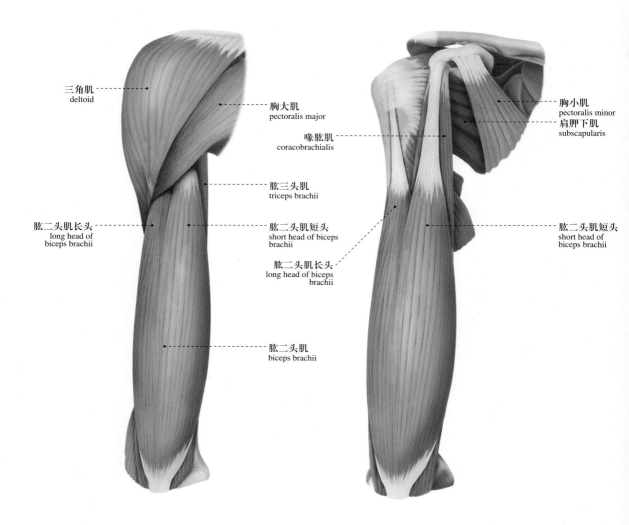

三角肌
deltoid

胸大肌
pectoralis major

喙肱肌
coracobrachialis

肱三头肌
triceps brachii

肱二头肌长头
long head of
biceps brachii

肱二头肌短头
short head of biceps
brachii

肱二头肌长头
long head of biceps
brachii

肱二头肌
biceps brachii

胸小肌
pectoralis minor

肩胛下肌
subscapularis

肱二头肌短头
short head of
biceps brachii

图 203　肩臂部肌（前面观 1）

Muscles of the shoulder and arm (anterior aspect 1)

图 204　肩臂部肌（前面观 2）

Muscles of the shoulder and arm (anterior aspect 2)

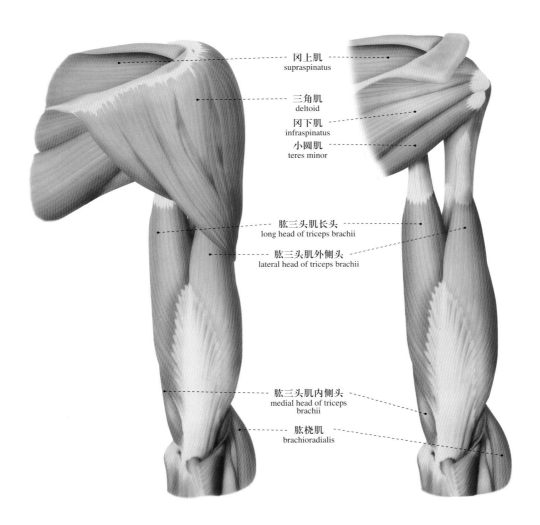

冈上肌
supraspinatus

三角肌
deltoid

冈下肌
infraspinatus

小圆肌
teres minor

肱三头肌长头
long head of triceps brachii

肱三头肌外侧头
lateral head of triceps brachii

肱三头肌内侧头
medial head of triceps
brachii

肱桡肌
brachioradialis

图 205　肩臂部肌（后面观 1）
Muscles of the shoulder and arm (posterior aspect 1)

图 206　肩臂部肌（后面观 2）
Muscles of the shoulder and arm (posterior aspect 2)

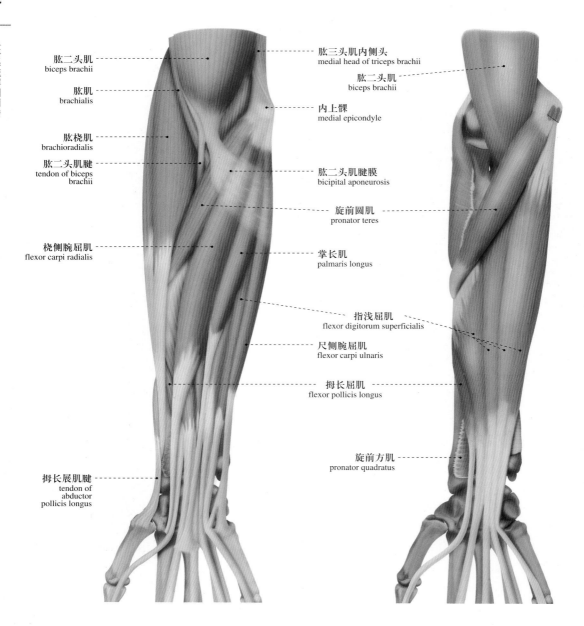

肱二头肌
biceps brachii

肱肌
brachialis

肱桡肌
brachioradialis

肱二头肌腱
tendon of biceps
brachii

桡侧腕屈肌
flexor carpi radialis

拇长展肌腱
tendon of
abductor
pollicis longus

肱三头肌内侧头
medial head of triceps brachii

肱二头肌
biceps brachii

内上髁
medial epicondyle

肱二头肌腱膜
bicipital aponeurosis

旋前圆肌
pronator teres

掌长肌
palmaris longus

指浅屈肌
flexor digitorum superficialis

尺侧腕屈肌
flexor carpi ulnaris

拇长屈肌
flexor pollicis longus

旋前方肌
pronator quadratus

图 207　肘前臂肌（前面观 1）
Muscles of the elbow and forearm (anterior aspect 1)

图 208　肘前臂肌（前面观 2）
Muscles of the elbow and forearm (anterior aspect 2)

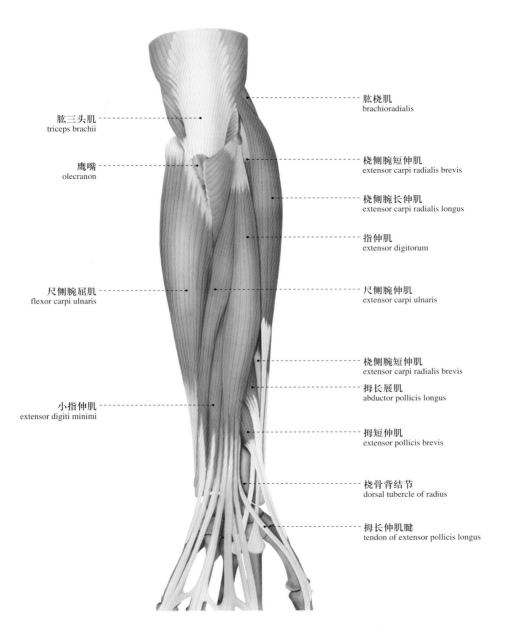

肱三头肌
triceps brachii

鹰嘴
olecranon

尺侧腕屈肌
flexor carpi ulnaris

小指伸肌
extensor digiti minimi

肱桡肌
brachioradialis

桡侧腕短伸肌
extensor carpi radialis brevis

桡侧腕长伸肌
extensor carpi radialis longus

指伸肌
extensor digitorum

尺侧腕伸肌
extensor carpi ulnaris

桡侧腕短伸肌
extensor carpi radialis brevis

拇长展肌
abductor pollicis longus

拇短伸肌
extensor pollicis brevis

桡骨背结节
dorsal tubercle of radius

拇长伸肌腱
tendon of extensor pollicis longus

图 209　前臂肌（后面观）
Forearm muscles (posterior aspect)

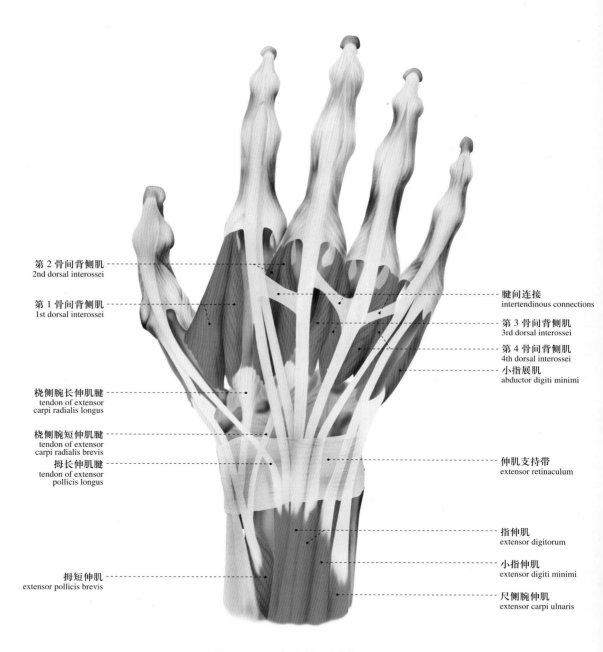

第 2 骨间背侧肌
2nd dorsal interossei

第 1 骨间背侧肌
1st dorsal interossei

桡侧腕长伸肌腱
tendon of extensor
carpi radialis longus

桡侧腕短伸肌腱
tendon of extensor
carpi radialis brevis

拇长伸肌腱
tendon of extensor
pollicis longus

拇短伸肌
extensor pollicis brevis

腱间连接
intertendinous connections

第 3 骨间背侧肌
3rd dorsal interossei

第 4 骨间背侧肌
4th dorsal interossei

小指展肌
abductor digiti minimi

伸肌支持带
extensor retinaculum

指伸肌
extensor digitorum

小指伸肌
extensor digiti minimi

尺侧腕伸肌
extensor carpi ulnaris

图 210 手部肌肉（背侧面）
Muscles of the hand (dorsal aspect)

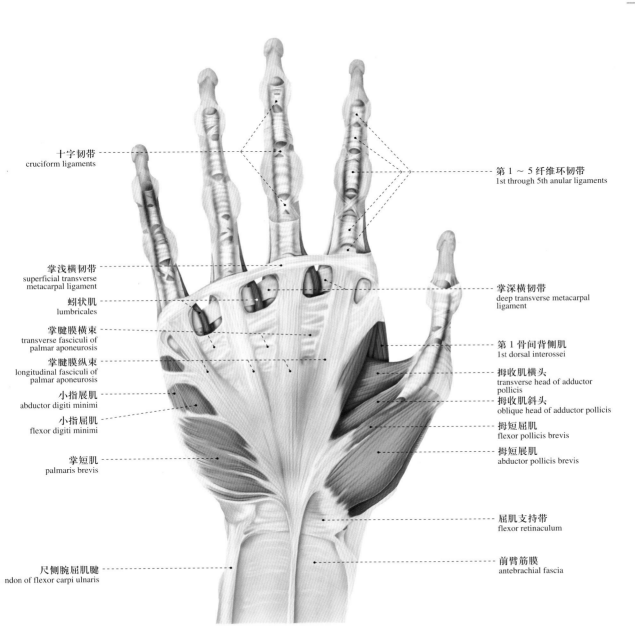

十字韧带
cruciform ligaments

掌浅横韧带
superficial transverse
metacarpal ligament

蚓状肌
lumbricales

掌腱膜横束
transverse fasciculi of
palmar aponeurosis

掌腱膜纵束
longitudinal fasciculi of
palmar aponeurosis

小指展肌
abductor digiti minimi

小指屈肌
flexor digiti minimi

掌短肌
palmaris brevis

尺侧腕屈肌腱
ndon of flexor carpi ulnaris

第 1 ～ 5 纤维环韧带
1st through 5th anular ligaments

掌深横韧带
deep transverse metacarpal
ligament

第 1 骨间背侧肌
1st dorsal interossei

拇收肌横头
transverse head of adductor
pollicis

拇收肌斜头
oblique head of adductor pollicis

拇短屈肌
flexor pollicis brevis

拇短展肌
abductor pollicis brevis

屈肌支持带
flexor retinaculum

前臂筋膜
antebrachial fascia

图 211　手部肌肉（掌侧面 1）
Muscles of the hand (palmar aspect 1)

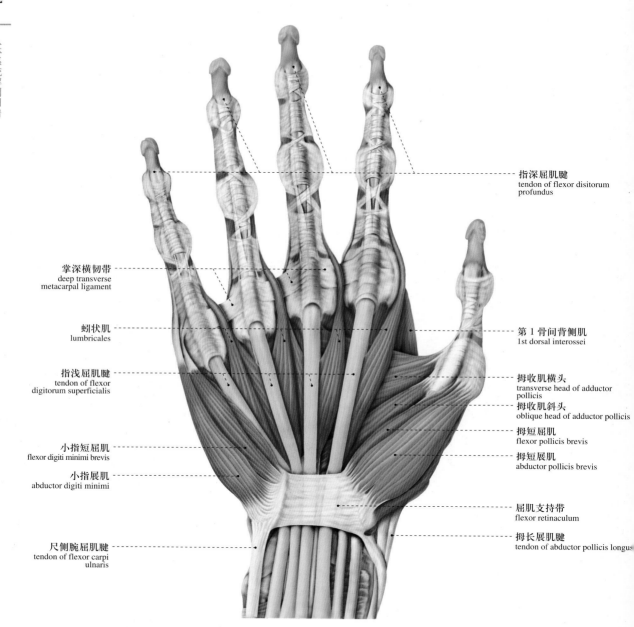

指深屈肌腱
tendon of flexor disitorum profundus

掌深横韧带
deep transverse metacarpal ligament

蚓状肌
lumbricales

指浅屈肌腱
tendon of flexor digitorum superficialis

小指短屈肌
flexor digiti minimi brevis

小指展肌
abductor digiti minimi

尺侧腕屈肌腱
tendon of flexor carpi ulnaris

第 1 骨间背侧肌
1st dorsal interossei

拇收肌横头
transverse head of adductor pollicis

拇收肌斜头
oblique head of adductor pollicis

拇短屈肌
flexor pollicis brevis

拇短展肌
abductor pollicis brevis

屈肌支持带
flexor retinaculum

拇长展肌腱
tendon of abductor pollicis longus

图 212　手部肌肉（掌侧面 2）
Muscles of the hand (palmar aspect 2)

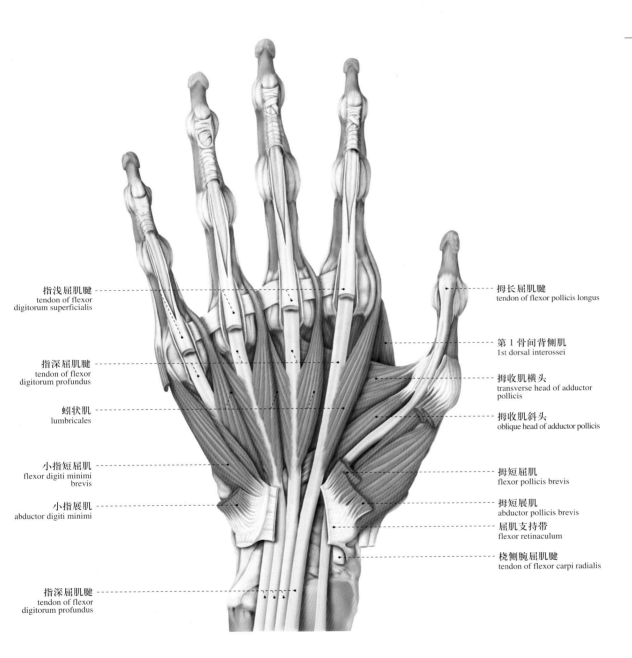

指浅屈肌腱
tendon of flexor
digitorum superficialis

指深屈肌腱
tendon of flexor
digitorum profundus

蚓状肌
lumbricales

小指短屈肌
flexor digiti minimi
brevis

小指展肌
abductor digiti minimi

指深屈肌腱
tendon of flexor
digitorum profundus

拇长屈肌腱
tendon of flexor pollicis longus

第 1 骨间背侧肌
1st dorsal interossei

拇收肌横头
transverse head of adductor
pollicis

拇收肌斜头
oblique head of adductor pollicis

拇短屈肌
flexor pollicis brevis

拇短展肌
abductor pollicis brevis

屈肌支持带
flexor retinaculum

桡侧腕屈肌腱
tendon of flexor carpi radialis

图 213　手部肌肉（掌侧面 3）
Muscles of the hand (palmar aspect 3)

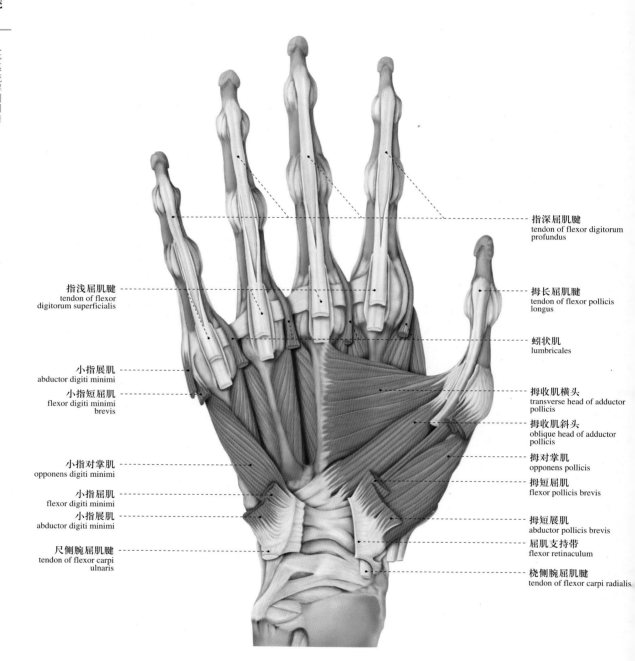

指深屈肌腱
tendon of flexor digitorum profundus

指浅屈肌腱
tendon of flexor digitorum superficialis

拇长屈肌腱
tendon of flexor pollicis longus

蚓状肌
lumbricales

小指展肌
abductor digiti minimi

小指短屈肌
flexor digiti minimi brevis

拇收肌横头
transverse head of adductor pollicis

拇收肌斜头
oblique head of adductor pollicis

小指对掌肌
opponens digiti minimi

拇对掌肌
opponens pollicis

小指屈肌
flexor digiti minimi

拇短屈肌
flexor pollicis brevis

小指展肌
abductor digiti minimi

拇短展肌
abductor pollicis brevis

尺侧腕屈肌腱
tendon of flexor carpi ulnaris

屈肌支持带
flexor retinaculum

桡侧腕屈肌腱
tendon of flexor carpi radialis

图 214　手部肌肉（掌侧面 4）
Muscles of the hand (palmar aspect 4)

第八节

下 肢 肌

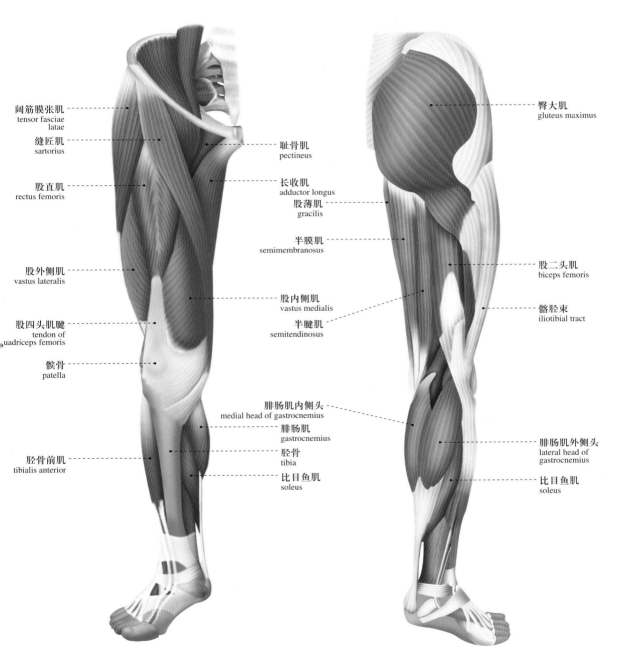

阔筋膜张肌
tensor fasciae latae

缝匠肌
sartorius

股直肌
rectus femoris

股外侧肌
vastus lateralis

股四头肌腱
tendon of quadriceps femoris

髌骨
patella

胫骨前肌
tibialis anterior

耻骨肌
pectineus

长收肌
adductor longus

股薄肌
gracilis

半膜肌
semimembranosus

股内侧肌
vastus medialis

半腱肌
semitendinosus

腓肠肌内侧头
medial head of gastrocnemius

腓肠肌
gastrocnemius

胫骨
tibia

比目鱼肌
soleus

臀大肌
gluteus maximus

股二头肌
biceps femoris

髂胫束
iliotibial tract

腓肠肌外侧头
lateral head of gastrocnemius

比目鱼肌
soleus

图 215　下肢肌（前面观）
Muscles of the lower limb (anterior aspect)

图 216　下肢肌（侧面观）
Muscles of the lower limb (lateral aspect)

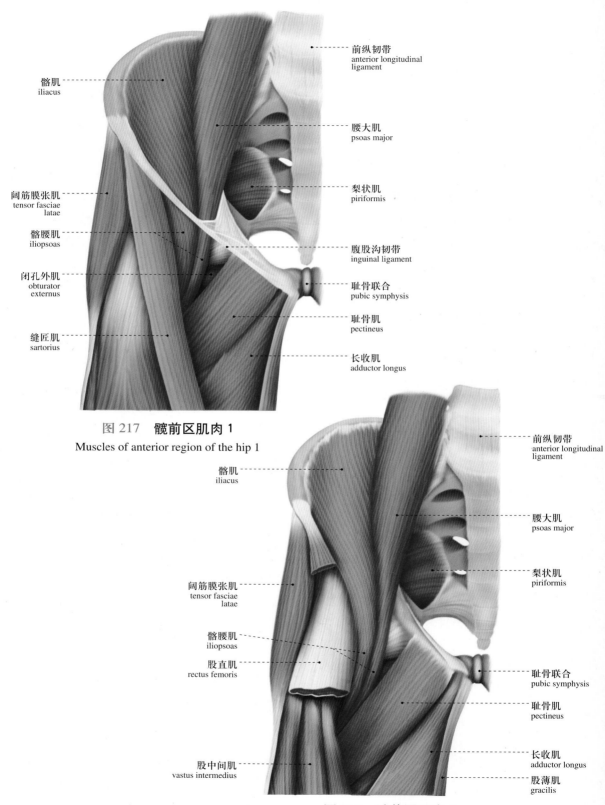

髂肌
iliacus

前纵韧带
anterior longitudinal
ligament

腰大肌
psoas major

阔筋膜张肌
tensor fasciae
latae

梨状肌
piriformis

髂腰肌
iliopsoas

腹股沟韧带
inguinal ligament

闭孔外肌
obturator
externus

耻骨联合
pubic symphysis

缝匠肌
sartorius

耻骨肌
pectineus

长收肌
adductor longus

图 217　髋前区肌肉 1
Muscles of anterior region of the hip 1

髂肌
iliacus

前纵韧带
anterior longitudinal
ligament

腰大肌
psoas major

阔筋膜张肌
tensor fasciae
latae

梨状肌
piriformis

髂腰肌
iliopsoas

股直肌
rectus femoris

耻骨联合
pubic symphysis

耻骨肌
pectineus

股中间肌
vastus intermedius

长收肌
adductor longus

股薄肌
gracilis

图 218　髋前区肌肉 2
Muscles of anterior region of the hip 2

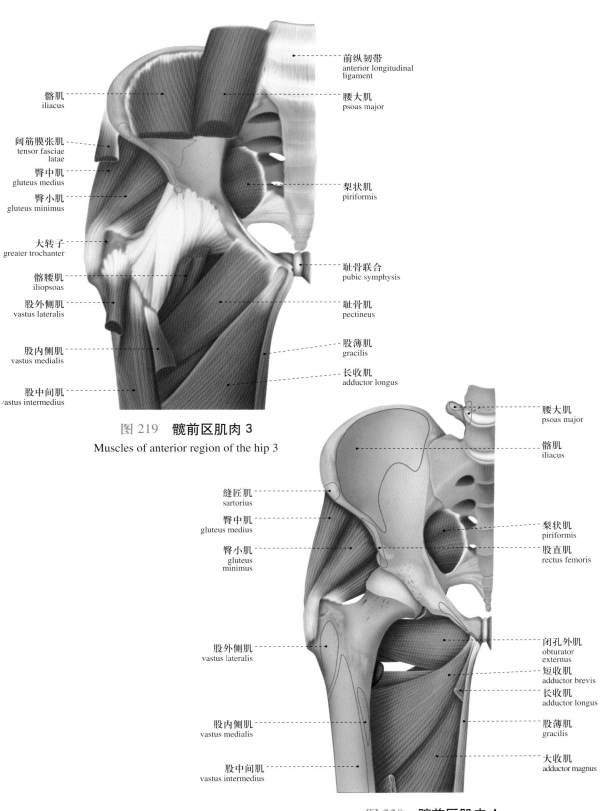

髂肌
iliacus

前纵韧带
anterior longitudinal
ligament

腰大肌
psoas major

阔筋膜张肌
tensor fasciae
latae

臀中肌
gluteus medius

臀小肌
gluteus minimus

梨状肌
piriformis

大转子
greater trochanter

髂腰肌
iliopsoas

耻骨联合
pubic symphysis

股外侧肌
vastus lateralis

耻骨肌
pectineus

股内侧肌
vastus medialis

股薄肌
gracilis

长收肌
adductor longus

股中间肌
vastus intermedius

图 219　髋前区肌肉 3

Muscles of anterior region of the hip 3

缝匠肌
sartorius

腰大肌
psoas major

臀中肌
gluteus medius

髂肌
iliacus

臀小肌
gluteus
minimus

梨状肌
piriformis

股直肌
rectus femoris

股外侧肌
vastus lateralis

闭孔外肌
obturator
externus

短收肌
adductor brevis

长收肌
adductor longus

股内侧肌
vastus medialis

股薄肌
gracilis

股中间肌
vastus intermedius

大收肌
adductor magnus

图 220　髋前区肌肉 4

Muscles of anterior region of the hip 4

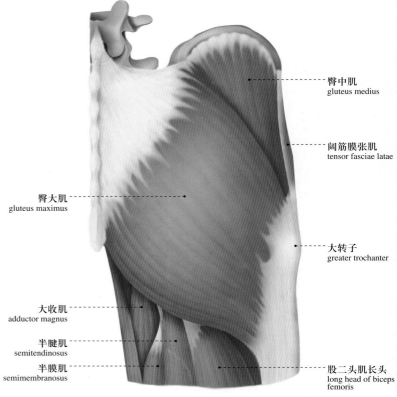

臀中肌
gluteus medius

阔筋膜张肌
tensor fasciae latae

臀大肌
gluteus maximus

大转子
greater trochanter

大收肌
adductor magnus

半腱肌
semitendinosus

半膜肌
semimembranosus

股二头肌长头
long head of biceps femoris

图 221　臀区肌肉 1
Muscles of the gluteal region 1

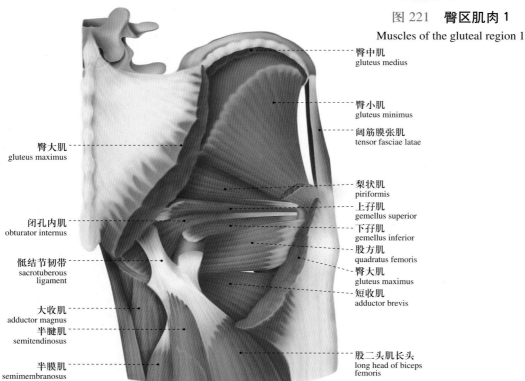

臀中肌
gluteus medius

臀小肌
gluteus minimus

阔筋膜张肌
tensor fasciae latae

梨状肌
piriformis

上孖肌
gemellus superior

下孖肌
gemellus inferior

股方肌
quadratus femoris

臀大肌
gluteus maximus

短收肌
adductor brevis

股二头肌长头
long head of biceps femoris

臀大肌
gluteus maximus

闭孔内肌
obturator internus

骶结节韧带
sacrotuberous ligament

大收肌
adductor magnus

半腱肌
semitendinosus

半膜肌
semimembranosus

图 222　臀区肌肉 2
Muscles of the gluteal region 2

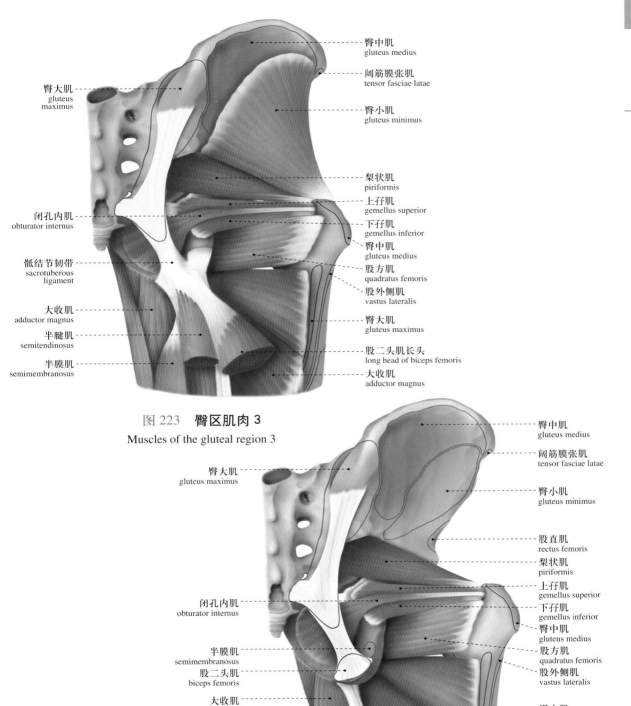

臀中肌
gluteus medius

阔筋膜张肌
tensor fasciae latae

臀大肌
gluteus
maximus

臀小肌
gluteus minimus

梨状肌
piriformis

上孖肌
gemellus superior

下孖肌
gemellus inferior

闭孔内肌
obturator internus

臀中肌
gluteus medius

骶结节韧带
sacrotuberous
ligament

股方肌
quadratus femoris

股外侧肌
vastus lateralis

大收肌
adductor magnus

臀大肌
gluteus maximus

半腱肌
semitendinosus

股二头肌长头
long head of biceps femoris

半膜肌
semimembranosus

大收肌
adductor magnus

图 223　臀区肌肉 3

Muscles of the gluteal region 3

臀大肌
gluteus maximus

臀中肌
gluteus medius

阔筋膜张肌
tensor fasciae latae

臀小肌
gluteus minimus

股直肌
rectus femoris

梨状肌
piriformis

上孖肌
gemellus superior

闭孔内肌
obturator internus

下孖肌
gemellus inferior

臀中肌
gluteus medius

股方肌
quadratus femoris

半膜肌
semimembranosus

股外侧肌
vastus lateralis

股二头肌
biceps femoris

臀大肌
gluteus maximus

大收肌
adductor magnus

大收肌
adductor magnus

图 224　臀区肌肉 4

Muscles of the gluteal region 4

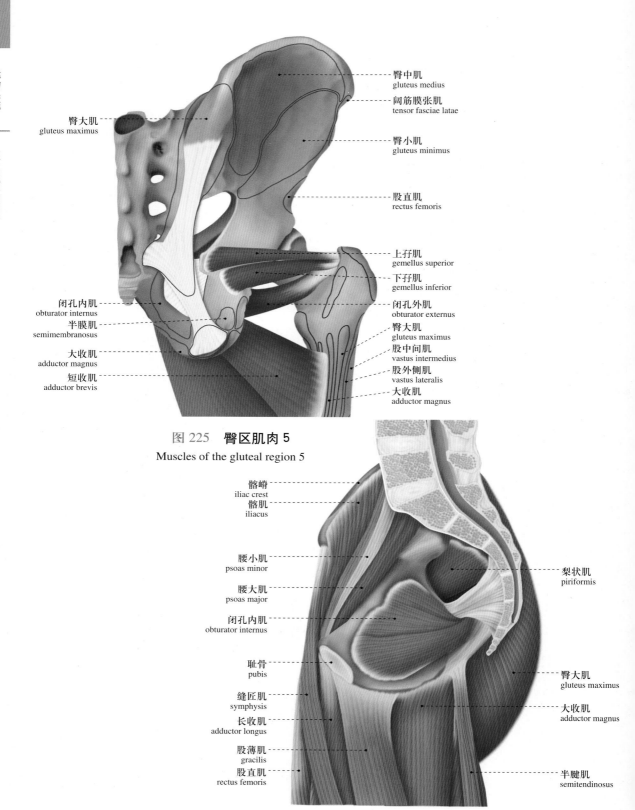

臀中肌
gluteus medius

阔筋膜张肌
tensor fasciae latae

臀小肌
gluteus minimus

股直肌
rectus femoris

上孖肌
gemellus superior

下孖肌
gemellus inferior

闭孔外肌
obturator externus

臀大肌
gluteus maximus

股中间肌
vastus intermedius

股外侧肌
vastus lateralis

大收肌
adductor magnus

臀大肌
gluteus maximus

闭孔内肌
obturator internus

半膜肌
semimembranosus

大收肌
adductor magnus

短收肌
adductor brevis

图 225　臀区肌肉 5
Muscles of the gluteal region 5

髂嵴
iliac crest

髂肌
iliacus

腰小肌
psoas minor

腰大肌
psoas major

闭孔内肌
obturator internus

耻骨
pubis

缝匠肌
symphysis

长收肌
adductor longus

股薄肌
gracilis

股直肌
rectus femoris

梨状肌
piriformis

臀大肌
gluteus maximus

大收肌
adductor magnus

半腱肌
semitendinosus

图 226　髋内侧面肌肉
Muscles of the medial aspect of the hip

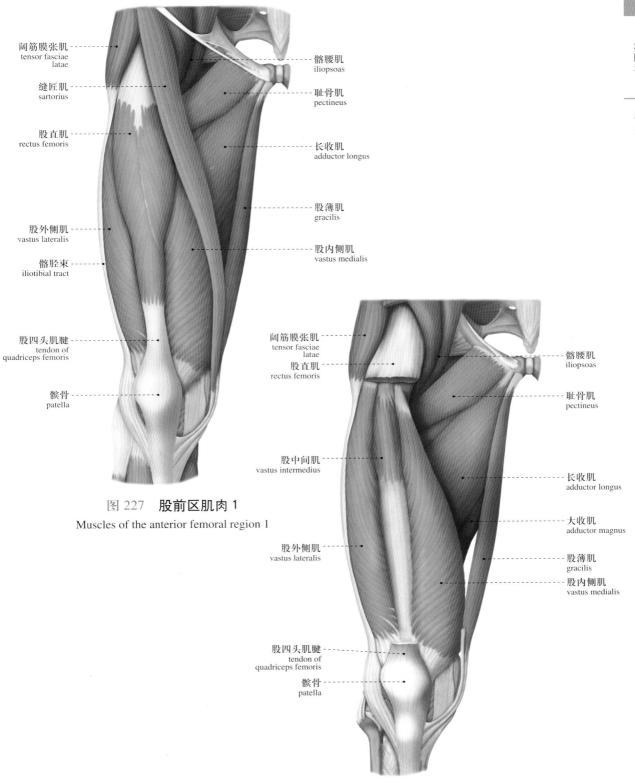

阔筋膜张肌
tensor fasciae
latae

缝匠肌
sartorius

股直肌
rectus femoris

股外侧肌
vastus lateralis

髂胫束
iliotibial tract

股四头肌腱
tendon of
quadriceps femoris

髌骨
patella

髂腰肌
iliopsoas

耻骨肌
pectineus

长收肌
adductor longus

股薄肌
gracilis

股内侧肌
vastus medialis

图 227　股前区肌肉 1
Muscles of the anterior femoral region 1

阔筋膜张肌
tensor fasciae
latae

股直肌
rectus femoris

股中间肌
vastus intermedius

股外侧肌
vastus lateralis

股四头肌腱
tendon of
quadriceps femoris

髌骨
patella

髂腰肌
iliopsoas

耻骨肌
pectineus

长收肌
adductor longus

大收肌
adductor magnus

股薄肌
gracilis

股内侧肌
vastus medialis

图 228　股前区肌肉 2
Muscles of the anterior femoral region 2

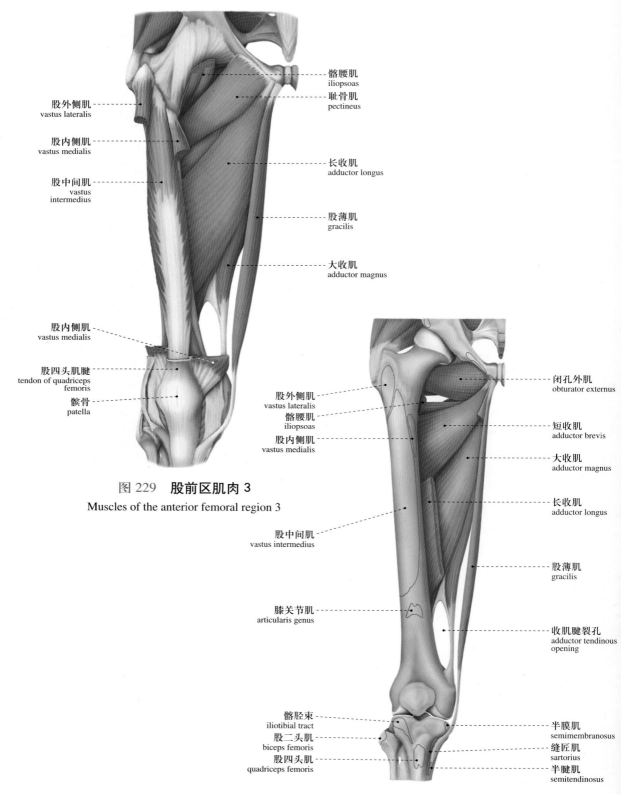

髂腰肌
iliopsoas

股外侧肌
vastus lateralis

耻骨肌
pectineus

股内侧肌
vastus medialis

股中间肌
vastus
intermedius

长收肌
adductor longus

股薄肌
gracilis

大收肌
adductor magnus

股内侧肌
vastus medialis

股四头肌腱
tendon of quadriceps
femoris

髌骨
patella

股外侧肌
vastus lateralis

髂腰肌
iliopsoas

股内侧肌
vastus medialis

股中间肌
vastus intermedius

图 229　股前区肌肉 3

Muscles of the anterior femoral region 3

闭孔外肌
obturator externus

短收肌
adductor brevis

大收肌
adductor magnus

长收肌
adductor longus

股薄肌
gracilis

收肌腱裂孔
adductor tendinous
opening

膝关节肌
articularis genus

髂胫束
iliotibial tract

股二头肌
biceps femoris

股四头肌
quadriceps femoris

半膜肌
semimembranosus

缝匠肌
sartorius

半腱肌
semitendinosus

图 230　股前区肌肉 4

Muscles of the anterior femoral region 4

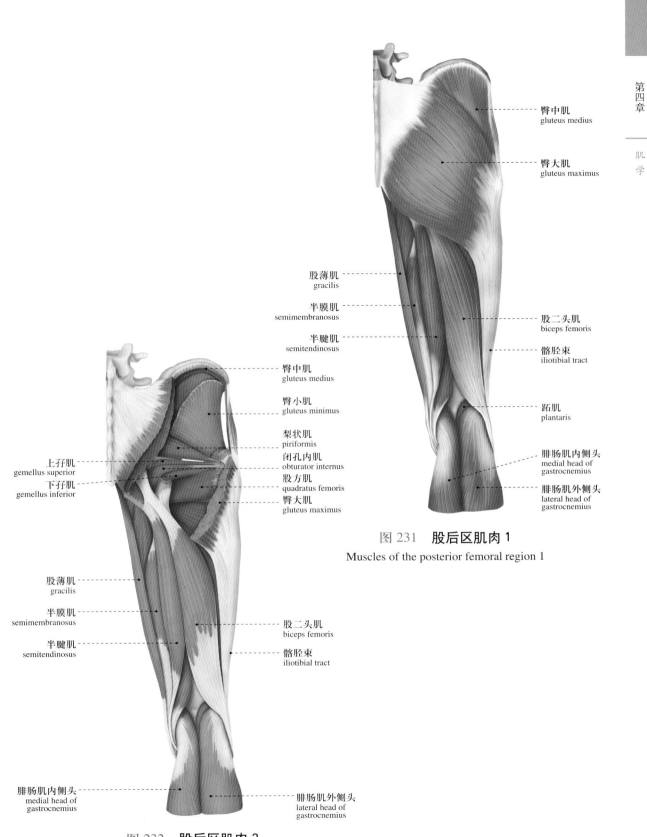

臀中肌
gluteus medius

臀大肌
gluteus maximus

股薄肌
gracilis

半膜肌
semimembranosus

半腱肌
semitendinosus

股二头肌
biceps femoris

髂胫束
iliotibial tract

跖肌
plantaris

腓肠肌内侧头
medial head of
gastrocnemius

腓肠肌外侧头
lateral head of
gastrocnemius

图 231　股后区肌肉 1
Muscles of the posterior femoral region 1

臀中肌
gluteus medius

臀小肌
gluteus minimus

梨状肌
piriformis

闭孔内肌
obturator internus

股方肌
quadratus femoris

臀大肌
gluteus maximus

上孖肌
gemellus superior

下孖肌
gemellus inferior

股薄肌
gracilis

半膜肌
semimembranosus

半腱肌
semitendinosus

股二头肌
biceps femoris

髂胫束
iliotibial tract

腓肠肌内侧头
medial head of
gastrocnemius

腓肠肌外侧头
lateral head of
gastrocnemius

图 232　股后区肌肉 2
Muscles of the posterior femoral region 2

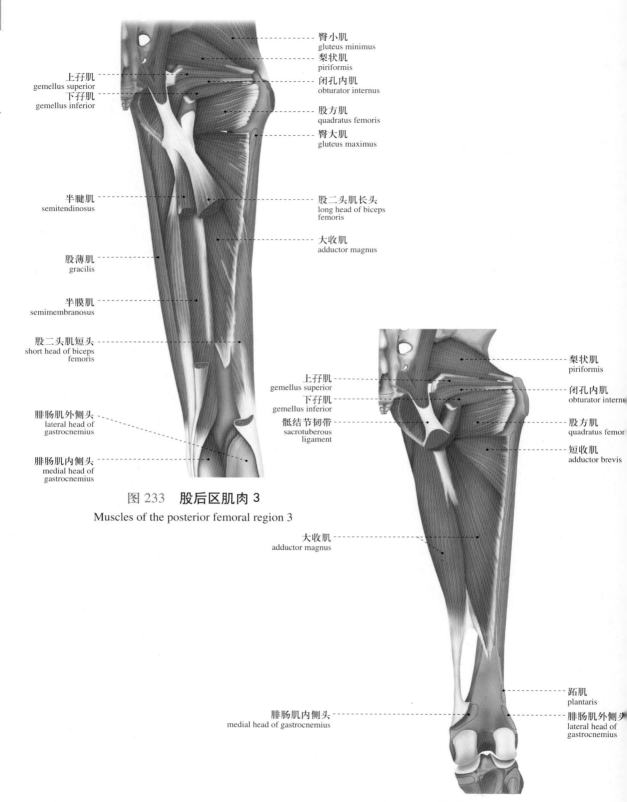

臀小肌
gluteus minimus

梨状肌
piriformis

上孖肌
gemellus superior

下孖肌
gemellus inferior

闭孔内肌
obturator internus

股方肌
quadratus femoris

臀大肌
gluteus maximus

半腱肌
semitendinosus

股二头肌长头
long head of biceps femoris

大收肌
adductor magnus

股薄肌
gracilis

半膜肌
semimembranosus

股二头肌短头
short head of biceps femoris

腓肠肌外侧头
lateral head of gastrocnemius

腓肠肌内侧头
medial head of gastrocnemius

图 233　股后区肌肉 3
Muscles of the posterior femoral region 3

梨状肌
piriformis

上孖肌
gemellus superior

下孖肌
gemellus inferior

闭孔内肌
obturator internus

骶结节韧带
sacrotuberous ligament

股方肌
quadratus femoris

短收肌
adductor brevis

大收肌
adductor magnus

跖肌
plantaris

腓肠肌内侧头
medial head of gastrocnemius

腓肠肌外侧头
lateral head of gastrocnemius

图 234　股后区肌肉 4
Muscles of the posterior femoral region 4

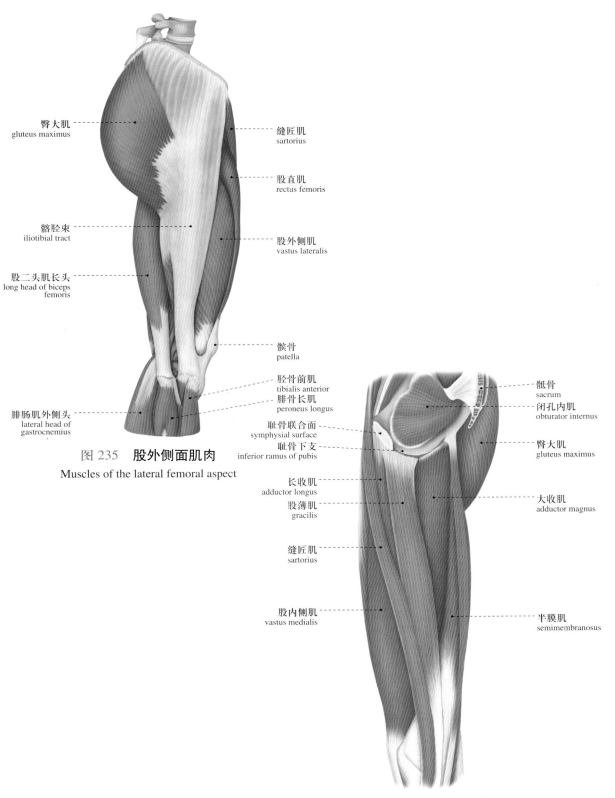

臀大肌
gluteus maximus

缝匠肌
sartorius

股直肌
rectus femoris

髂胫束
iliotibial tract

股外侧肌
vastus lateralis

股二头肌长头
long head of biceps femoris

髌骨
patella

胫骨前肌
tibialis anterior

腓骨长肌
peroneus longus

腓肠肌外侧头
lateral head of gastrocnemius

图 235　股外侧面肌肉
Muscles of the lateral femoral aspect

骶骨
sacrum

闭孔内肌
obturator internus

臀大肌
gluteus maximus

大收肌
adductor magnus

半膜肌
semimembranosus

耻骨联合面
symphysial surface

耻骨下支
inferior ramus of pubis

长收肌
adductor longus

股薄肌
gracilis

缝匠肌
sartorius

股内侧肌
vastus medialis

图 236　股内侧面肌肉
Muscles of the medial femoral aspect

125

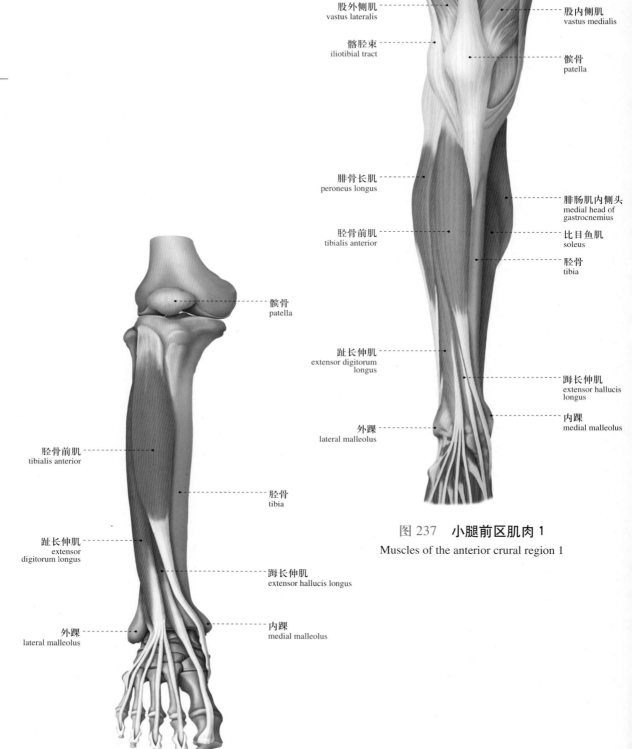

股外侧肌
vastus lateralis

股内侧肌
vastus medialis

髂胫束
iliotibial tract

髌骨
patella

腓骨长肌
peroneus longus

腓肠肌内侧头
medial head of gastrocnemius

比目鱼肌
soleus

胫骨前肌
tibialis anterior

胫骨
tibia

趾长伸肌
extensor digitorum longus

蹬长伸肌
extensor hallucis longus

内踝
medial malleolus

外踝
lateral malleolus

图 237　小腿前区肌肉 1
Muscles of the anterior crural region 1

髌骨
patella

胫骨前肌
tibialis anterior

胫骨
tibia

趾长伸肌
extensor digitorum longus

蹬长伸肌
extensor hallucis longus

外踝
lateral malleolus

内踝
medial malleolus

图 238　小腿前区肌肉 2
Muscles of the anterior crural region 2

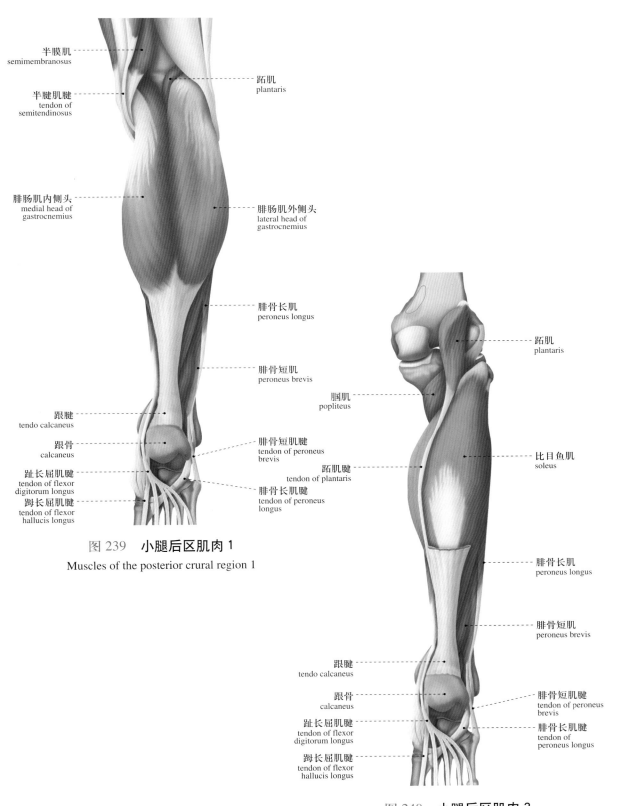

半膜肌
semimembranosus

半腱肌腱
tendon of
semitendinosus

腓肠肌内侧头
medial head of
gastrocnemius

跖肌
plantaris

腓肠肌外侧头
lateral head of
gastrocnemius

腓骨长肌
peroneus longus

腓骨短肌
peroneus brevis

跟腱
tendo calcaneus

跟骨
calcaneus

趾长屈肌腱
tendon of flexor
digitorum longus

踇长屈肌腱
tendon of flexor
hallucis longus

腓骨短肌腱
tendon of peroneus
brevis

跖肌腱
tendon of plantaris

腓骨长肌腱
tendon of peroneus
longus

图 239　小腿后区肌肉 1
Muscles of the posterior crural region 1

跖肌
plantaris

腘肌
popliteus

比目鱼肌
soleus

腓骨长肌
peroneus longus

腓骨短肌
peroneus brevis

跟腱
tendo calcaneus

跟骨
calcaneus

趾长屈肌腱
tendon of flexor
digitorum longus

踇长屈肌腱
tendon of flexor
hallucis longus

腓骨短肌腱
tendon of peroneus
brevis

腓骨长肌腱
tendon of
peroneus longus

图 240　小腿后区肌肉 2
Muscles of the posterior crural region 2

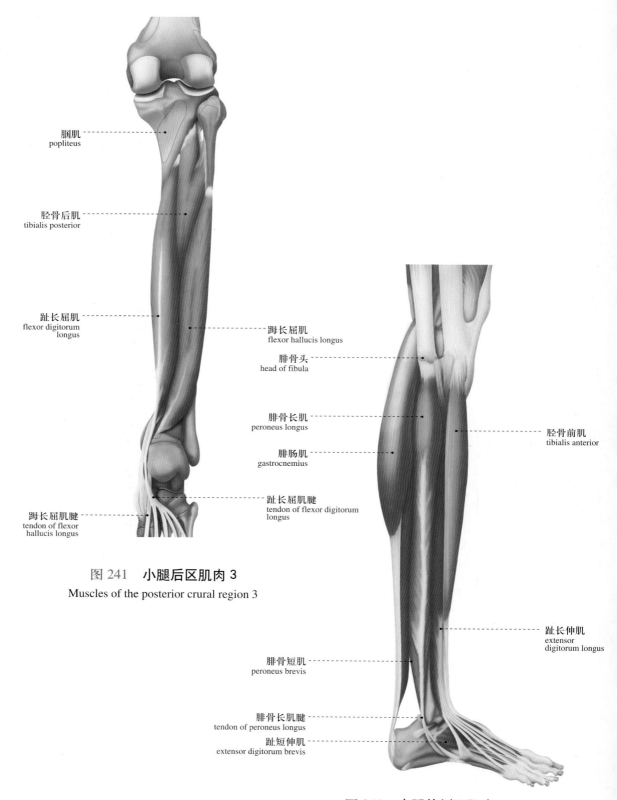

腘肌
popliteus

胫骨后肌
tibialis posterior

趾长屈肌
flexor digitorum
longus

踇长屈肌
flexor hallucis longus

腓骨头
head of fibula

腓骨长肌
peroneus longus

腓肠肌
gastrocnemius

趾长屈肌腱
tendon of flexor digitorum
longus

踇长屈肌腱
tendon of flexor
hallucis longus

图 241　小腿后区肌肉 3

Muscles of the posterior crural region 3

胫骨前肌
tibialis anterior

趾长伸肌
extensor
digitorum longus

腓骨短肌
peroneus brevis

腓骨长肌腱
tendon of peroneus longus

趾短伸肌
extensor digitorum brevis

图 242　小腿外侧面肌肉

Muscles of the lateral crural aspect

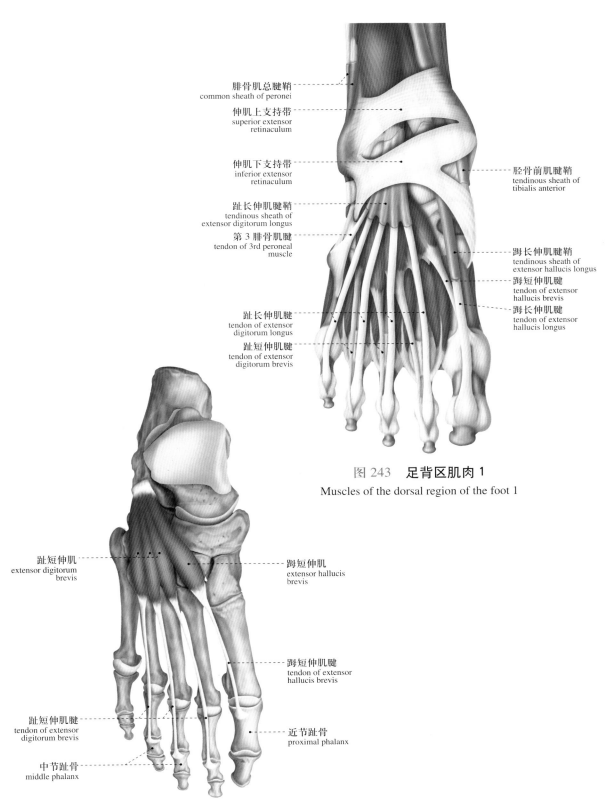

腓骨肌总腱鞘
common sheath of peronei

伸肌上支持带
superior extensor
retinaculum

伸肌下支持带
inferior extensor
retinaculum

趾长伸肌腱鞘
tendinous sheath of
extensor digitorum longus

第 3 腓骨肌腱
tendon of 3rd peroneal
muscle

趾长伸肌腱
tendon of extensor
digitorum longus

趾短伸肌腱
tendon of extensor
digitorum brevis

胫骨前肌腱鞘
tendinous sheath of
tibialis anterior

拇长伸肌腱鞘
tendinous sheath of
extensor hallucis longus

拇短伸肌腱
tendon of extensor
hallucis brevis

拇长伸肌腱
tendon of extensor
hallucis longus

图 243　足背区肌肉 1
Muscles of the dorsal region of the foot 1

趾短伸肌
extensor digitorum
brevis

拇短伸肌
extensor hallucis
brevis

拇短伸肌腱
tendon of extensor
hallucis brevis

趾短伸肌腱
tendon of extensor
digitorum brevis

近节趾骨
proximal phalanx

中节趾骨
middle phalanx

图 244　足背区肌肉 2
Muscles of the dorsal region of the foot 2

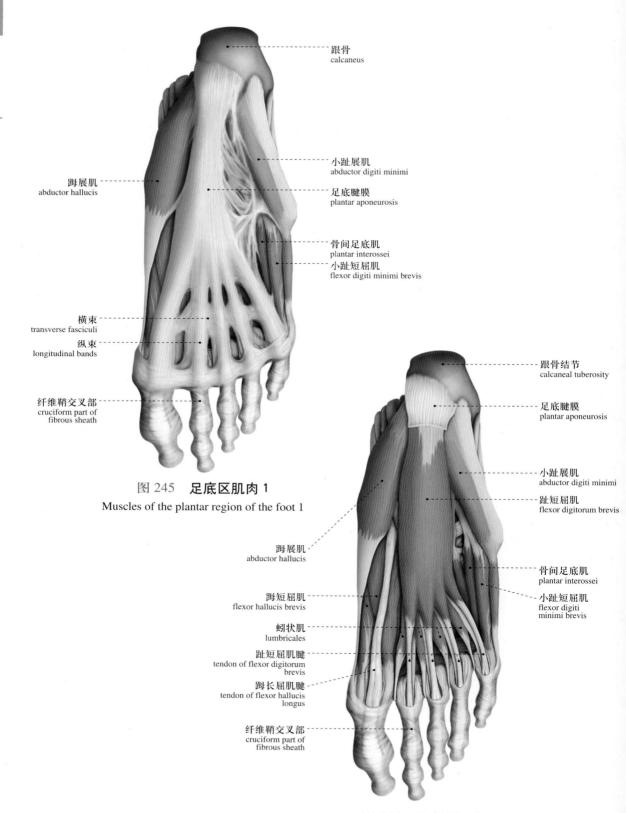

跟骨
calcaneus

小趾展肌
abductor digiti minimi

足底腱膜
plantar aponeurosis

骨间足底肌
plantar interossei

小趾短屈肌
flexor digiti minimi brevis

蹈展肌
abductor hallucis

横束
transverse fasciculi

纵束
longitudinal bands

纤维鞘交叉部
cruciform part of
fibrous sheath

图 245　足底区肌肉 1

Muscles of the plantar region of the foot 1

跟骨结节
calcaneal tuberosity

足底腱膜
plantar aponeurosis

小趾展肌
abductor digiti minimi

趾短屈肌
flexor digitorum brevis

骨间足底肌
plantar interossei

小趾短屈肌
flexor digiti
minimi brevis

蹈展肌
abductor hallucis

蹈短屈肌
flexor hallucis brevis

蚓状肌
lumbricales

趾短屈肌腱
tendon of flexor digitorum
brevis

蹈长屈肌腱
tendon of flexor hallucis
longus

纤维鞘交叉部
cruciform part of
fibrous sheath

图 246　足底区肌肉 2

Muscles of the plantar region of the foot 2

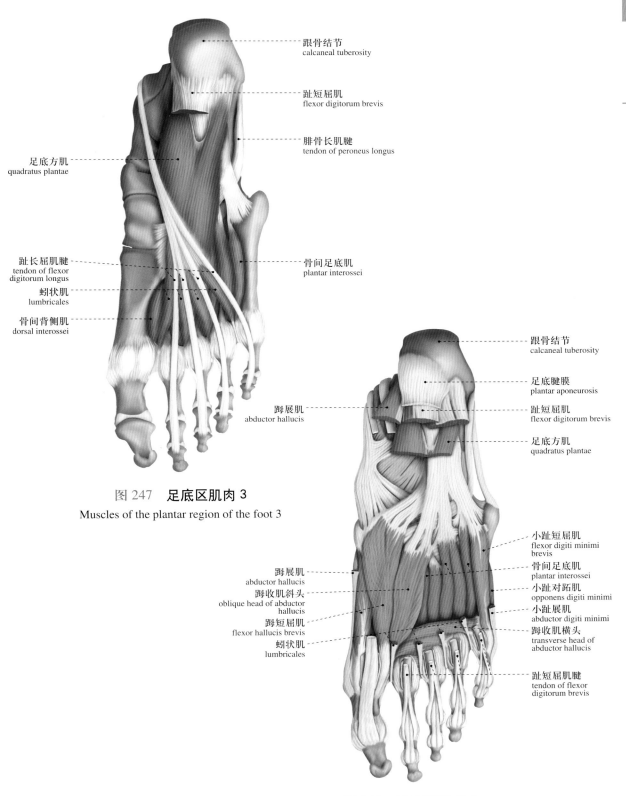

跟骨结节
calcaneal tuberosity

趾短屈肌
flexor digitorum brevis

腓骨长肌腱
tendon of peroneus longus

足底方肌
quadratus plantae

趾长屈肌腱
tendon of flexor
digitorum longus

蚓状肌
lumbricales

骨间背侧肌
dorsal interossei

骨间足底肌
plantar interossei

蹋展肌
abductor hallucis

图 247　足底区肌肉 3

Muscles of the plantar region of the foot 3

跟骨结节
calcaneal tuberosity

足底腱膜
plantar aponeurosis

趾短屈肌
flexor digitorum brevis

足底方肌
quadratus plantae

小趾短屈肌
flexor digiti minimi
brevis

骨间足底肌
plantar interossei

小趾对跖肌
opponens digiti minimi

小趾展肌
abductor digiti minimi

蹋收肌横头
transverse head of
abductor hallucis

趾短屈肌腱
tendon of flexor
digitorum brevis

蹋展肌
abductor hallucis

蹋收肌斜头
oblique head of abductor
hallucis

蹋短屈肌
flexor hallucis brevis

蚓状肌
lumbricales

图 248　足底区肌肉 4

Muscles of the plantar region of the foot 4

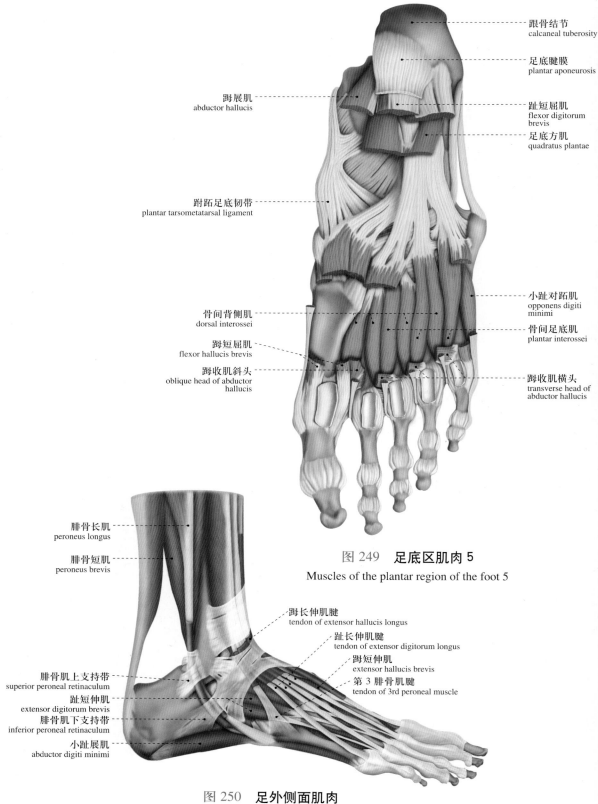

跟骨结节
calcaneal tuberosity

足底腱膜
plantar aponeurosis

跗展肌
abductor hallucis

趾短屈肌
flexor digitorum brevis

足底方肌
quadratus plantae

跗跖足底韧带
plantar tarsometatarsal ligament

小趾对跖肌
opponens digiti minimi

骨间背侧肌
dorsal interossei

骨间足底肌
plantar interossei

跗短屈肌
flexor hallucis brevis

跗收肌斜头
oblique head of abductor hallucis

跗收肌横头
transverse head of abductor hallucis

图 249　足底区肌肉 5

Muscles of the plantar region of the foot 5

腓骨长肌
peroneus longus

腓骨短肌
peroneus brevis

跗长伸肌腱
tendon of extensor hallucis longus

趾长伸肌腱
tendon of extensor digitorum longus

跗短伸肌
extensor hallucis brevis

第 3 腓骨肌腱
tendon of 3rd peroneal muscle

腓骨肌上支持带
superior peroneal retinaculum

趾短伸肌
extensor digitorum brevis

腓骨肌下支持带
inferior peroneal retinaculum

小趾展肌
abductor digiti minimi

图 250　足外侧面肌肉

Muscles of the lateral aspect of the foot

第一节

消化系统模式图

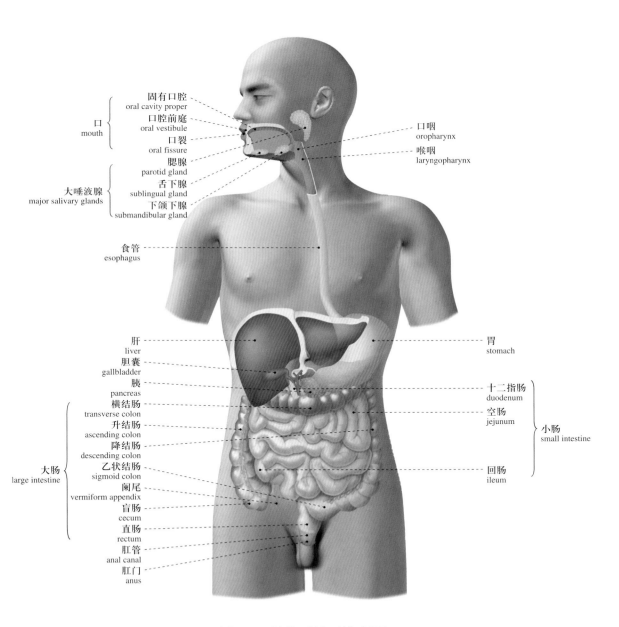

口 mouth
固有口腔 oral cavity proper
口腔前庭 oral vestibule
口裂 oral fissure

大唾液腺 major salivary glands
腮腺 parotid gland
舌下腺 sublingual gland
下颌下腺 submandibular gland

食管 esophagus

口咽 oropharynx
喉咽 laryngopharynx

肝 liver
胆囊 gallbladder
胰 pancreas
横结肠 transverse colon
升结肠 ascending colon
降结肠 descending colon
乙状结肠 sigmoid colon
阑尾 vermiform appendix
盲肠 cecum
直肠 rectum
肛管 anal canal
肛门 anus

大肠 large intestine

胃 stomach
十二指肠 duodenum
空肠 jejunum
回肠 ileum

小肠 small intestine

图 251　消化系统（模式图）
Alimentary system (diagram)

133

第二节

口 腔

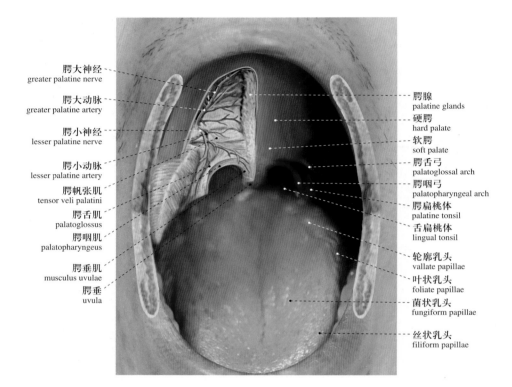

图 252　口腔及扁桃体动脉

Oral cavity and the arteries of the palatine tonsil

腭大神经
greater palatine nerve

腭大动脉
greater palatine artery

腭小神经
lesser palatine nerve

腭小动脉
lesser palatine artery

腭帆张肌
tensor veli palatini

腭舌肌
palatoglossus

腭咽肌
palatopharyngeus

腭垂肌
musculus uvulae

腭垂
uvula

腭腺
palatine glands

硬腭
hard palate

软腭
soft palate

腭舌弓
palatoglossal arch

腭咽弓
palatopharyngeal arch

腭扁桃体
palatine tonsil

舌扁桃体
lingual tonsil

轮廓乳头
vallate papillae

叶状乳头
foliate papillae

菌状乳头
fungiform papillae

丝状乳头
filiform papillae

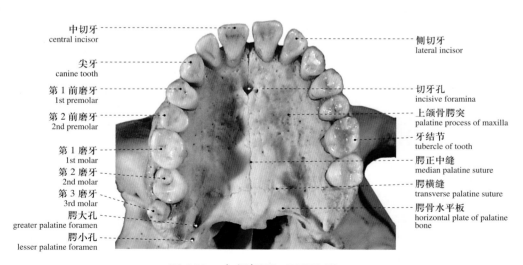

图 253　上颌恒牙（下面观）

Maxillary permanent tooth (inferior aspect)

中切牙
central incisor

尖牙
canine tooth

第1前磨牙
1st premolar

第2前磨牙
2nd premolar

第1磨牙
1st molar

第2磨牙
2nd molar

第3磨牙
3rd molar

腭大孔
greater palatine foramen

腭小孔
lesser palatine foramen

侧切牙
lateral incisor

切牙孔
incisive foramina

上颌骨腭突
palatine process of maxilla

牙结节
tubercle of tooth

腭正中缝
median palatine suture

腭横缝
transverse palatine suture

腭骨水平板
horizontal plate of palatine bone

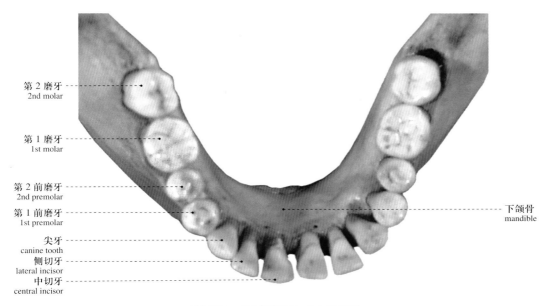

第 2 磨牙
2nd molar

第 1 磨牙
1st molar

第 2 前磨牙
2nd premolar

第 1 前磨牙
1st premolar

尖牙
canine tooth

侧切牙
lateral incisor

中切牙
central incisor

下颌骨
mandible

图 254　下颌恒牙（上面观）
Mandibular permanent tooth (superior aspect)

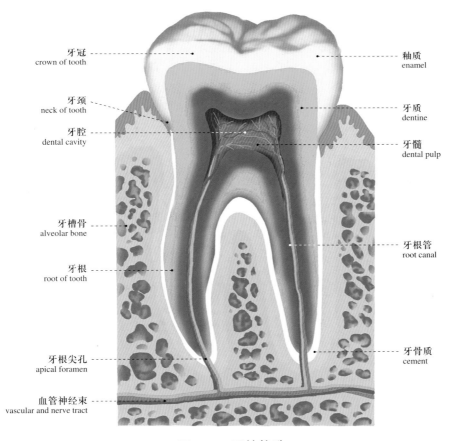

牙冠
crown of tooth

牙颈
neck of tooth

牙腔
dental cavity

牙槽骨
alveolar bone

牙根
root of tooth

牙根尖孔
apical foramen

血管神经束
vascular and nerve tract

釉质
enamel

牙质
dentine

牙髓
dental pulp

牙根管
root canal

牙骨质
cement

图 255　牙的构造
Structure of the teeth

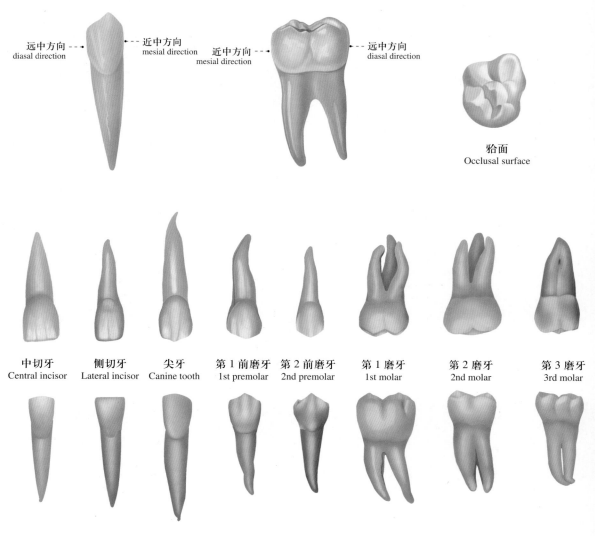

远中方向
diasal direction

近中方向
mesial direction

近中方向
mesial direction

远中方向
diasal direction

殆面
Occlusal surface

中切牙
Central incisor

侧切牙
Lateral incisor

尖牙
Canine tooth

第 1 前磨牙
1st premolar

第 2 前磨牙
2nd premolar

第 1 磨牙
1st molar

第 2 磨牙
2nd molar

第 3 磨牙
3rd molar

图 256　上下颌恒牙（左侧）
Maxillary and mandibular permanent tooth (left)

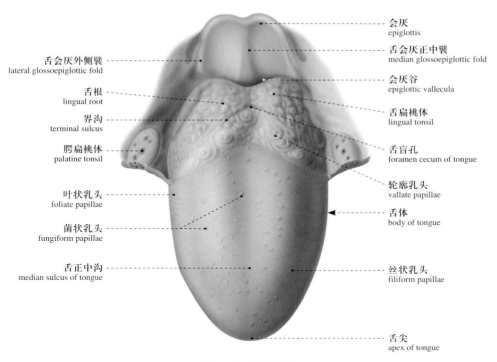

会厌
epiglottis

舌会厌正中襞
median glossoepiglottic fold

会厌谷
epiglottic vallecula

舌扁桃体
lingual tonsil

舌盲孔
foramen cecum of tongue

轮廓乳头
vallate papillae

舌体
body of tongue

丝状乳头
filiform papillae

舌尖
apex of tongue

舌会厌外侧襞
lateral glossoepiglottic fold

舌根
lingual root

界沟
terminal sulcus

腭扁桃体
palatine tonsil

叶状乳头
foliate papillae

菌状乳头
fungiform papillae

舌正中沟
median sulcus of tongue

图 257　舌背面
Dorsum of the tongue

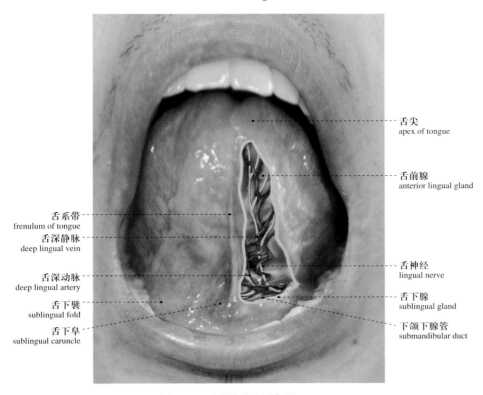

舌尖
apex of tongue

舌前腺
anterior lingual gland

舌神经
lingual nerve

舌下腺
sublingual gland

下颌下腺管
submandibular duct

舌系带
frenulum of tongue

舌深静脉
deep lingual vein

舌深动脉
deep lingual artery

舌下襞
sublingual fold

舌下阜
sublingual caruncle

图 258　舌的血管神经
Blood vessels and nerves of the tongue

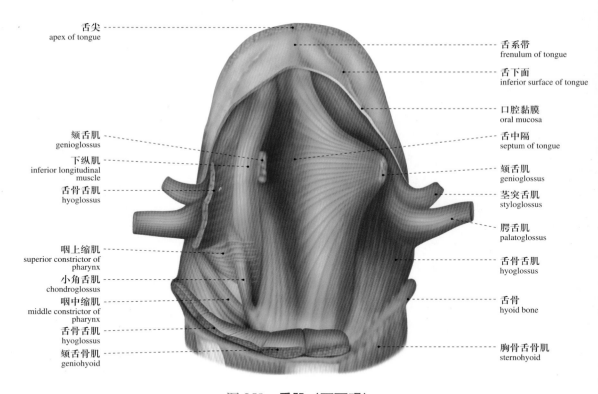

舌尖
apex of tongue

舌系带
frenulum of tongue

舌下面
inferior surface of tongue

口腔黏膜
oral mucosa

颏舌肌
genioglossus

舌中隔
septum of tongue

下纵肌
inferior longitudinal muscle

颏舌肌
genioglossus

舌骨舌肌
hyoglossus

茎突舌肌
styloglossus

腭舌肌
palatoglossus

咽上缩肌
superior constrictor of pharynx

舌骨舌肌
hyoglossus

小角舌肌
chondroglossus

舌骨
hyoid bone

咽中缩肌
middle constrictor of pharynx

舌骨舌肌
hyoglossus

胸骨舌骨肌
sternohyoid

颏舌骨肌
geniohyoid

图 259　舌肌（下面观）
Muscles of the tongue (inferior aspect)

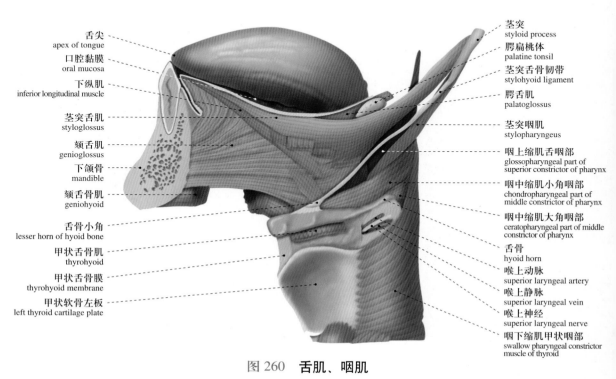

舌尖
apex of tongue

茎突
styloid process

腭扁桃体
palatine tonsil

口腔黏膜
oral mucosa

茎突舌骨韧带
stylohyoid ligament

下纵肌
inferior longitudinal muscle

腭舌肌
palatoglossus

茎突舌肌
styloglossus

茎突咽肌
stylopharyngeus

颏舌肌
genioglossus

咽上缩肌舌咽部
glossopharyngeal part of superior constrictor of pharynx

下颌骨
mandible

颏舌骨肌
geniohyoid

咽中缩肌小角咽部
chondropharyngeal part of middle constrictor of pharynx

舌骨小角
lesser horn of hyoid bone

咽中缩肌大角咽部
ceratopharyngeal part of middle constrictor of pharynx

甲状舌骨肌
thyrohyoid

舌骨
hyoid horn

甲状舌骨膜
thyrohyoid membrane

喉上动脉
superior laryngeal artery

甲状软骨左板
left thyroid cartilage plate

喉上静脉
superior laryngeal vein

喉上神经
superior laryngeal nerve

咽下缩肌甲状咽部
swallow pharyngeal constrictor muscle of thyroid

图 260　舌肌、咽肌
Muscles of the tongue and pharynx

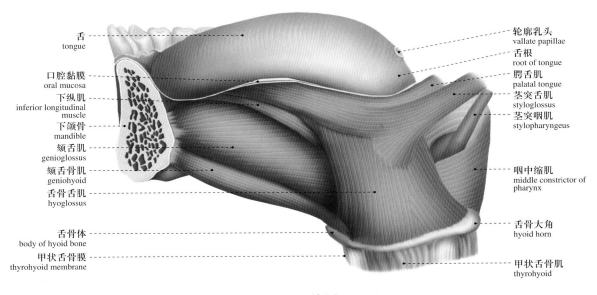

舌 tongue
口腔黏膜 oral mucosa
下纵肌 inferior longitudinal muscle
下颌骨 mandible
颏舌肌 genioglossus
颏舌骨肌 geniohyoid
舌骨舌肌 hyoglossus
舌骨体 body of hyoid bone
甲状舌骨膜 thyrohyoid membrane

轮廓乳头 vallate papillae
舌根 root of tongue
腭舌肌 palatal tongue
茎突舌肌 styloglossus
茎突咽肌 stylopharyngeus
咽中缩肌 middle constrictor of pharynx
舌骨大角 hyoid horn
甲状舌骨肌 thyrohyoid

图 261　舌肌（外侧面观 1）

Muscles of the tongue (lateral aspect 1)

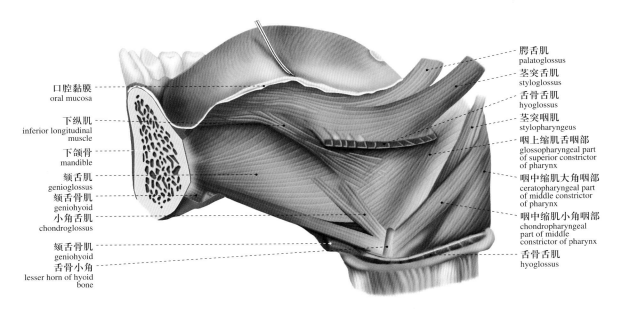

口腔黏膜 oral mucosa
下纵肌 inferior longitudinal muscle
下颌骨 mandible
颏舌肌 genioglossus
颏舌骨肌 geniohyoid
小角舌肌 chondroglossus
颏舌骨肌 geniohyoid
舌骨小角 lesser horn of hyoid bone

腭舌肌 palatoglossus
茎突舌肌 styloglossus
舌骨舌肌 hyoglossus
茎突咽肌 stylopharyngeus
咽上缩肌舌咽部 glossopharyngeal part of superior constrictor of pharynx
咽中缩肌大角咽部 ceratopharyngeal part of middle constrictor of pharynx
咽中缩肌小角咽部 chondropharyngeal part of middle constrictor of pharynx
舌骨舌肌 hyoglossus

图 262　舌肌（外侧面观 2）

Muscles of the tongue (lateral aspect 2)

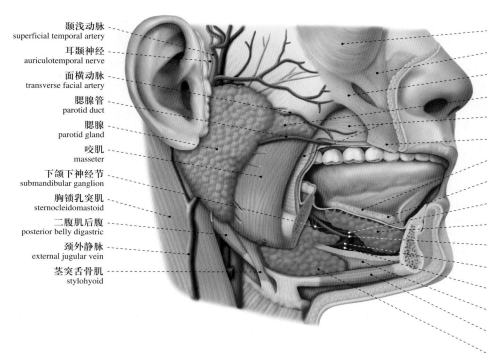

颞浅动脉
superficial temporal artery

耳颞神经
auriculotemporal nerve

面横动脉
transverse facial artery

腮腺管
parotid duct

腮腺
parotid gland

咬肌
masseter

下颌下神经节
submandibular ganglion

胸锁乳突肌
sternocleidomastoid

二腹肌后腹
posterior belly digastric

颈外静脉
external jugular vein

茎突舌骨肌
stylohyoid

眼轮匝肌
orbicularis oculi

提上唇肌
levator labii superioris

颧肌
musculus zygomaticus

副腮腺
accessory parotid gland

颊肌
buccinator

口轮匝肌
orbicularis oris

舌下襞
sublingual fold

舌下阜
sublingual caruncle

下颌下腺管
submandibular duct

舌下腺
sublingual gland

舌神经
lingual nerve

舌动脉
lingual artery

舌静脉
lingual vein

下颌舌骨肌
mylohyoid

二腹肌
digastric

下颌下腺
submandibular gland

图 263　腮腺、下颌下腺及舌下腺（外侧面观）

Parotid, submandibular and sublingual glands (lateral aspect)

咽

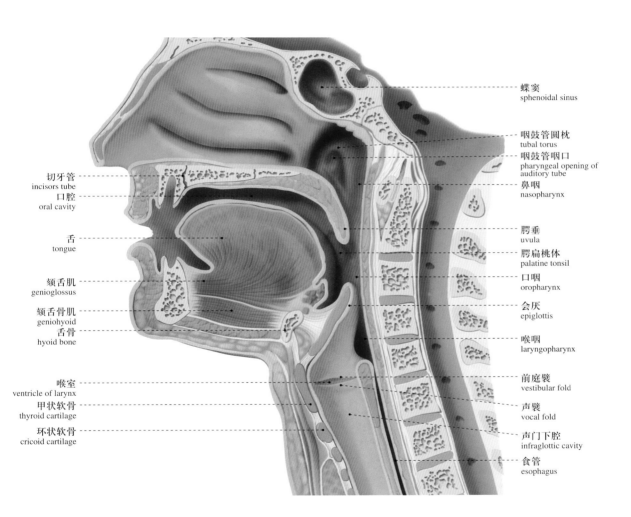

蝶窦
sphenoidal sinus

咽鼓管圆枕
tubal torus

咽鼓管咽口
pharyngeal opening of
auditory tube

鼻咽
nasopharynx

腭垂
uvula

腭扁桃体
palatine tonsil

口咽
oropharynx

会厌
epiglottis

喉咽
laryngopharynx

前庭襞
vestibular fold

声襞
vocal fold

声门下腔
infraglottic cavity

食管
esophagus

切牙管
incisors tube

口腔
oral cavity

舌
tongue

颏舌肌
genioglossus

颏舌骨肌
geniohyoid

舌骨
hyoid bone

喉室
ventricle of larynx

甲状软骨
thyroid cartilage

环状软骨
cricoid cartilage

图 264　鼻腔、口腔、咽和喉（正中矢状断面观）
Nasal cavity, oral cavity, pharynx and larynx (midsagittal section aspect)

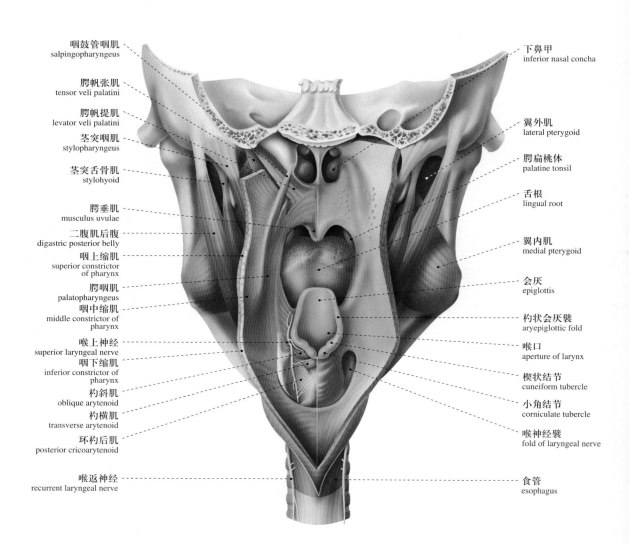

咽鼓管咽肌
salpingopharyngeus

腭帆张肌
tensor veli palatini

腭帆提肌
levator veli palatini

茎突咽肌
stylopharyngeus

茎突舌骨肌
stylohyoid

腭垂肌
musculus uvulae

二腹肌后腹
digastric posterior belly

咽上缩肌
superior constrictor
of pharynx

腭咽肌
palatopharyngeus

咽中缩肌
middle constrictor of
pharynx

喉上神经
superior laryngeal nerve

咽下缩肌
inferior constrictor of
pharynx

杓斜肌
oblique arytenoid

杓横肌
transverse arytenoid

环杓后肌
posterior cricoarytenoid

喉返神经
recurrent laryngeal nerve

下鼻甲
inferior nasal concha

翼外肌
lateral pterygoid

腭扁桃体
palatine tonsil

舌根
lingual root

翼内肌
medial pterygoid

会厌
epiglottis

杓状会厌襞
aryepiglottic fold

喉口
aperture of larynx

楔状结节
cuneiform tubercle

小角结节
corniculate tubercle

喉神经襞
fold of laryngeal nerve

食管
esophagus

图 265　咽腔（后面观）
Pharyngeal cavity (posterior aspect)

第四节

食 管

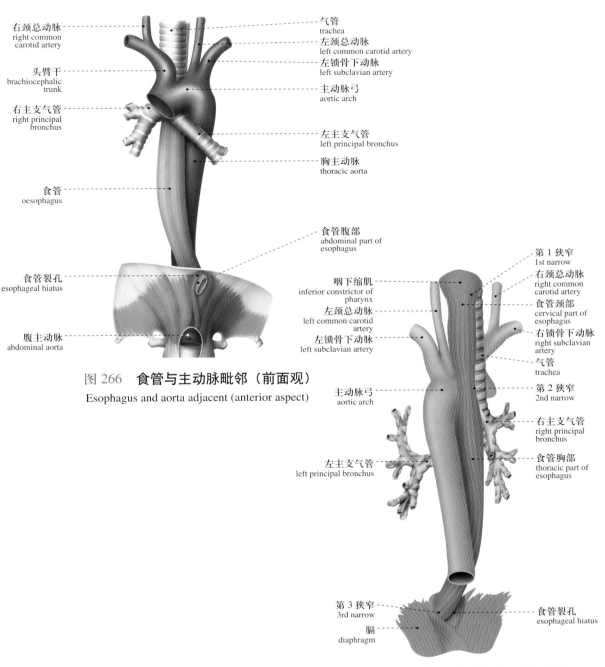

右颈总动脉
right common
carotid artery

头臂干
brachiocephalic
trunk

右主支气管
right principal
bronchus

食管
oesophagus

食管裂孔
esophageal hiatus

腹主动脉
abdominal aorta

气管
trachea

左颈总动脉
left common carotid artery

左锁骨下动脉
left subclavian artery

主动脉弓
aortic arch

左主支气管
left principal bronchus

胸主动脉
thoracic aorta

食管腹部
abdominal part of
esophagus

图 266 食管与主动脉毗邻（前面观）
Esophagus and aorta adjacent (anterior aspect)

咽下缩肌
inferior constrictor of
pharynx

左颈总动脉
left common carotid
artery

左锁骨下动脉
left subclavian artery

主动脉弓
aortic arch

左主支气管
left principal bronchus

第 1 狭窄
1st narrow

右颈总动脉
right common
carotid artery

食管颈部
cervical part of
esophagus

右锁骨下动脉
right subclavian
artery

气管
trachea

第 2 狭窄
2nd narrow

右主支气管
right principal
bronchus

食管胸部
thoracic part of
esophagus

第 3 狭窄
3rd narrow

膈
diaphragm

食管裂孔
esophageal hiatus

图 267 主动脉、食管与气管毗邻（后面观）
Aorta, esophagus and trachea adjacent (posterior aspect)

第五节

胃

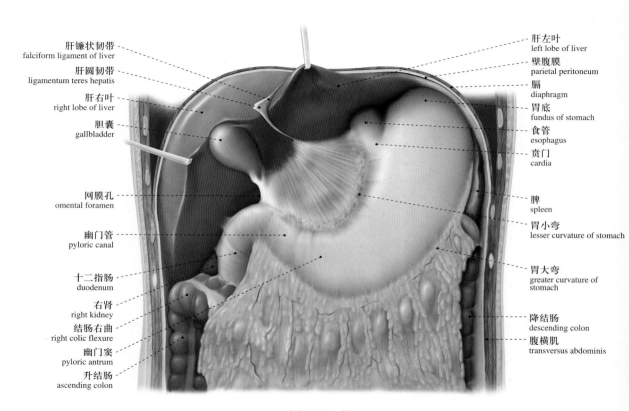

肝镰状韧带
falciform ligament of liver

肝圆韧带
ligamentum teres hepatis

肝右叶
right lobe of liver

胆囊
gallbladder

网膜孔
omental foramen

幽门管
pyloric canal

十二指肠
duodenum

右肾
right kidney

结肠右曲
right colic flexure

幽门窦
pyloric antrum

升结肠
ascending colon

肝左叶
left lobe of liver

壁腹膜
parietal peritoneum

膈
diaphragm

胃底
fundus of stomach

食管
esophagus

贲门
cardia

脾
spleen

胃小弯
lesser curvature of stomach

胃大弯
greater curvature of stomach

降结肠
descending colon

腹横肌
transversus abdominis

图 268　胃
Stomach

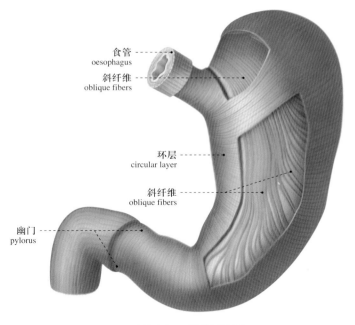

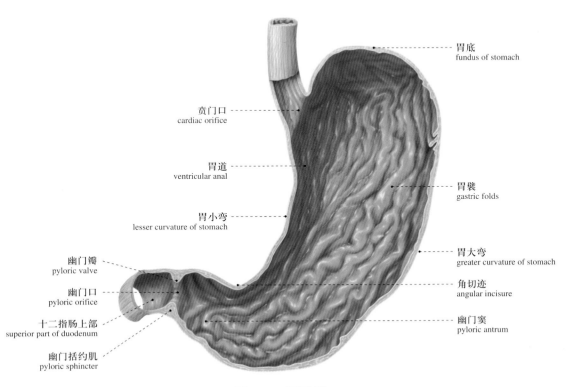

食管
oesophagus

斜纤维
oblique fibers

环层
circular layer

斜纤维
oblique fibers

幽门
pylorus

图 269　胃的肌层
Muscle layer of the stomach

胃底
fundus of stomach

贲门口
cardiac orifice

胃道
ventricular anal

胃小弯
lesser curvature of stomach

胃襞
gastric folds

幽门瓣
pyloric valve

幽门口
pyloric orifice

十二指肠上部
superior part of duodenum

幽门括约肌
pyloric sphincter

胃大弯
greater curvature of stomach

角切迹
angular incisure

幽门窦
pyloric antrum

图 270　胃黏膜
Gastric mucosa

第六节

小 肠

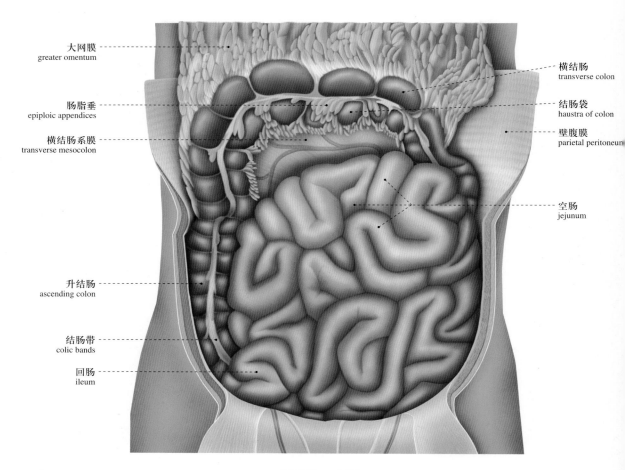

大网膜 greater omentum	横结肠 transverse colon
肠脂垂 epiploic appendices	结肠袋 haustra of colon
横结肠系膜 transverse mesocolon	壁腹膜 parietal peritoneum
	空肠 jejunum
升结肠 ascending colon	
结肠带 colic bands	
回肠 ileum	

图 271　小肠
Small intestine

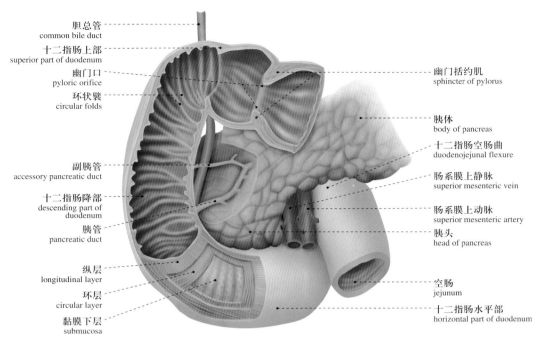

胆总管
common bile duct

十二指肠上部
superior part of duodenum

幽门口
pyloric orifice

环状襞
circular folds

副胰管
accessory pancreatic duct

十二指肠降部
descending part of
duodenum

胰管
pancreatic duct

纵层
longitudinal layer

环层
circular layer

黏膜下层
submucosa

幽门括约肌
sphincter of pylorus

胰体
body of pancreas

十二指肠空肠曲
duodenojejunal flexure

肠系膜上静脉
superior mesenteric vein

肠系膜上动脉
superior mesenteric artery

胰头
head of pancreas

空肠
jejunum

十二指肠水平部
horizontal part of duodenum

图 272　十二指肠的构造
Construction of the duodenum

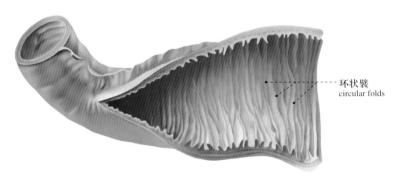

环状襞
circular folds

图 273　空肠（内面观）
Jejunum (internal aspect)

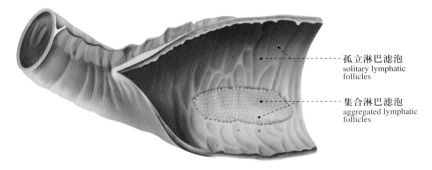

孤立淋巴滤泡
solitary lymphatic
follicles

集合淋巴滤泡
aggregated lymphatic
follicles

图 274　回肠（内面观）
Ileum (internal aspect)

147

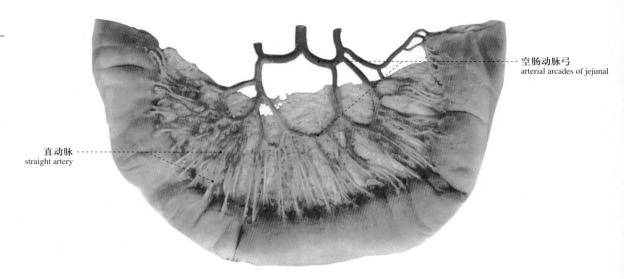

空肠动脉弓
arterial arcades of jejunal

直动脉
straight artery

图 275　空肠动脉弓
Arterial arcades of the jejunal

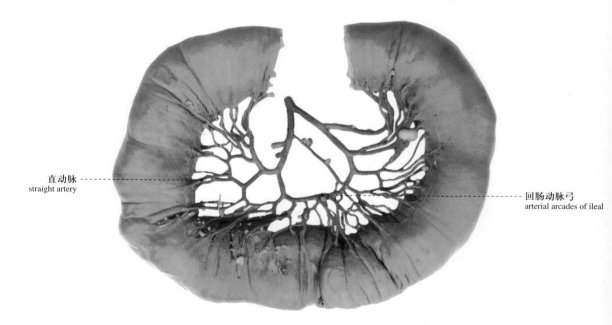

直动脉
straight artery

回肠动脉弓
arterial arcades of ileal

图 276　回肠动脉弓
Arterial arcades of the ileum

大 肠

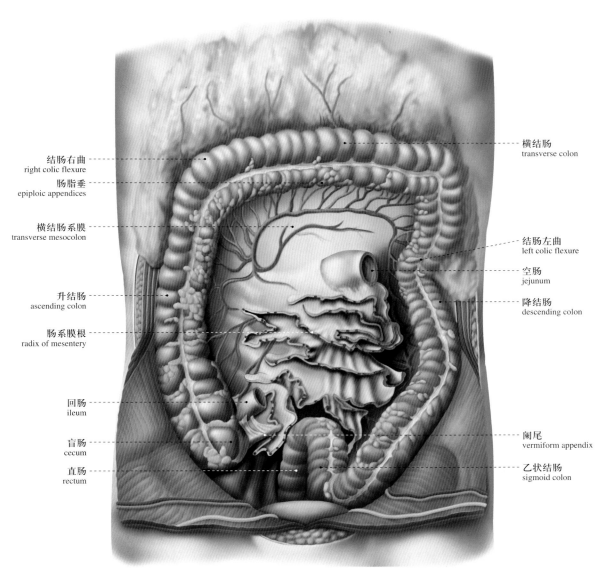

结肠右曲
right colic flexure

肠脂垂
epiploic appendices

横结肠系膜
transverse mesocolon

升结肠
ascending colon

肠系膜根
radix of mesentery

回肠
ileum

盲肠
cecum

直肠
rectum

横结肠
transverse colon

结肠左曲
left colic flexure

空肠
jejunum

降结肠
descending colon

阑尾
vermiform appendix

乙状结肠
sigmoid colon

图 277　结肠 1
Colon 1

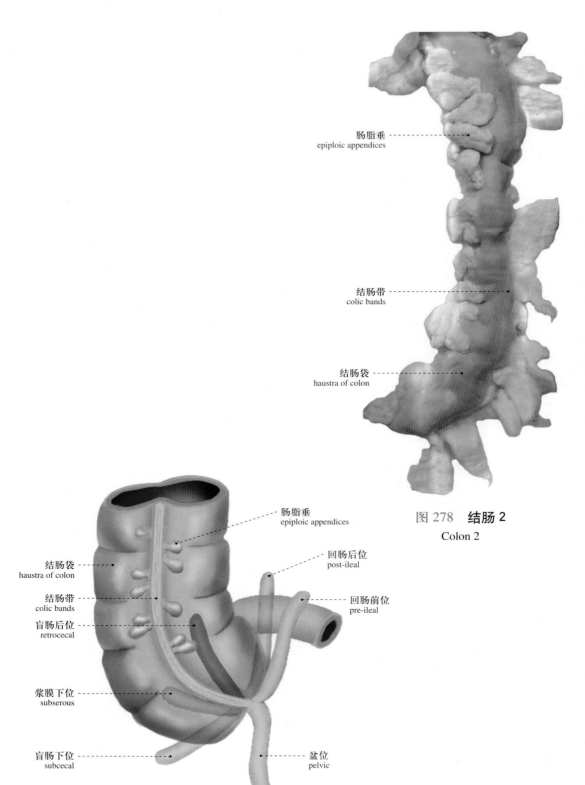

肠脂垂
epiploic appendices

结肠带
colic bands

结肠袋
haustra of colon

图 278　**结肠 2**
Colon 2

肠脂垂
epiploic appendices

结肠袋
haustra of colon

结肠带
colic bands

盲肠后位
retrocecal

浆膜下位
subserous

盲肠下位
subcecal

回肠后位
post-ileal

回肠前位
pre-ileal

盆位
pelvic

图 279　**阑尾位置**
Position of the vermiform appendix

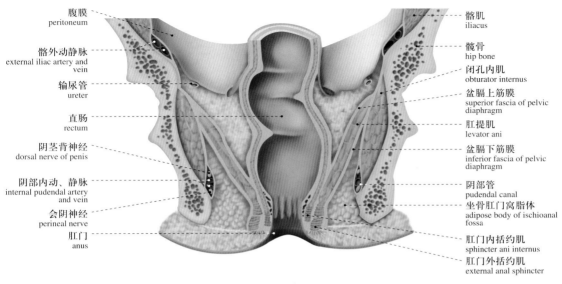

腹膜
peritoneum

髂外动静脉
external iliac artery and vein

输尿管
ureter

直肠
rectum

阴茎背神经
dorsal nerve of penis

阴部内动、静脉
internal pudendal artery and vein

会阴神经
perineal nerve

肛门
anus

髂肌
iliacus

髋骨
hip bone

闭孔内肌
obturator internus

盆膈上筋膜
superior fascia of pelvic diaphragm

肛提肌
levator ani

盆膈下筋膜
inferior fascia of pelvic diaphragm

阴部管
pudendal canal

坐骨肛门窝脂体
adipose body of ischioanal fossa

肛门内括约肌
sphincter ani internus

肛门外括约肌
external anal sphincter

图 280　直肠（男性骨盆冠状切面）
Rectum (coronal section of male pelvis)

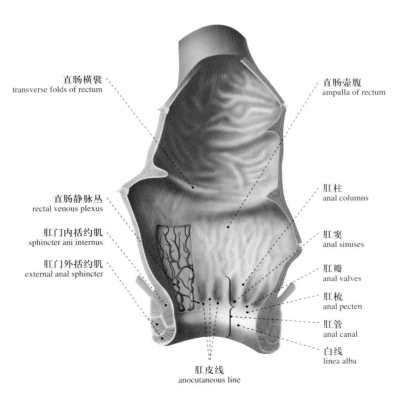

直肠横襞
transverse folds of rectum

直肠静脉丛
rectal venous plexus

肛门内括约肌
sphincter ani internus

肛门外括约肌
external anal sphincter

肛皮线
anocutaneous line

直肠壶腹
ampulla of rectum

肛柱
anal columns

肛窦
anal sinuses

肛瓣
anal valves

肛梳
anal pecten

肛管
anal canal

白线
linea alba

图 281　直肠（内面观）
Rectum (internal aspect)

第八节

肝

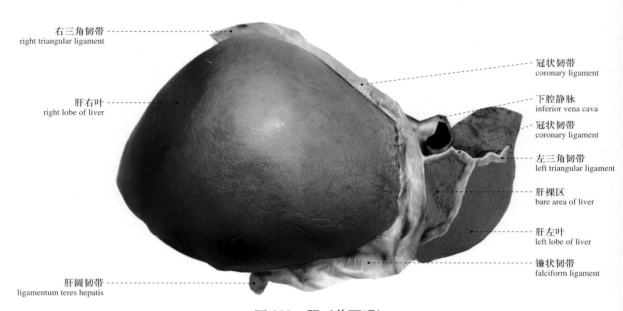

右三角韧带
right triangular ligament

肝右叶
right lobe of liver

肝圆韧带
ligamentum teres hepatis

冠状韧带
coronary ligament

下腔静脉
inferior vena cava

冠状韧带
coronary ligament

左三角韧带
left triangular ligament

肝裸区
bare area of liver

肝左叶
left lobe of liver

镰状韧带
falciform ligament

图 282　肝（前面观）
Liver (anterior aspect)

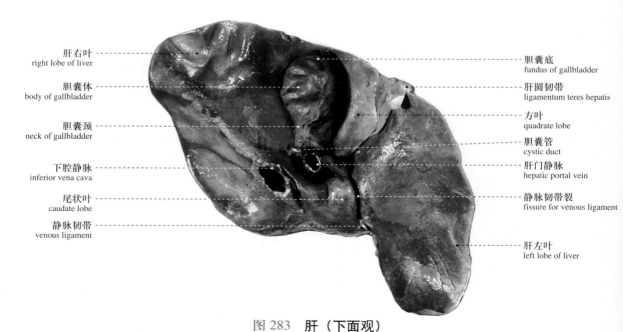

肝右叶
right lobe of liver

胆囊体
body of gallbladder

胆囊颈
neck of gallbladder

下腔静脉
inferior vena cava

尾状叶
caudate lobe

静脉韧带
venous ligament

胆囊底
fundus of gallbladder

肝圆韧带
ligamentum teres hepatis

方叶
quadrate lobe

胆囊管
cystic duct

肝门静脉
hepatic portal vein

静脉韧带裂
fissure for venous ligament

肝左叶
left lobe of liver

图 283　肝（下面观）
Liver (inferior aspect)

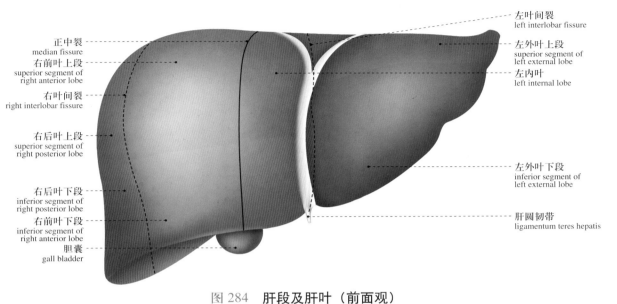

正中裂
median fissure

右前叶上段
superior segment of
right anterior lobe

右叶间裂
right interlobar fissure

右后叶上段
superior segment of
right posterior lobe

右后叶下段
inferior segment of
right posterior lobe

右前叶下段
inferior segment of
right anterior lobe

胆囊
gall bladder

左叶间裂
left interlobar fissure

左外叶上段
superior segment of
left external lobe

左内叶
left internal lobe

左外叶下段
inferior segment of
left external lobe

肝圆韧带
ligamentum teres hepatis

图 284　肝段及肝叶（前面观）
Hepatic segments and lobes (anterior aspect)

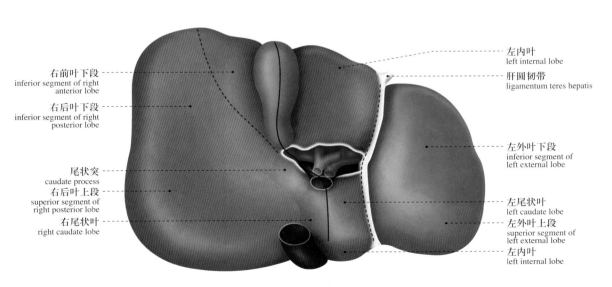

右前叶下段
inferior segment of right
anterior lobe

右后叶下段
inferior segment of right
posterior lobe

尾状突
caudate process

右后叶上段
superior segment of
right posterior lobe

右尾状叶
right caudate lobe

左内叶
left internal lobe

肝圆韧带
ligamentum teres hepatis

左外叶下段
inferior segment of
left external lobe

左尾状叶
left caudate lobe

左外叶上段
superior segment of
left external lobe

左内叶
left internal lobe

图 285　肝段及肝叶（下面观）
Hepatic segments and lobes (posterior aspect)

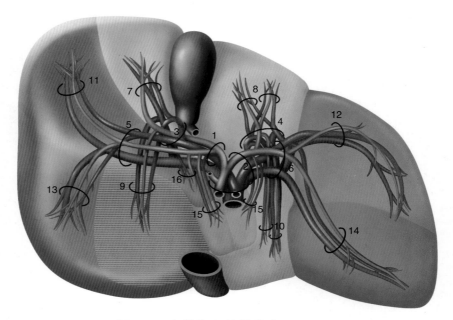

图 286　血管和肝管的分布

Distribution of the blood vessels and the hepatic ducts

1. 右支；2. 左支；3. 前段；4. 内侧段；5. 后段；6. 外侧段；7. 前上区；8. 内侧下区；9. 前上区；10. 内侧上区；11. 后下区；12. 下外侧区；13. 后上区；14. 外侧区；15. 尾叶；16. 尾状突

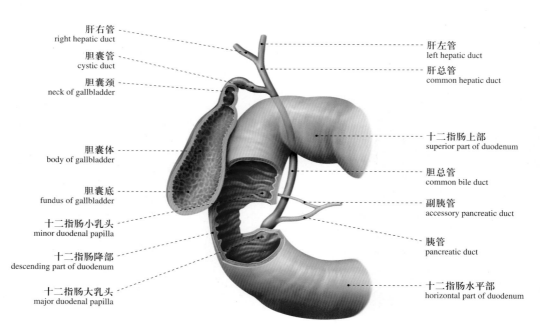

肝右管
right hepatic duct

胆囊管
cystic duct

胆囊颈
neck of gallbladder

胆囊体
body of gallbladder

胆囊底
fundus of gallbladder

十二指肠小乳头
minor duodenal papilla

十二指肠降部
descending part of duodenum

十二指肠大乳头
major duodenal papilla

肝左管
left hepatic duct

肝总管
common hepatic duct

十二指肠上部
superior part of duodenum

胆总管
common bile duct

副胰管
accessory pancreatic duct

胰管
pancreatic duct

十二指肠水平部
horizontal part of duodenum

图 287　肝外胆管

Extrahepatic bile ducts

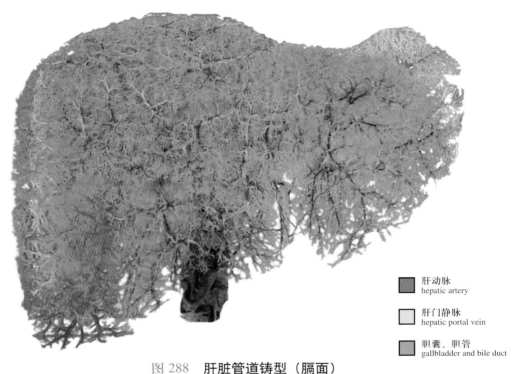

肝动脉
hepatic artery

肝门静脉
hepatic portal vein

胆囊、胆管
gallbladder and bile duct

图 288　肝脏管道铸型（膈面）
Cast of the hepatic duct (diaphragmatic aspect)

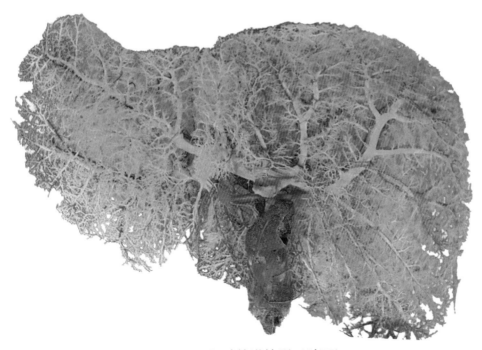

图 289　肝脏管道铸型（脏面）
Cast of the hepatic duct (visceral aspect)

胰

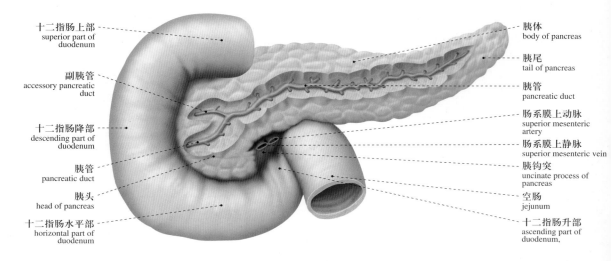

十二指肠上部
superior part of
duodenum

胰体
body of pancreas

副胰管
accessory pancreatic
duct

胰尾
tail of pancreas

胰管
pancreatic duct

十二指肠降部
descending part of
duodenum

肠系膜上动脉
superior mesenteric
artery

肠系膜上静脉
superior mesenteric vein

胰管
pancreatic duct

胰钩突
uncinate process of
pancreas

胰头
head of pancreas

空肠
jejunum

十二指肠水平部
horizontal part of
duodenum

十二指肠升部
ascending part of
duodenum,

图 290　胰的构造
Structure of the pancreas

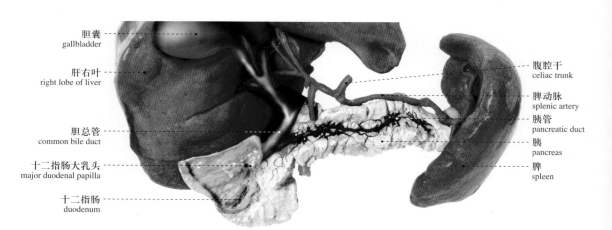

胆囊
gallbladder

肝右叶
right lobe of liver

腹腔干
celiac trunk

脾动脉
splenic artery

胰管
pancreatic duct

胆总管
common bile duct

胰
pancreas

十二指肠大乳头
major duodenal papilla

脾
spleen

十二指肠
duodenum

图 291　胰管
Pancreatic duct

第一节
呼吸系统模式图

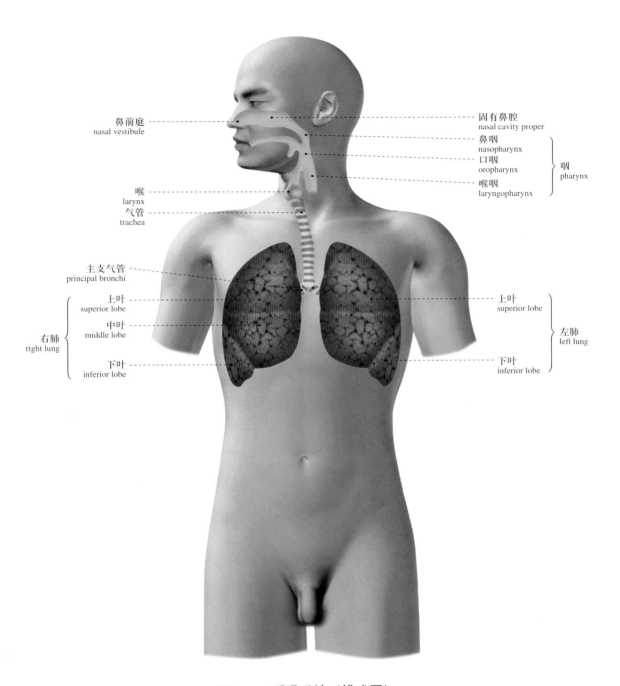

鼻前庭
nasal vestibule

固有鼻腔
nasal cavity proper

鼻咽
nasopharynx

口咽
oropharynx

喉咽
laryngopharynx

咽
pharynx

喉
larynx

气管
trachea

主支气管
principal bronchi

上叶
superior lobe

中叶
middle lobe

下叶
inferior lobe

右肺
right lung

上叶
superior lobe

下叶
inferior lobe

左肺
left lung

图 292　呼吸系统（模式图）
Respiratory system (diagram)

第二节

鼻

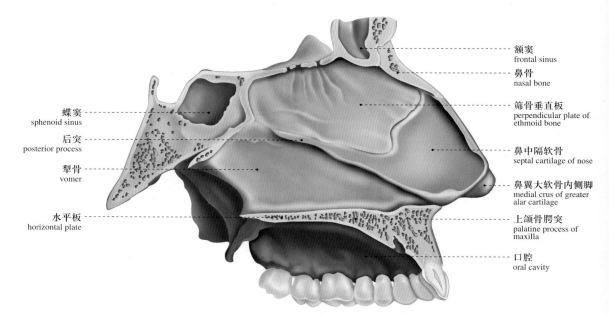

额窦
frontal sinus

鼻骨
nasal bone

筛骨垂直板
perpendicular plate of
ethmoid bone

鼻中隔软骨
septal cartilage of nose

鼻翼大软骨内侧脚
medial crus of greater
alar cartilage

上颌骨腭突
palatine process of
maxilla

口腔
oral cavity

蝶窦
sphenoid sinus

后突
posterior process

犁骨
vomer

水平板
horizontal plate

图 293　鼻中隔（右侧面观）
Nasal septum (right lateral aspect)

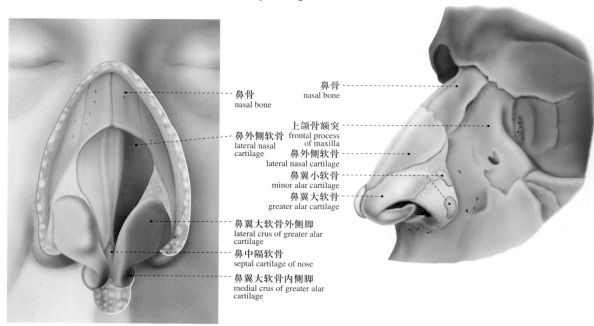

鼻骨
nasal bone

鼻外侧软骨
lateral nasal
cartilage

鼻翼大软骨外侧脚
lateral crus of greater
alar cartilage

鼻中隔软骨
septal cartilage of nose

鼻翼大软骨内侧脚
medial crus of greater alar
cartilage

鼻骨
nasal bone

上颌骨额突
frontal process
of maxilla

鼻外侧软骨
lateral nasal cartilage

鼻翼小软骨
minor alar cartilage

鼻翼大软骨
greater alar cartilage

图 294　鼻的骨骼（前面观）
Nose bones (anterior aspect)

图 295　鼻的骨骼（左外侧面观）
Nasal bones (left lateral aspect)

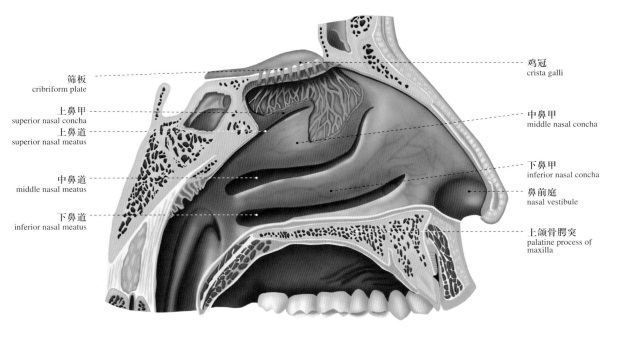

筛板
cribriform plate

上鼻甲
superior nasal concha

上鼻道
superior nasal meatus

中鼻道
middle nasal meatus

下鼻道
inferior nasal meatus

鸡冠
crista galli

中鼻甲
middle nasal concha

下鼻甲
inferior nasal concha

鼻前庭
nasal vestibule

上颌骨腭突
palatine process of maxilla

图 296　鼻腔外侧壁（内侧面观 1）
Lateral wall of the nasal cavity (medial aspect 1)

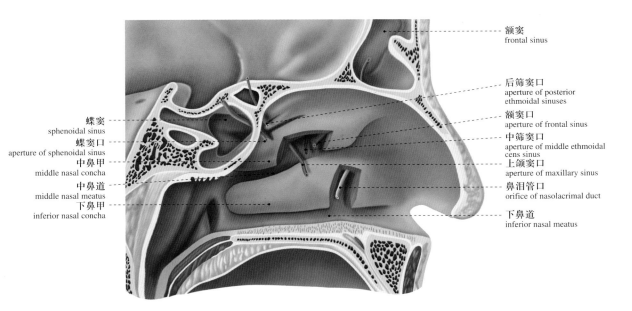

蝶窦
sphenoidal sinus

蝶窦口
aperture of sphenoidal sinus

中鼻甲
middle nasal concha

中鼻道
middle nasal meatus

下鼻甲
inferior nasal concha

额窦
frontal sinus

后筛窦口
aperture of posterior ethmoidal sinuses

额窦口
aperture of frontal sinus

中筛窦口
aperture of middle ethmoidal cens sinus

上颌窦口
aperture of maxillary sinus

鼻泪管口
orifice of nasolacrimal duct

下鼻道
inferior nasal meatus

图 297　鼻腔外侧壁（内侧面观 2）
Lateral wall of the nasal cavity (medial aspect 2)

喉

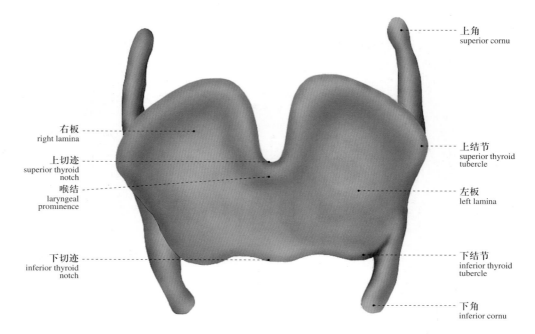

图 298　甲状软骨（前面观）
Thyroid cartilage (anterior aspect)

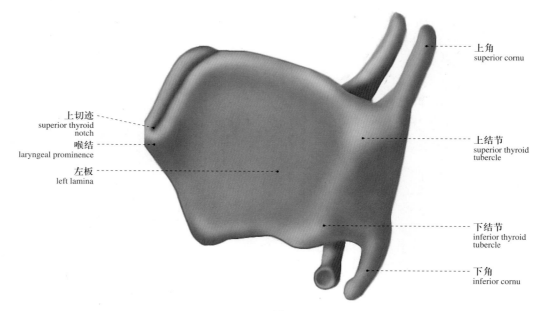

图 299　甲状软骨（外侧面观）
Thyroid cartilage (lateral aspect)

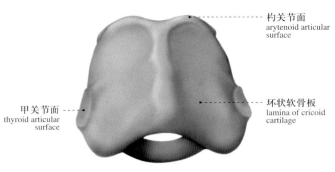

杓关节面
arytenoid articular
surface

环状软骨板
lamina of cricoid
cartilage

甲关节面
thyroid articular
surface

图 300　环状软骨（后面观）
Cricoid cartilage (posterior aspect)

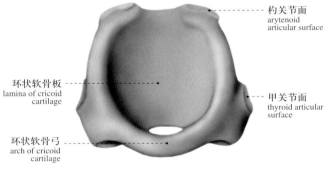

杓关节面
arytenoid
articular surface

环状软骨板
lamina of cricoid
cartilage

甲关节面
thyroid articular
surface

环状软骨弓
arch of cricoid
cartilage

图 301　环状软骨（前上面观）
Cricoid cartilage (anterior superior aspect)

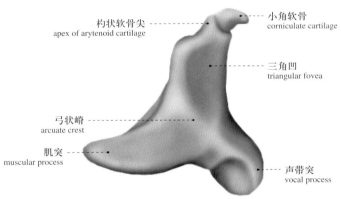

杓状软骨尖
apex of arytenoid cartilage

小角软骨
corniculate cartilage

三角凹
triangular fovea

弓状嵴
arcuate crest

肌突
muscular process

声带突
vocal process

图 302　环状软骨（外侧面观）
Cricoid cartilage (lateral aspect)

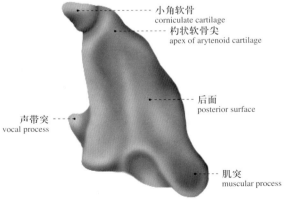

小角软骨
corniculate cartilage

杓状软骨尖
apex of arytenoid cartilage

后面
posterior surface

声带突
vocal process

肌突
muscular process

图 303　杓状软骨（后面观）
Arytenoid cartilage (posterior aspect)

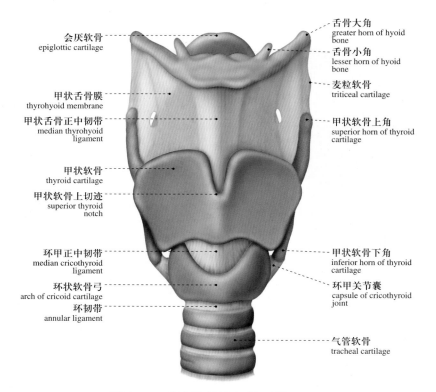

会厌软骨
epiglottic cartilage

甲状舌骨膜
thyrohyoid membrane

甲状舌骨正中韧带
median thyrohyoid
ligament

甲状软骨
thyroid cartilage

甲状软骨上切迹
superior thyroid
notch

环甲正中韧带
median cricothyroid
ligament

环状软骨弓
arch of cricoid cartilage

环韧带
annular ligament

舌骨大角
greater horn of hyoid
bone

舌骨小角
lesser horn of hyoid
bone

麦粒软骨
triticeal cartilage

甲状软骨上角
superior horn of thyroid
cartilage

甲状软骨下角
inferior horn of thyroid
cartilage

环甲关节囊
capsule of cricothyroid
joint

气管软骨
tracheal cartilage

图 304　喉的软骨及韧带（前面观）
Cartilages and ligaments of larynx (anterior aspect)

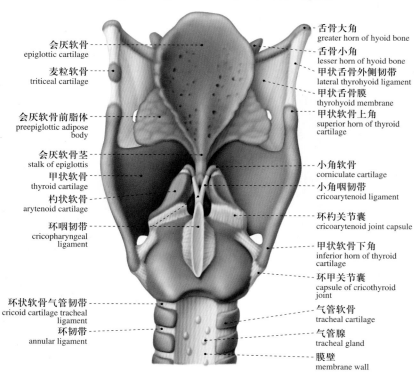

会厌软骨
epiglottic cartilage

麦粒软骨
triticeal cartilage

会厌软骨前脂体
preepiglottic adipose
body

会厌软骨茎
stalk of epiglottis

甲状软骨
thyroid cartilage

杓状软骨
arytenoid cartilage

环咽韧带
cricopharyngeal
ligament

环状软骨气管韧带
cricoid cartilage tracheal
ligament

环韧带
annular ligament

舌骨大角
greater horn of hyoid bone

舌骨小角
lesser horn of hyoid bone

甲状舌骨外侧韧带
lateral thyrohyoid ligament

甲状舌骨膜
thyrohyoid membrane

甲状软骨上角
superior horn of thyroid
cartilage

小角软骨
corniculate cartilage

小角咽韧带
cricoarytenoid ligament

环杓关节囊
cricoarytenoid joint capsule

甲状软骨下角
inferior horn of thyroid
cartilage

环甲关节囊
capsule of cricothyroid
joint

气管软骨
tracheal cartilage

气管腺
tracheal gland

膜壁
membrane wall

图 305　喉的软骨及韧带（后面观）
Cartilages and ligaments of larynx (posterior aspect)

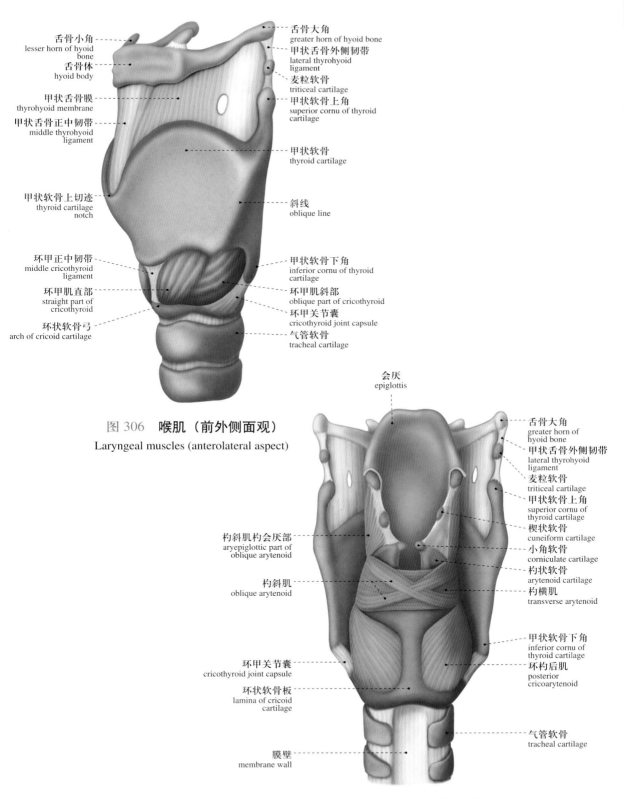

舌骨小角
lesser horn of hyoid bone
舌骨体
hyoid body
甲状舌骨膜
thyrohyoid membrane
甲状舌骨正中韧带
middle thyrohyoid ligament

甲状软骨上切迹
thyroid cartilage notch

环甲正中韧带
middle cricothyroid ligament
环甲肌直部
straight part of cricothyroid
环状软骨弓
arch of cricoid cartilage

舌骨大角
greater horn of hyoid bone
甲状舌骨外侧韧带
lateral thyrohyoid ligament
麦粒软骨
triticeal cartilage
甲状软骨上角
superior cornu of thyroid cartilage
甲状软骨
thyroid cartilage

斜线
oblique line

甲状软骨下角
inferior cornu of thyroid cartilage
环甲肌斜部
oblique part of cricothyroid
环甲关节囊
cricothyroid joint capsule
气管软骨
tracheal cartilage

图 306　喉肌（前外侧面观）
Laryngeal muscles (anterolateral aspect)

会厌
epiglottis

舌骨大角
greater horn of hyoid bone
甲状舌骨外侧韧带
lateral thyrohyoid ligament
麦粒软骨
triticeal cartilage
甲状软骨上角
superior cornu of thyroid cartilage
楔状软骨
cuneiform cartilage
小角软骨
corniculate cartilage
杓状软骨
arytenoid cartilage
杓横肌
transverse arytenoid

杓斜肌杓会厌部
aryepiglottic part of oblique arytenoid
杓斜肌
oblique arytenoid

甲状软骨下角
inferior cornu of thyroid cartilage
环杓后肌
posterior cricoarytenoid

环甲关节囊
cricothyroid joint capsule
环状软骨板
lamina of cricoid cartilage

膜壁
membrane wall

气管软骨
tracheal cartilage

图 307　喉肌（后面观）
Laryngeal muscles (posterior aspect)

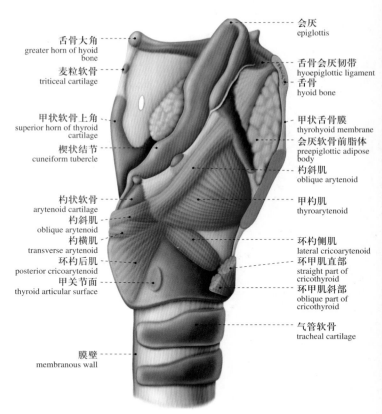

会厌
epiglottis

舌骨大角
greater horn of hyoid bone

麦粒软骨
triticeal cartilage

舌骨会厌韧带
hyoepiglottic ligament

舌骨
hyoid bone

甲状软骨上角
superior horn of thyroid cartilage

甲状舌骨膜
thyrohyoid membrane

会厌软骨前脂体
preepiglottic adipose body

楔状结节
cuneiform tubercle

杓斜肌
oblique arytenoid

杓状软骨
arytenoid cartilage

甲杓肌
thyroarytenoid

杓斜肌
oblique arytenoid

杓横肌
transverse arytenoid

环杓侧肌
lateral cricoarytenoid

环杓后肌
posterior cricoarytenoid

环甲肌直部
straight part of cricothyroid

甲关节面
thyroid articular surface

环甲肌斜部
oblique part of cricothyroid

气管软骨
tracheal cartilage

膜壁
membranous wall

图 308　喉肌（后斜面观）
Laryngeal muscles (after oblique aspect)

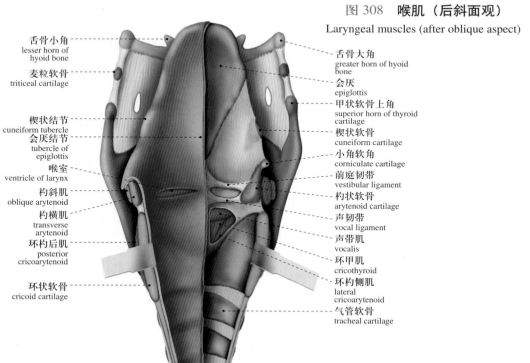

舌骨小角
lesser horn of hyoid bone

麦粒软骨
triticeal cartilage

楔状结节
cuneiform tubercle

会厌结节
tubercle of epiglottis

喉室
ventricle of larynx

杓斜肌
oblique arytenoid

杓横肌
transverse arytenoid

环杓后肌
posterior cricoarytenoid

环状软骨
cricoid cartilage

舌骨大角
greater horn of hyoid bone

会厌
epiglottis

甲状软骨上角
superior horn of thyroid cartilage

楔状软骨
cuneiform cartilage

小角软骨
corniculate cartilage

前庭韧带
vestibular ligament

杓状软骨
arytenoid cartilage

声韧带
vocal ligament

声带肌
vocalis

环甲肌
cricothyroid

环杓侧肌
lateral cricoarytenoid

气管软骨
tracheal cartilage

图 309　喉后正中切开（后面观）
Laryngeal posterior midline incision (posterior aspect)

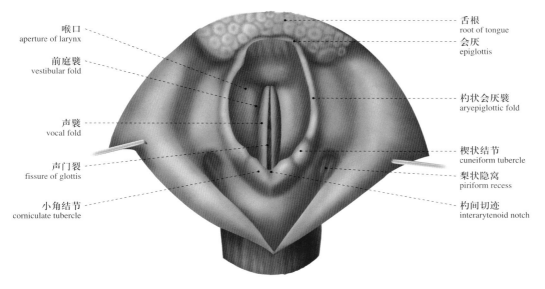

喉口
aperture of larynx

前庭襞
vestibular fold

声襞
vocal fold

声门裂
fissure of glottis

小角结节
corniculate tubercle

舌根
root of tongue

会厌
epiglottis

杓状会厌襞
aryepiglottic fold

楔状结节
cuneiform tubercle

梨状隐窝
piriform recess

杓间切迹
interarytenoid notch

图 310　喉口（后面观）
Aperture of larynx (posterior aspect)

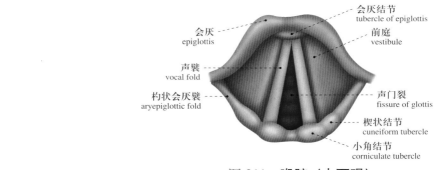

会厌
epiglottis

声襞
vocal fold

杓状会厌襞
aryepiglottic fold

会厌结节
tubercle of epiglottis

前庭
vestibule

声门裂
fissure of glottis

楔状结节
cuneiform tubercle

小角结节
corniculate tubercle

图 311　喉腔（上面观）
Laryngeal cavity (superior aspect)

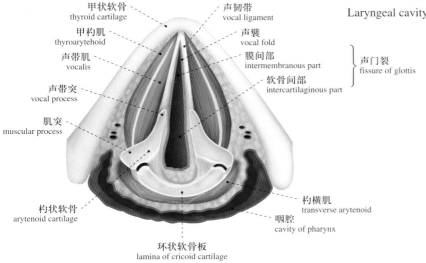

甲状软骨
thyroid cartilage

甲杓肌
thyroarytehoid

声带肌
vocalis

声带突
vocal process

肌突
muscular process

杓状软骨
arytenoid cartilage

声韧带
vocal ligament

声襞
vocal fold

膜间部
intermembranous part

软骨间部
intercartilaginous part

声门裂
fissure of glottis

杓横肌
transverse arytenoid

咽腔
cavity of pharynx

环状软骨板
lamina of cricoid cartilage

图 312　喉横切面（通过声带）
Transverse section of larynx (through the level of vocal folds)

165

第四节

气管与支气管

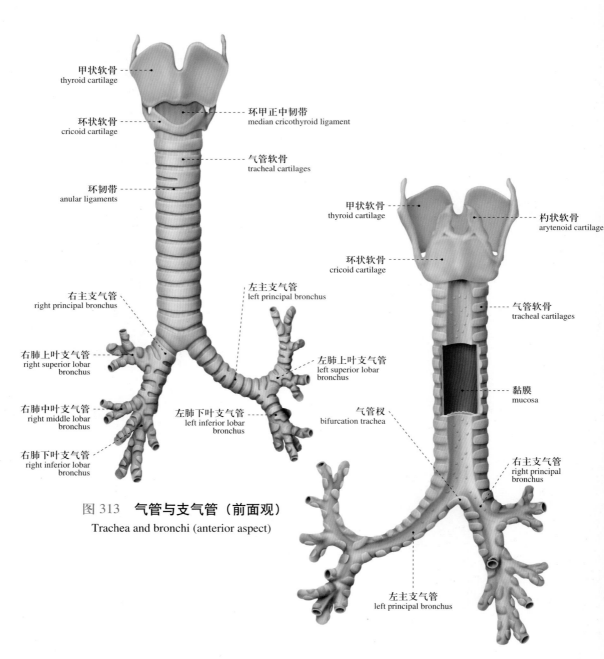

甲状软骨
thyroid cartilage

环甲正中韧带
median cricothyroid ligament

环状软骨
cricoid cartilage

气管软骨
tracheal cartilages

环韧带
anular ligaments

甲状软骨
thyroid cartilage

杓状软骨
arytenoid cartilage

环状软骨
cricoid cartilage

右主支气管
right principal bronchus

左主支气管
left principal bronchus

气管软骨
tracheal cartilages

右肺上叶支气管
right superior lobar
bronchus

左肺上叶支气管
left superior lobar
bronchus

黏膜
mucosa

右肺中叶支气管
right middle lobar
bronchus

左肺下叶支气管
left inferior lobar
bronchus

气管杈
bifurcation trachea

右主支气管
right principal
bronchus

右肺下叶支气管
right inferior lobar
bronchus

图 313 **气管与支气管（前面观）**
Trachea and bronchi (anterior aspect)

左主支气管
left principal bronchus

图 314 **气管与支气管（后面观）**
Trachea and bronchi (posterior aspect)

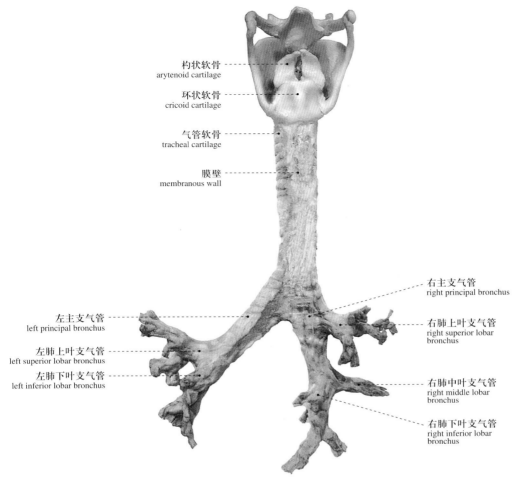

杓状软骨
arytenoid cartilage

环状软骨
cricoid cartilage

气管软骨
tracheal cartilage

膜壁
membranous wall

右主支气管
right principal bronchus

左主支气管
left principal bronchus

右肺上叶支气管
right superior lobar
bronchus

左肺上叶支气管
left superior lobar bronchus

左肺下叶支气管
left inferior lobar bronchus

右肺中叶支气管
right middle lobar
bronchus

右肺下叶支气管
right inferior lobar
bronchus

图 315　气管和支气管局解（后面观）
Topography of the trachea and the bronchi (posterior aspect)

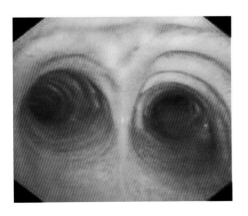

图 316　气管镜像（隆嵴）
Bronchoscope image (carina)

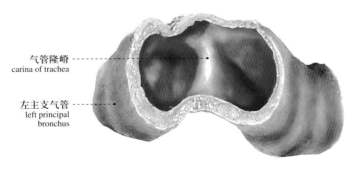

气管隆嵴
carina of trachea

左主支气管
left principal
bronchus

图 317　气管隆嵴
Carina of the trachea

第五节

肺

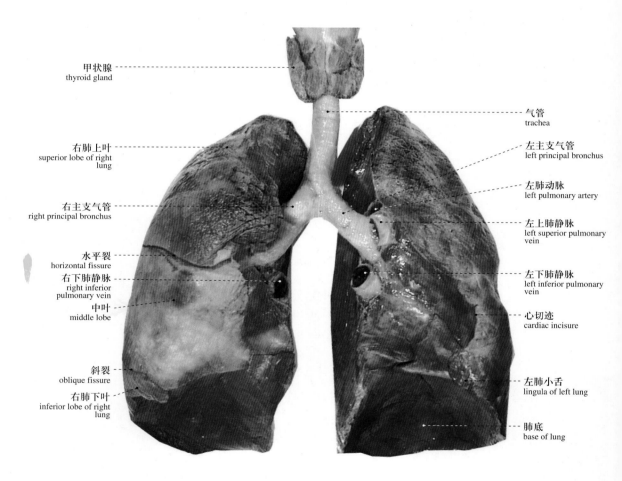

甲状腺
thyroid gland

右肺上叶
superior lobe of right lung

右主支气管
right principal bronchus

水平裂
horizontal fissure

右下肺静脉
right inferior pulmonary vein

中叶
middle lobe

斜裂
oblique fissure

右肺下叶
inferior lobe of right lung

气管
trachea

左主支气管
left principal bronchus

左肺动脉
left pulmonary artery

左上肺静脉
left superior pulmonary vein

左下肺静脉
left inferior pulmonary vein

心切迹
cardiac incisure

左肺小舌
lingula of left lung

肺底
base of lung

图 318　肺（前面观）

Lungs (anterior aspect)

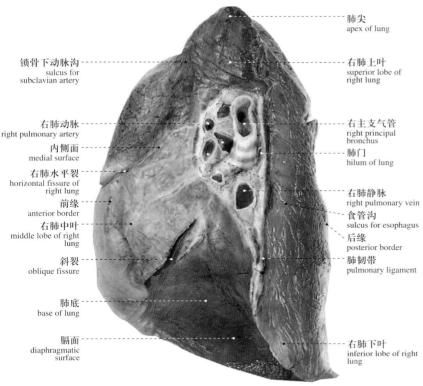

肺尖
apex of lung

锁骨下动脉沟
sulcus for
subclavian artery

右肺上叶
superior lobe of
right lung

右肺动脉
right pulmonary artery

右主支气管
right principal
bronchus

内侧面
medial surface

肺门
hilum of lung

右肺水平裂
horizontal fissure of
right lung

右肺静脉
right pulmonary vein

前缘
anterior border

食管沟
sulcus for esophagus

右肺中叶
middle lobe of right
lung

后缘
posterior border

斜裂
oblique fissure

肺韧带
pulmonary ligament

肺底
base of lung

膈面
diaphragmatic
surface

右肺下叶
inferior lobe of right
lung

图 319　右肺（内侧面观）
Right lung (medial aspect)

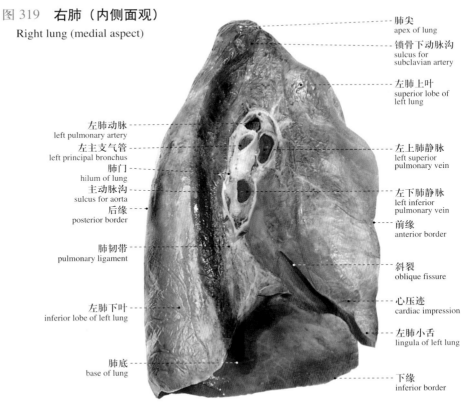

肺尖
apex of lung

锁骨下动脉沟
sulcus for
subclavian artery

左肺上叶
superior lobe of
left lung

左肺动脉
left pulmonary artery

左主支气管
left principal bronchus

左上肺静脉
left superior
pulmonary vein

肺门
hilum of lung

主动脉沟
sulcus for aorta

左下肺静脉
left inferior
pulmonary vein

后缘
posterior border

前缘
anterior border

肺韧带
pulmonary ligament

斜裂
oblique fissure

左肺下叶
inferior lobe of left lung

心压迹
cardiac impression

左肺小舌
lingula of left lung

肺底
base of lung

下缘
inferior border

图 320　左肺（内侧面观）
Left lung (medial aspect)

左肺
上叶
Ⅰ + Ⅱ：尖后段
Ⅲ：前段
Ⅳ：上舌段
Ⅴ：下舌段

下叶
Ⅵ：上段
Ⅷ：前底段
Ⅸ：外侧底段
Ⅹ：后底段

右肺
上叶
Ⅰ：尖段
Ⅱ：后段
Ⅲ：前段

中叶
Ⅳ：外侧段
Ⅴ：内侧段

下叶
Ⅵ：上段
Ⅶ：内侧底段
Ⅷ：前底段
Ⅸ：外侧底段
Ⅹ：后底段

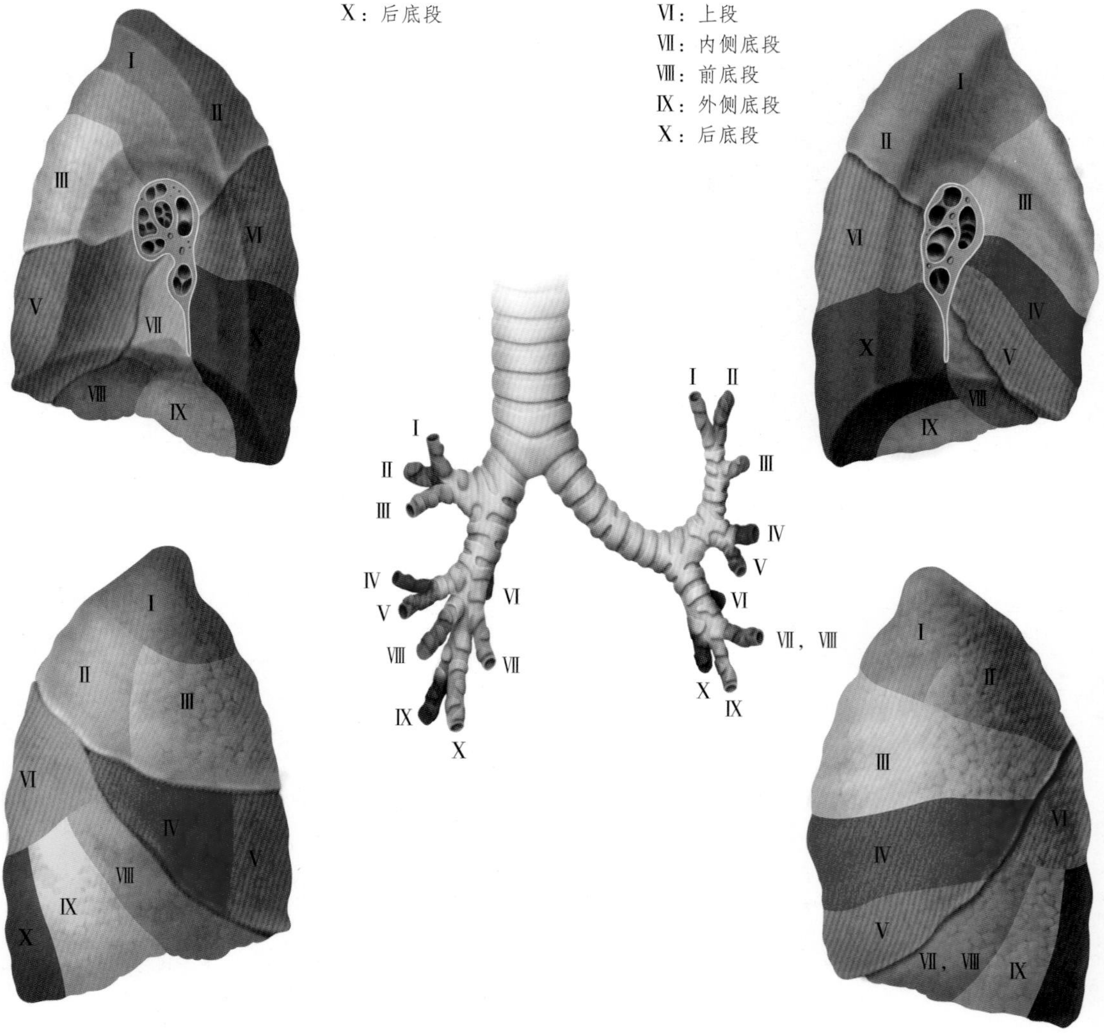

图 321　**肺的节段性结构**
Segmental architecture of the lungs

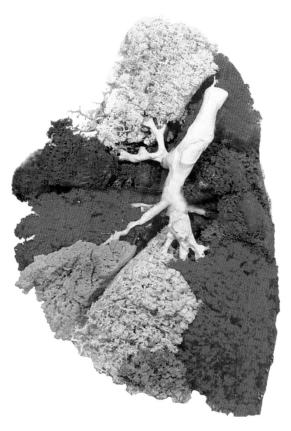

图 322　支气管肺段铸型（内侧面观）
Cast of the bronchopulmonary segments (medial aspect)

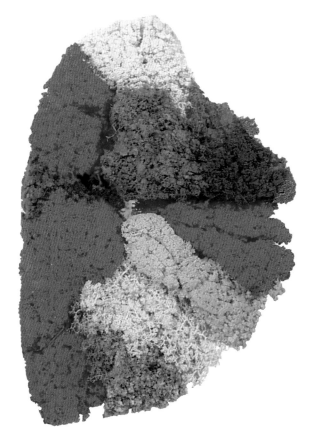

图 323　支气管肺段铸型（外侧面观）
Cast of the bronchopulmonary segments (lateral aspect)

第六节

胸 膜

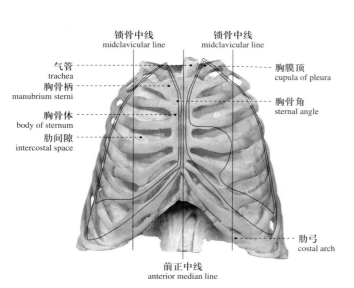

锁骨中线
midclavicular line

锁骨中线
midclavicular line

腋中线
midaxillary line

气管
trachea

胸骨柄
manubrium sterni

胸骨体
body of sternum

肋间隙
intercostal space

胸膜顶
cupula of pleura

胸骨角
sternal angle

肋弓
costal arch

前正中线
anterior median line

肺下缘
inferior border of lung

胸膜下线
inferior line of pleura

图 324　胸膜及肺体表投影（前面观）
Body surface projection of the pleura and the lung (anterior aspect)

图 325　胸膜及肺体表投影（左侧面观）
Body surface projection of the pleura and the lung (left lateral aspect)

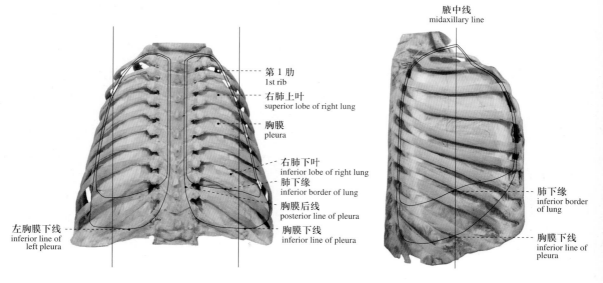

第 1 肋
1st rib

右肺上叶
superior lobe of right lung

胸膜
pleura

右肺下叶
inferior lobe of right lung

肺下缘
inferior border of lung

胸膜后线
posterior line of pleura

胸膜下线
inferior line of pleura

左胸膜下线
inferior line of left pleura

腋中线
midaxillary line

肺下缘
inferior border of lung

胸膜下线
inferior line of pleura

图 326　胸膜及肺体表投影（后面观）
Body surface projection of the pleura and the lung (posterior aspect)

图 327　胸膜及肺体表投影（右侧面观）
Body surface projection of the pleura and the lung (right lateral aspect)

第七节

纵　隔

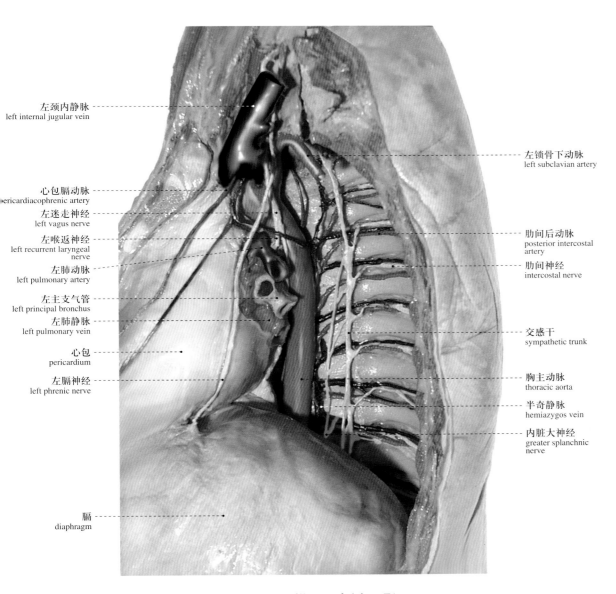

左颈内静脉
left internal jugular vein

心包膈动脉
pericardiacophrenic artery

左迷走神经
left vagus nerve

左喉返神经
left recurrent laryngeal nerve

左肺动脉
left pulmonary artery

左主支气管
left principal bronchus

左肺静脉
left pulmonary vein

心包
pericardium

左膈神经
left phrenic nerve

膈
diaphragm

左锁骨下动脉
left subclavian artery

肋间后动脉
posterior intercostal artery

肋间神经
intercostal nerve

交感干
sympathetic trunk

胸主动脉
thoracic aorta

半奇静脉
hemiazygos vein

内脏大神经
greater splanchnic nerve

图 328　纵隔（左侧面观）
Mediastinum (left latera aspect)

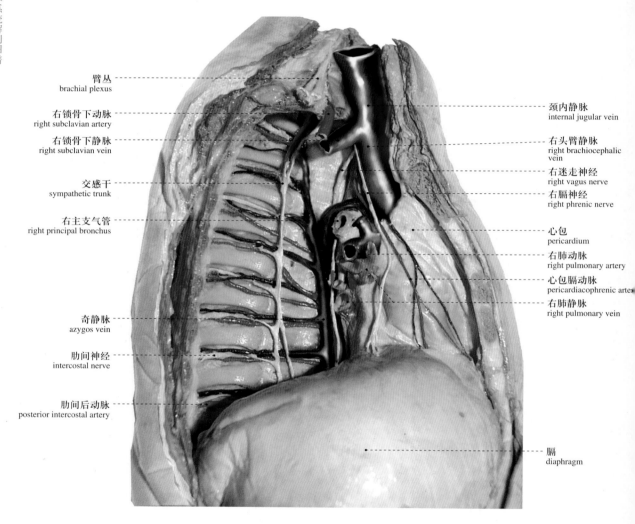

臂丛
brachial plexus

右锁骨下动脉
right subclavian artery

右锁骨下静脉
right subclavian vein

交感干
sympathetic trunk

右主支气管
right principal bronchus

奇静脉
azygos vein

肋间神经
intercostal nerve

肋间后动脉
posterior intercostal artery

颈内静脉
internal jugular vein

右头臂静脉
right brachiocephalic vein

右迷走神经
right vagus nerve

右膈神经
right phrenic nerve

心包
pericardium

右肺动脉
right pulmonary artery

心包膈动脉
pericardiacophrenic artery

右肺静脉
right pulmonary vein

膈
diaphragm

图 329　纵隔（右侧面观）
Mediastinum (right lateral aspect)

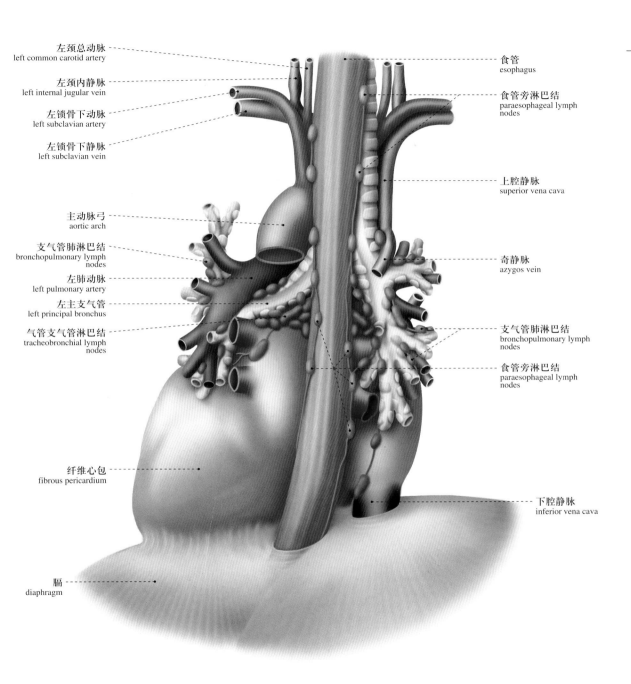

左颈总动脉
left common carotid artery

左颈内静脉
left internal jugular vein

左锁骨下动脉
left subclavian artery

左锁骨下静脉
left subclavian vein

主动脉弓
aortic arch

支气管肺淋巴结
bronchopulmonary lymph nodes

左肺动脉
left pulmonary artery

左主支气管
left principal bronchus

气管支气管淋巴结
tracheobronchial lymph nodes

纤维心包
fibrous pericardium

膈
diaphragm

食管
esophagus

食管旁淋巴结
paraesophageal lymph nodes

上腔静脉
superior vena cava

奇静脉
azygos vein

支气管肺淋巴结
bronchopulmonary lymph nodes

食管旁淋巴结
paraesophageal lymph nodes

下腔静脉
inferior vena cava

图 330 胸部淋巴结（后面观）
Thoracic lymph nodes (posterior aspect)

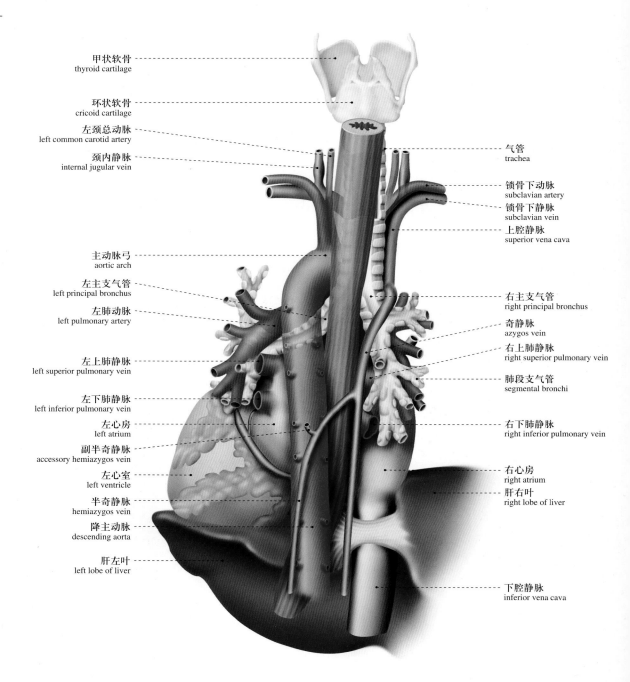

甲状软骨
thyroid cartilage

环状软骨
cricoid cartilage

左颈总动脉
left common carotid artery

颈内静脉
internal jugular vein

气管
trachea

锁骨下动脉
subclavian artery

锁骨下静脉
subclavian vein

上腔静脉
superior vena cava

主动脉弓
aortic arch

左主支气管
left principal bronchus

左肺动脉
left pulmonary artery

右主支气管
right principal bronchus

奇静脉
azygos vein

右上肺静脉
right superior pulmonary vein

左上肺静脉
left superior pulmonary vein

肺段支气管
segmental bronchi

左下肺静脉
left inferior pulmonary vein

右下肺静脉
right inferior pulmonary vein

左心房
left atrium

副半奇静脉
accessory hemiazygos vein

左心室
left ventricle

右心房
right atrium

肝右叶
right lobe of liver

半奇静脉
hemiazygos vein

降主动脉
descending aorta

肝左叶
left lobe of liver

下腔静脉
inferior vena cava

图 331　纵隔的内容（后面观）
Contents of the mediastinum (posterior aspect)

泌尿系统模式图

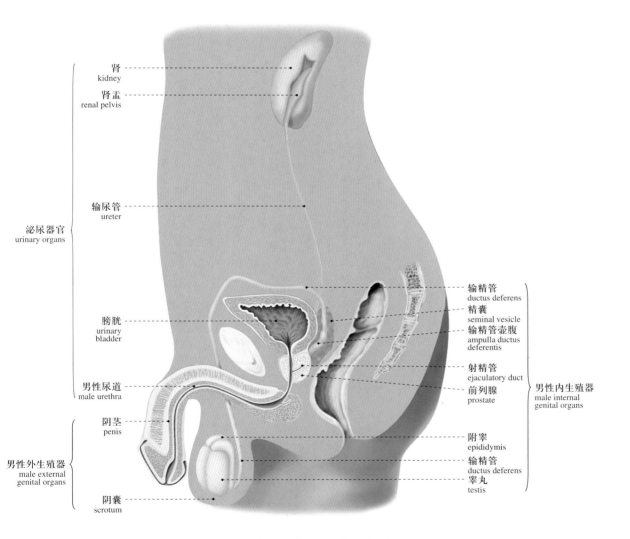

肾
kidney

肾盂
renal pelvis

输尿管
ureter

泌尿器官
urinary organs

膀胱
urinary
bladder

男性尿道
male urethra

阴茎
penis

男性外生殖器
male external
genital organs

阴囊
scrotum

输精管
ductus deferens

精囊
seminal vesicle

输精管壶腹
ampulla ductus
deferentis

射精管
ejaculatory duct

前列腺
prostate

男性内生殖器
male internal
genital organs

附睾
epididymis

输精管
ductus deferens

睾丸
testis

图 332　男性泌尿生殖系统（内侧面观）
Male urogenital system（medial aspect）

肾

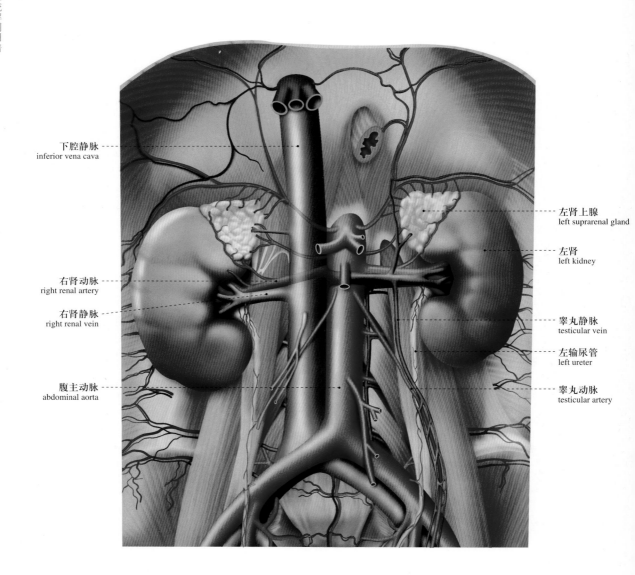

下腔静脉
inferior vena cava

左肾上腺
left suprarenal gland

左肾
left kidney

右肾动脉
right renal artery

右肾静脉
right renal vein

睾丸静脉
testicular vein

左输尿管
left ureter

腹主动脉
abdominal aorta

睾丸动脉
testicular artery

图 333　肾
Kidney

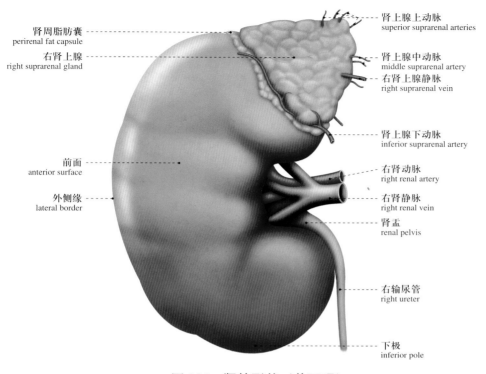

肾周脂肪囊
perirenal fat capsule

右肾上腺
right suprarenal gland

前面
anterior surface

外侧缘
lateral border

肾上腺上动脉
superior suprarenal arteries

肾上腺中动脉
middle suprarenal artery

右肾上腺静脉
right suprarenal vein

肾上腺下动脉
inferior suprarenal artery

右肾动脉
right renal artery

右肾静脉
right renal vein

肾盂
renal pelvis

右输尿管
right ureter

下极
inferior pole

图 334　肾的形状（前面观）
Shape of the kidney (anterior aspect)

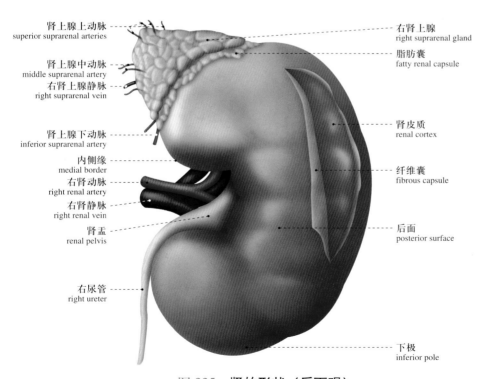

肾上腺上动脉
superior suprarenal arteries

肾上腺中动脉
middle suprarenal artery

右肾上腺静脉
right suprarenal vein

肾上腺下动脉
inferior suprarenal artery

内侧缘
medial border

右肾动脉
right renal artery

右肾静脉
right renal vein

肾盂
renal pelvis

右尿管
right ureter

右肾上腺
right suprarenal gland

脂肪囊
fatty renal capsule

肾皮质
renal cortex

纤维囊
fibrous capsule

后面
posterior surface

下极
inferior pole

图 335　肾的形状（后面观）
Shape of the kidney (posterior aspect)

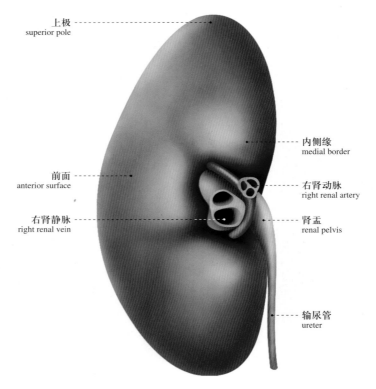

上极
superior pole

内侧缘
medial border

前面
anterior surface

右肾动脉
right renal artery

右肾静脉
right renal vein

肾盂
renal pelvis

输尿管
ureter

图 336　肾的形状（内侧面观）

Shape of the kidney (medial aspect)

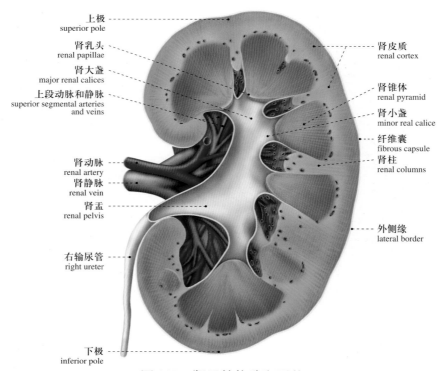

上极
superior pole

肾乳头
renal papillae

肾大盏
major renal calices

上段动脉和静脉
superior segmental arteries
and veins

肾动脉
renal artery

肾静脉
renal vein

肾盂
renal pelvis

右输尿管
right ureter

下极
inferior pole

肾皮质
renal cortex

肾锥体
renal pyramid

肾小盏
minor real calice

纤维囊
fibrous capsule

肾柱
renal columns

外侧缘
lateral border

图 337　肾盂的构造和形状

Structure and shape of the renal pelvis

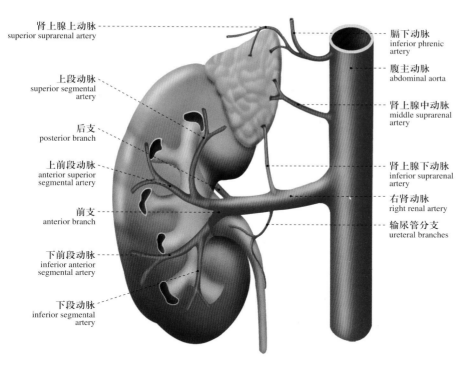

图 338　肾动脉分支到各肾段的关系

Relationship of the renal arterial branches to the renal segments

肾上腺上动脉
superior suprarenal artery

上段动脉
superior segmental
artery

后支
posterior branch

上前段动脉
anterior superior
segmental artery

前支
anterior branch

下前段动脉
inferior anterior
segmental artery

下段动脉
inferior segmental
artery

膈下动脉
inferior phrenic
artery

腹主动脉
abdominal aorta

肾上腺中动脉
middle suprarenal
artery

肾上腺下动脉
inferior suprarenal
artery

右肾动脉
right renal artery

输尿管分支
ureteral branches

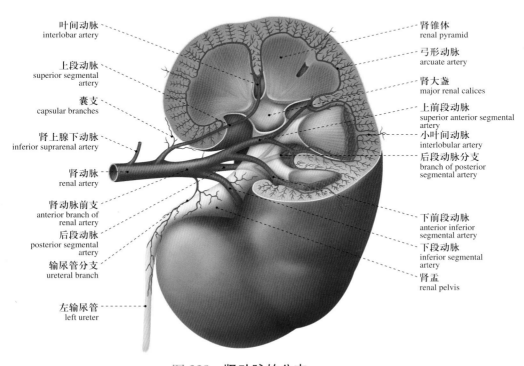

叶间动脉
interlobar artery

上段动脉
superior segmental
artery

囊支
capsular branches

肾上腺下动脉
inferior suprarenal artery

肾动脉
renal artery

肾动脉前支
anterior branch of
renal artery

后段动脉
posterior segmental
artery

输尿管分支
ureteral branch

左输尿管
left ureter

肾锥体
renal pyramid

弓形动脉
arcuate artery

肾大盏
major renal calices

上前段动脉
superior anterior segmental
artery

小叶间动脉
interlobular artery

后段动脉分支
branch of posterior
segmental artery

下前段动脉
anterior inferior
segmental artery

下段动脉
inferior segmental
artery

肾盂
renal pelvis

图 339　肾动脉的分支

Branches of renal artery

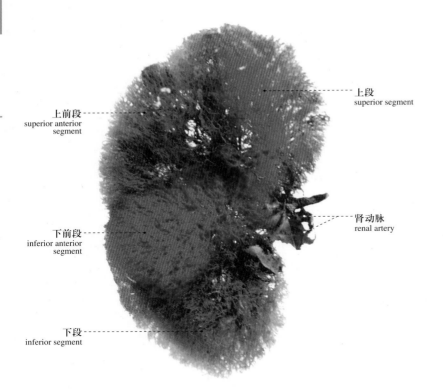

上段
superior segment

上前段
superior anterior
segment

下前段
inferior anterior
segment

下段
inferior segment

肾动脉
renal artery

图 340　肾段铸型 （前面观）
Cast of the renal segments (anterior aspect)

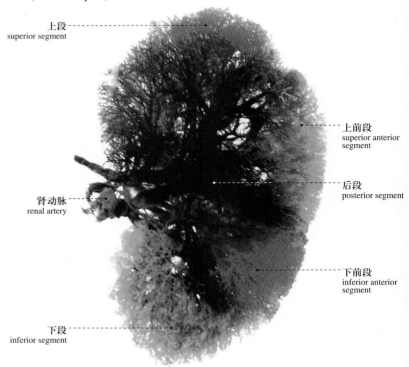

上段
superior segment

上前段
superior anterior
segment

后段
posterior segment

下前段
inferior anterior
segment

下段
inferior segment

肾动脉
renal artery

图 341　肾段铸型 （后面观）
Cast of the renal segments (posterior aspect)

第三节

输 尿 管

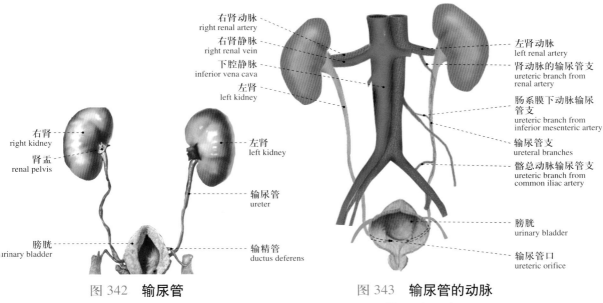

右肾动脉
right renal artery

右肾静脉
right renal vein

下腔静脉
inferior vena cava

左肾
left kidney

左肾动脉
left renal artery

肾动脉的输尿管支
ureteric branch from
renal artery

肠系膜下动脉输尿
管支
ureteric branch from
inferior mesenteric artery

输尿管支
ureteral branches

髂总动脉输尿管支
ureteric branch from
common iliac artery

膀胱
urinary bladder

输尿管口
ureteric orifice

右肾
right kidney

肾盂
renal pelvis

左肾
left kidney

输尿管
ureter

膀胱
urinary bladder

输精管
ductus deferens

图 342　输尿管
Ureter

图 343　输尿管的动脉
Ureteral arteries

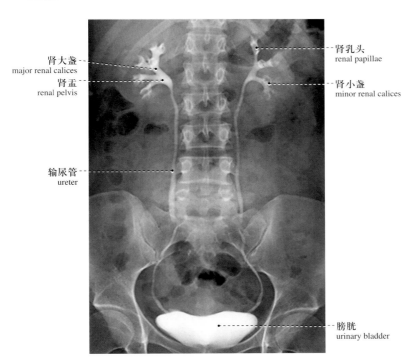

肾大盏
major renal calices

肾盂
renal pelvis

输尿管
ureter

肾乳头
renal papillae

肾小盏
minor renal calices

膀胱
urinary bladder

图 344　泌尿系造影
Ureteropyelography

膀 胱

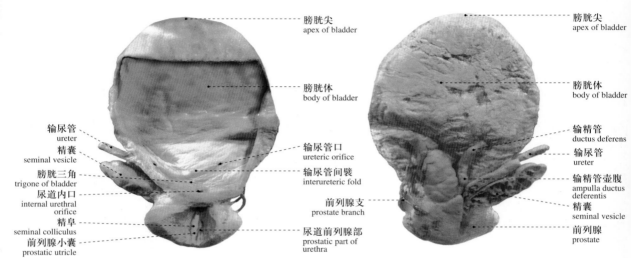

膀胱尖
apex of bladder

膀胱体
body of bladder

输尿管
ureter

精囊
seminal vesicle

膀胱三角
trigone of bladder

尿道内口
internal urethral orifice

精阜
seminal colliculus

前列腺小囊
prostatic utricle

输尿管口
ureteric orifice

输尿管间襞
interureteric fold

前列腺支
prostate branch

尿道前列腺部
prostatic part of urethra

图 345　膀胱
Bladder

膀胱尖
apex of bladder

膀胱体
body of bladder

输精管
ductus deferens

输尿管
ureter

输精管壶腹
ampulla ductus deferentis

精囊
seminal vesicle

前列腺
prostate

图 346　膀胱、输尿管、精囊和前列腺
Bladder, ureter, seminal vesicle and prostate

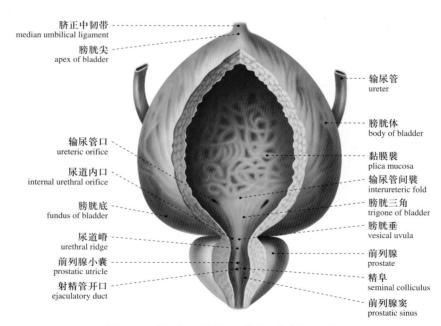

脐正中韧带
median umbilical ligament

膀胱尖
apex of bladder

输尿管口
ureteric orifice

尿道内口
internal urethral orifice

膀胱底
fundus of bladder

尿道嵴
urethral ridge

前列腺小囊
prostatic utricle

射精管开口
ejaculatory duct

输尿管
ureter

膀胱体
body of bladder

黏膜襞
plica mucosa

输尿管间襞
interureteric fold

膀胱三角
trigone of bladder

膀胱垂
vesical uvula

前列腺
prostate

精阜
seminal colliculus

前列腺窦
prostatic sinus

图 347　膀胱及男性尿道前列腺部（前面观）
Bladder and the prostatic part of the male urethra (anterior aspect)

第一节

男性生殖系统

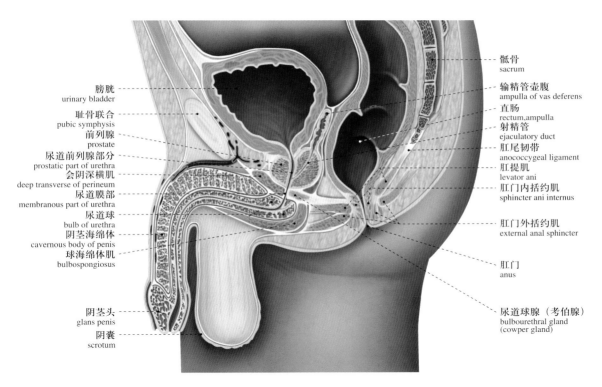

膀胱
urinary bladder

耻骨联合
pubic symphysis

前列腺
prostate

尿道前列腺部分
prostatic part of urethra

会阴深横肌
deep transverse of perineum

尿道膜部
membranous part of urethra

尿道球
bulb of urethra

阴茎海绵体
cavernous body of penis

球海绵体肌
bulbospongiosus

阴茎头
glans penis

阴囊
scrotum

骶骨
sacrum

输精管壶腹
ampulla of vas deferens

直肠
rectum,ampulla

射精管
ejaculatory duct

肛尾韧带
anococcygeal ligament

肛提肌
levator ani

肛门内括约肌
sphincter ani internus

肛门外括约肌
external anal sphincter

肛门
anus

尿道球腺（考伯腺）
bulbourethral gland
(cowper gland)

图 348　男性生殖器官（矢状断）
Male reproductive organs (sagittal aspect)

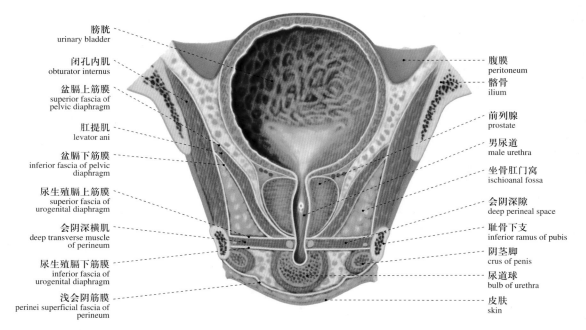

膀胱
urinary bladder

闭孔内肌
obturator internus

盆膈上筋膜
superior fascia of
pelvic diaphragm

肛提肌
levator ani

盆膈下筋膜
inferior fascia of pelvic
diaphragm

尿生殖膈上筋膜
superior fascia of
urogenital diaphragm

会阴深横肌
deep transverse muscle
of perineum

尿生殖膈下筋膜
inferior fascia of
urogenital diaphragm

浅会阴筋膜
perinei superficial fascia of
perineum

腹膜
peritoneum

髂骨
ilium

前列腺
prostate

男尿道
male urethra

坐骨肛门窝
ischioanal fossa

会阴深隙
deep perineal space

耻骨下支
inferior ramus of pubis

阴茎脚
crus of penis

尿道球
bulb of urethra

皮肤
skin

图 349 男性骨盆冠状切面（尿生殖膈及盆膈）
Coronal section of male pelvis (urogenital diaphragm and pelvic diaphragm)

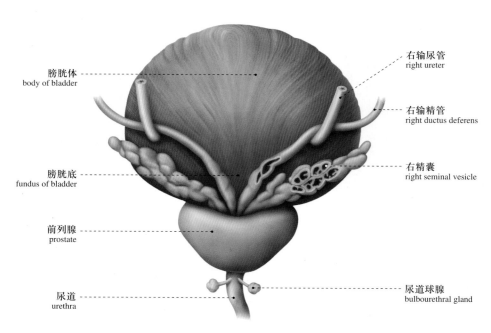

膀胱体
body of bladder

膀胱底
fundus of bladder

前列腺
prostate

尿道
urethra

右输尿管
right ureter

右输精管
right ductus deferens

右精囊
right seminal vesicle

尿道球腺
bulbourethral gland

图 350 性腺
Sex glands

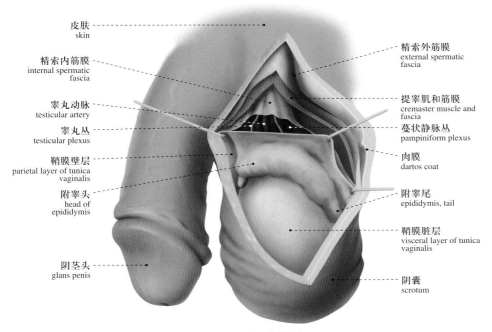

皮肤
skin

精索内筋膜
internal spermatic fascia

睾丸动脉
testicular artery

睾丸丛
testicular plexus

鞘膜壁层
parietal layer of tunica vaginalis

附睾头
head of epididymis

阴茎头
glans penis

精索外筋膜
external spermatic fascia

提睾肌和筋膜
cremaster muscle and fascia

蔓状静脉丛
pampiniform plexus

肉膜
dartos coat

附睾尾
epididymis, tail

鞘膜脏层
visceral layer of tunica vaginalis

阴囊
scrotum

图 351　阴囊结构
Structure of the scrotum

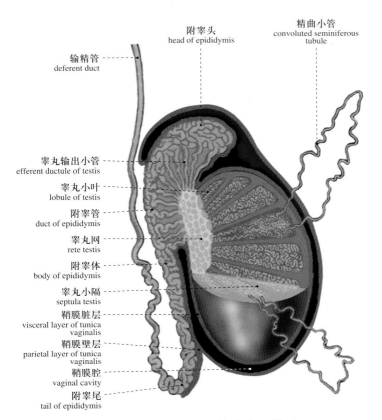

输精管
deferent duct

附睾头
head of epididymis

精曲小管
convoluted seminiferous tubule

睾丸输出小管
efferent ductule of testis

睾丸小叶
lobule of testis

附睾管
duct of epididymis

睾丸网
rete testis

附睾体
body of epididymis

睾丸小隔
septula testis

鞘膜脏层
visceral layer of tunica vaginalis

鞘膜壁层
parietal layer of tunica vaginalis

鞘膜腔
vaginal cavity

附睾尾
tail of epididymis

图 352　睾丸及附睾的结构（模式图）
Structure of the testis and the epididymis (diagram)

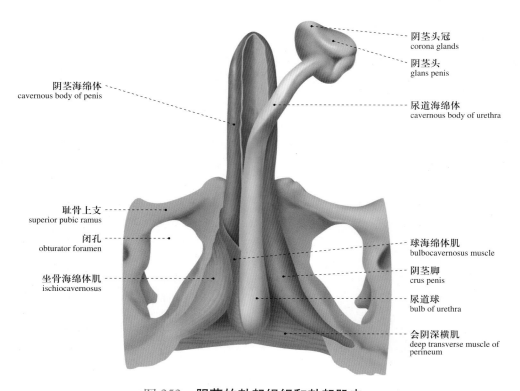

阴茎头冠
corona glands

阴茎头
glans penis

阴茎海绵体
cavernous body of penis

尿道海绵体
cavernous body of urethra

耻骨上支
superior pubic ramus

闭孔
obturator foramen

坐骨海绵体肌
ischiocavernosus

球海绵体肌
bulbocavernosus muscle

阴茎脚
crus penis

尿道球
bulb of urethra

会阴深横肌
deep transverse muscle of perineum

图 353　阴茎的勃起组织和勃起肌肉

Erectile tissues and erectile muscles of the penis

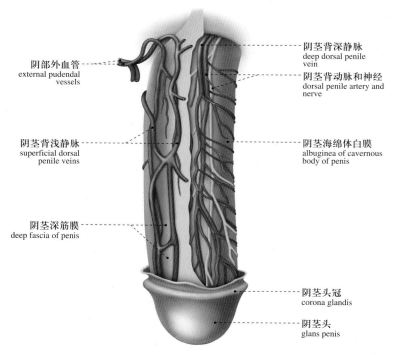

阴部外血管
external pudendal vessels

阴茎背深静脉
deep dorsal penile vein

阴茎背动脉和神经
dorsal penile artery and nerve

阴茎背浅静脉
superficial dorsal penile veins

阴茎海绵体白膜
albuginea of cavernous body of penis

阴茎深筋膜
deep fascia of penis

阴茎头冠
corona glandis

阴茎头
glans penis

图 354　阴茎背部血管和神经

Dorsal blood vessels and nerves of the penis

女性生殖系统

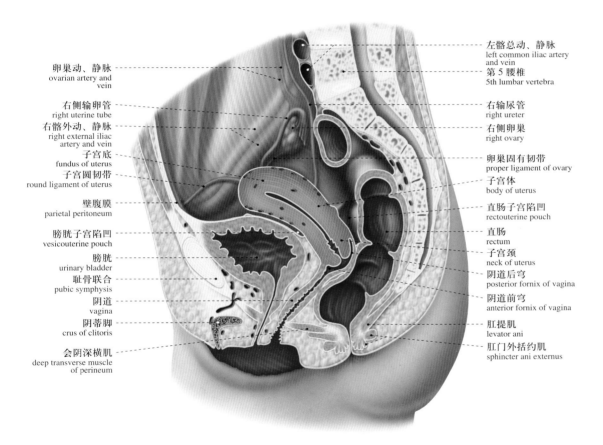

卵巢动、静脉
ovarian artery and vein

右侧输卵管
right uterine tube

右髂外动、静脉
right external iliac artery and vein

子宫底
fundus of uterus

子宫圆韧带
round ligament of uterus

壁腹膜
parietal peritoneum

膀胱子宫陷凹
vesicouterine pouch

膀胱
urinary bladder

耻骨联合
pubic symphysis

阴道
vagina

阴蒂脚
crus of clitoris

会阴深横肌
deep transverse muscle of perineum

左髂总动、静脉
left common iliac artery and vein

第 5 腰椎
5th lumbar vertebra

右输尿管
right ureter

右侧卵巢
right ovary

卵巢固有韧带
proper ligament of ovary

子宫体
body of uterus

直肠子宫陷凹
rectouterine pouch

直肠
rectum

子宫颈
neck of uterus

阴道后穹
posterior fornix of vagina

阴道前穹
anterior fornix of vagina

肛提肌
levator ani

肛门外括约肌
sphincter ani externus

图 355　女性生殖器官（矢状断）

Female reproductive organs (sagittal aspect)

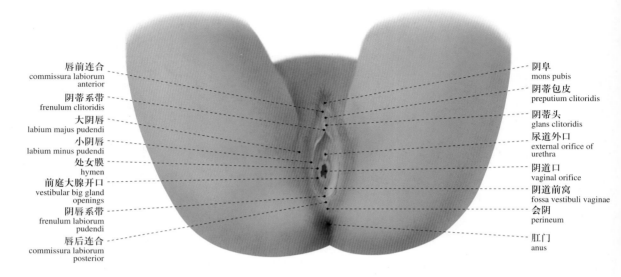

唇前连合
commissura labiorum
anterior

阴蒂系带
frenulum clitoridis

大阴唇
labium majus pudendi

小阴唇
labium minus pudendi

处女膜
hymen

前庭大腺开口
vestibular big gland
openings

阴唇系带
frenulum labiorum
pudendi

唇后连合
commissura labiorum
posterior

阴阜
mons pubis

阴蒂包皮
preputium clitoridis

阴蒂头
glans clitoridis

尿道外口
external orifice of
urethra

阴道口
vaginal orifice

阴道前窝
fossa vestibuli vaginae

会阴
perineum

肛门
anus

图 356 女性外生殖器
External genital organs of the female

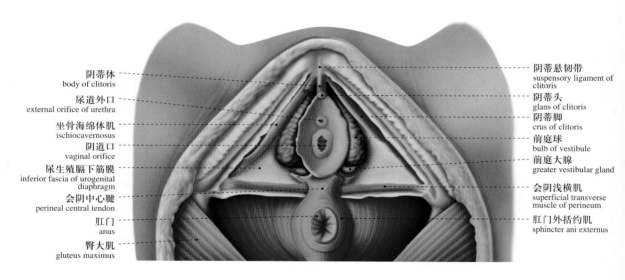

阴蒂体
body of clitoris

尿道外口
external orifice of urethra

坐骨海绵体肌
ischiocavernosus

阴道口
vaginal orifice

尿生殖膈下筋膜
inferior fascia of urogenital
diaphragm

会阴中心腱
perineal central tendon

肛门
anus

臀大肌
gluteus maximus

阴蒂悬韧带
suspensory ligament of
clitoris

阴蒂头
glans of clitoris

阴蒂脚
crus of clitoris

前庭球
bulb of vestibule

前庭大腺
greater vestibular gland

会阴浅横肌
superficial transverse
muscle of perineum

肛门外括约肌
sphincter ani externus

图 357 阴蒂、前庭球及前庭大腺
Clitoris, bulb of the vestibule and the greater vestibular glands

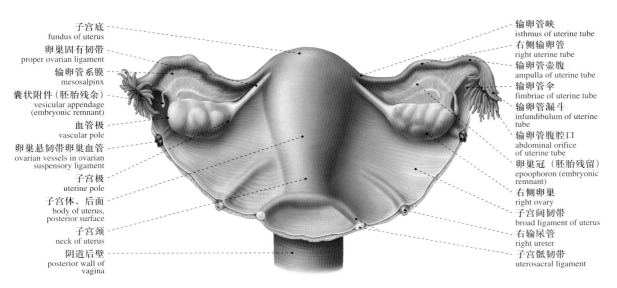

子宫底
fundus of uterus

卵巢固有韧带
proper ovarian ligament

输卵管系膜
mesosalpinx

囊状附件（胚胎残余）
vesicular appendage
(embryonic remnant)

血管极
vascular pole

卵巢悬韧带卵巢血管
ovarian vessels in ovarian
suspensory ligament

子宫极
uterine pole

子宫体，后面
body of uterus,
posterior surface

子宫颈
neck of uterus

阴道后壁
posterior wall of
vagina

输卵管峡
isthmus of uterine tube

右侧输卵管
right uterine tube

输卵管壶腹
ampulla of uterine tube

输卵管伞
fimbriae of uterine tube

输卵管漏斗
infundibulum of uterine
tube

输卵管腹腔口
abdominal orifice
of uterine tube

卵巢冠（胚胎残留）
epoophoron (embryonic
remnant)

右侧卵巢
right ovary

子宫阔韧带
broad ligament of uterus

右输尿管
right ureter

子宫骶韧带
uterosacral ligament

图 358　子宫及附件（后上面观）
Uterus and the adnexa (posterosuperior aspect)

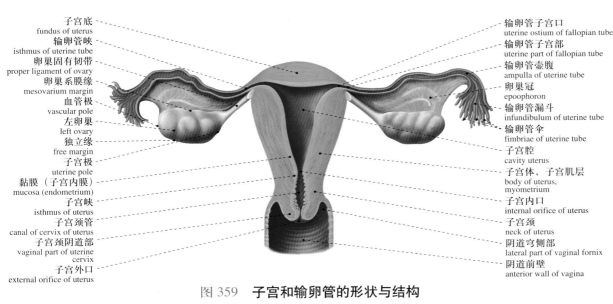

子宫底
fundus of uterus

输卵管峡
isthmus of uterine tube

卵巢固有韧带
proper ligament of ovary

卵巢系膜缘
mesovarium margin

血管极
vascular pole

左卵巢
left ovary

独立缘
free margin

子宫极
uterine pole

黏膜（子宫内膜）
mucosa (endometrium)

子宫峡
isthmus of uterus

子宫颈管
canal of cervix of uterus

子宫颈阴道部
vaginal part of uterine
cervix

子宫外口
external orifice of uterus

输卵管子宫口
uterine ostium of fallopian tube

输卵管子宫部
uterine part of fallopian tube

输卵管壶腹
ampulla of uterine tube

卵巢冠
epoophoron

输卵管漏斗
infundibulum of uterine tube

输卵管伞
fimbriae of uterine tube

子宫腔
cavity uterus

子宫体，子宫肌层
body of uterus,
myometrium

子宫内口
internal orifice of uterus

子宫颈
neck of uterus

阴道穹侧部
lateral part of vaginal fornix

阴道前壁
anterior wall of vagina

图 359　子宫和输卵管的形状与结构
Shape and structure of the uterus and the uterine tubes

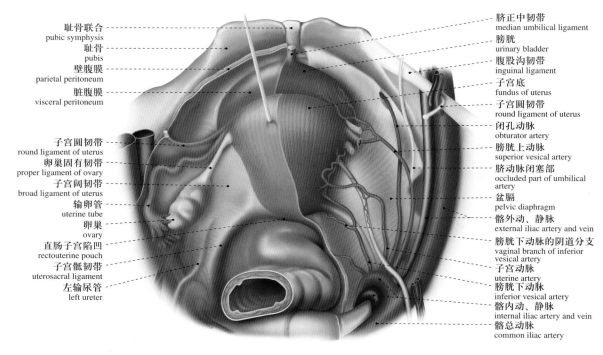

耻骨联合 pubic symphysis
耻骨 pubis
壁腹膜 parietal peritoneum
脏腹膜 visceral peritoneum

子宫圆韧带 round ligament of uterus
卵巢固有韧带 proper ligament of ovary
子宫阔韧带 broad ligament of uterus
输卵管 uterine tube
卵巢 ovary
直肠子宫陷凹 rectouterine pouch
子宫骶韧带 uterosacral ligament
左输尿管 left ureter

脐正中韧带 median umbilical ligament
膀胱 urinary bladder
腹股沟韧带 inguinal ligament
子宫底 fundus of uterus
子宫圆韧带 round ligament of uterus
闭孔动脉 obturator artery
膀胱上动脉 superior vesical artery
脐动脉闭塞部 occluded part of umbilical artery
盆膈 pelvic diaphragm
髂外动、静脉 external iliac artery and vein
膀胱下动脉的阴道分支 vaginal branch of inferior vesical artery
子宫动脉 uterine artery
膀胱下动脉 inferior vesical artery
髂内动、静脉 internal iliac artery and vein
髂总动脉 common iliac artery

图 360　**女性盆腔输尿管的进程**

Course of the ureter in the female pelvis

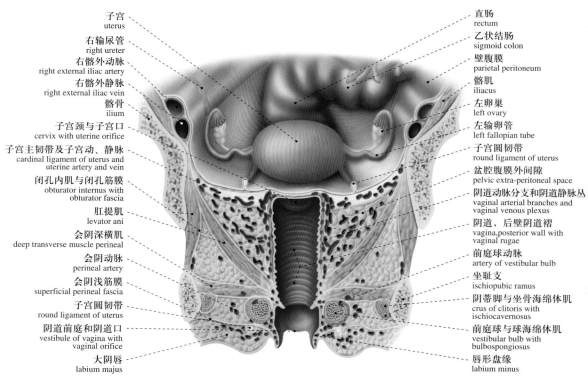

子宫 uterus
右输尿管 right ureter
右髂外动脉 right external iliac artery
右髂外静脉 right external iliac vein
髂骨 ilium
子宫颈与子宫口 cervix with uterine orifice
子宫主韧带及子宫动、静脉 cardinal ligament of uterus and uterine artery and vein
闭孔内肌与闭孔筋膜 obturator internus with obturator fascia
肛提肌 levator ani
会阴深横肌 deep transverse muscle perineal
会阴动脉 perineal artery
会阴浅筋膜 superficial perineal fascia
子宫圆韧带 round ligament of uterus
阴道前庭和阴道口 vestibule of vagina with vaginal orifice
大阴唇 labium majus

直肠 rectum
乙状结肠 sigmoid colon
壁腹膜 parietal peritoneum
髂肌 iliacus
左卵巢 left ovary
左输卵管 left fallopian tube
子宫圆韧带 round ligament of uterus
盆腔腹膜外间隙 pelvic extra-peritoneal space
阴道动脉分支和阴道静脉丛 vaginal arterial branches and vaginal venous plexus
阴道，后壁阴道褶 vagina,posterior wall with vaginal rugae
前庭球动脉 artery of vestibular bulb
坐耻支 ischiopubic ramus
阴蒂脚与坐骨海绵体肌 crus of clitoris with ischiocavernosus
前庭球与球海绵体肌 vestibular bulb with bulbospongiosus
唇形盘缘 labium minus

图 361　**子宫和阴道周围腹膜、筋膜和结缔组织间隙（冠状断）**

Peritoneum,fasciae, and connective-tissue spaces around the uterus and vagina (coronal aspect)

女性乳房

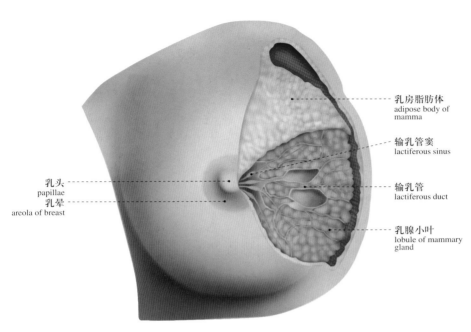

乳房脂肪体
adipose body of mamma

输乳管窦
lactiferous sinus

输乳管
lactiferous duct

乳头
papillae
乳晕
areola of breast

乳腺小叶
lobule of mammary gland

图 362　乳房结构
Mamma structure

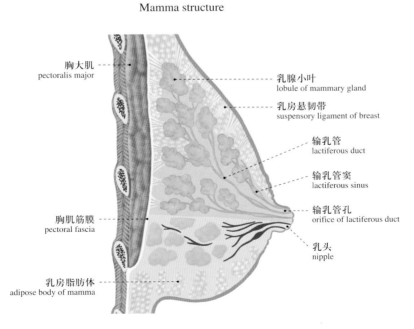

胸大肌
pectoralis major

乳腺小叶
lobule of mammary gland

乳房悬韧带
suspensory ligament of breast

输乳管
lactiferous duct

输乳管窦
lactiferous sinus

输乳管孔
orifice of lactiferous duct

胸肌筋膜
pectoral fascia

乳头
nipple

乳房脂肪体
adipose body of mamma

图 363　乳房矢状切面（模式图）
Sagittal section of the mamma (diagram)

第一节

概　述

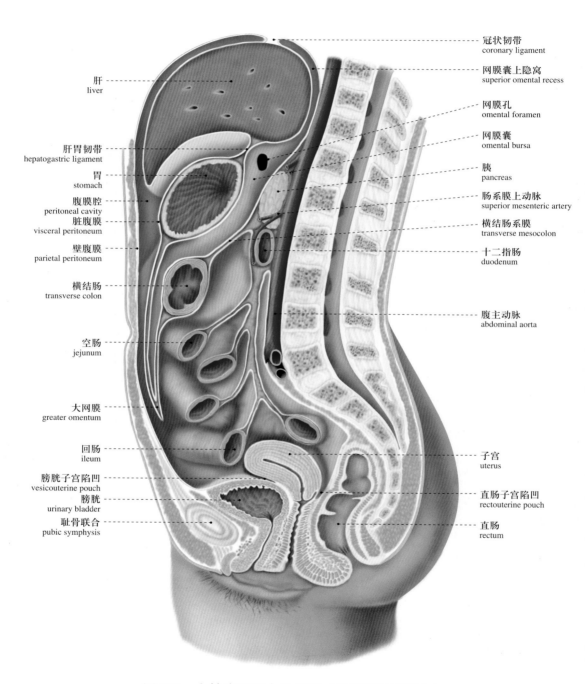

肝
liver

肝胃韧带
hepatogastric ligament

胃
stomach

腹膜腔
peritoneal cavity

脏腹膜
visceral peritoneum

壁腹膜
parietal peritoneum

横结肠
transverse colon

空肠
jejunum

大网膜
greater omentum

回肠
ileum

膀胱子宫陷凹
vesicouterine pouch

膀胱
urinary bladder

耻骨联合
pubic symphysis

冠状韧带
coronary ligament

网膜囊上隐窝
superior omental recess

网膜孔
omental foramen

网膜囊
omental bursa

胰
pancreas

肠系膜上动脉
superior mesenteric artery

横结肠系膜
transverse mesocolon

十二指肠
duodenum

腹主动脉
abdominal aorta

子宫
uterus

直肠子宫陷凹
rectouterine pouch

直肠
rectum

图 364　女性腹腔正中矢状断（示腹膜垂直配布）
Median sagittal section of female abdominal cavity (show vertical arrangement of peritoneum)

第二节

腹膜与腹盆腔脏器的关系

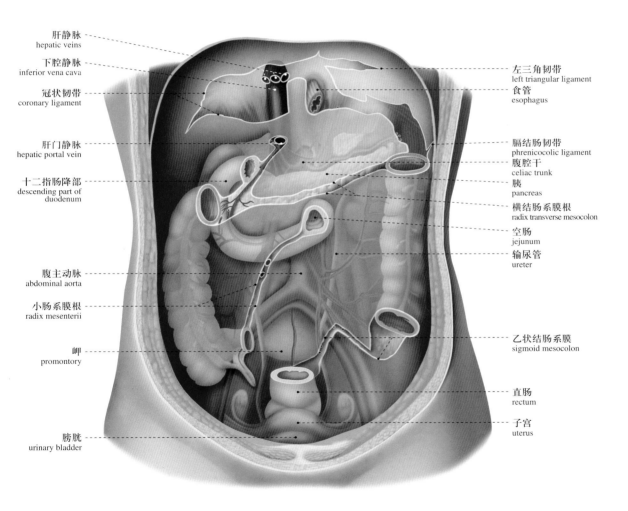

肝静脉
hepatic veins

下腔静脉
inferior vena cava

冠状韧带
coronary ligament

肝门静脉
hepatic portal vein

十二指肠降部
descending part of
duodenum

腹主动脉
abdominal aorta

小肠系膜根
radix mesenterii

岬
promontory

膀胱
urinary bladder

左三角韧带
left triangular ligament

食管
esophagus

膈结肠韧带
phrenicocolic ligament

腹腔干
celiac trunk

胰
pancreas

横结肠系膜根
radix transverse mesocolon

空肠
jejunum

输尿管
ureter

乙状结肠系膜
sigmoid mesocolon

直肠
rectum

子宫
uterus

图 365　腹后壁腹膜的配布
Arrangement of the peritoneum on the posterior abdominal wall

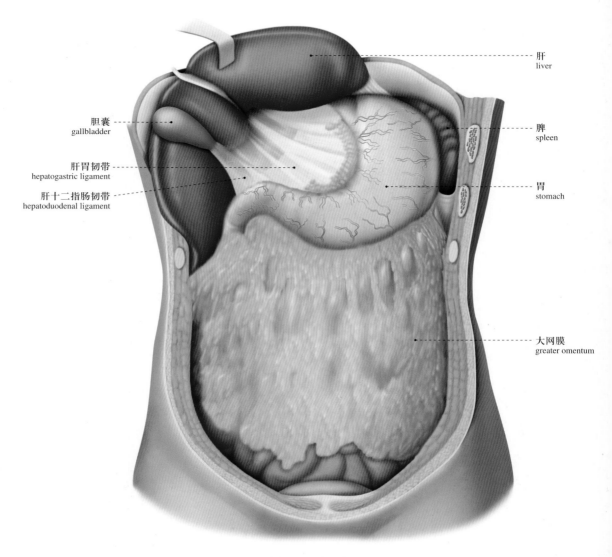

肝
liver

胆囊
gallbladder

脾
spleen

肝胃韧带
hepatogastric ligament

肝十二指肠韧带
hepatoduodenal ligament

胃
stomach

大网膜
greater omentum

图 366　网膜
Omentum

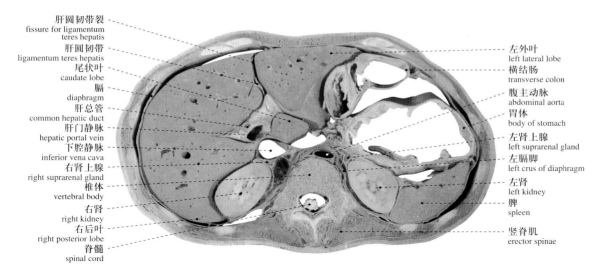

肝圆韧带裂
fissure for ligamentum teres hepatis

肝圆韧带
ligamentum teres hepatis

尾状叶
caudate lobe

膈
diaphragm

肝总管
common hepatic duct

肝门静脉
hepatic portal vein

下腔静脉
inferior vena cava

右肾上腺
right suprarenal gland

椎体
vertebral body

右肾
right kidney

右后叶
right posterior lobe

脊髓
spinal cord

左外叶
left lateral lobe

横结肠
transverse colon

腹主动脉
abdominal aorta

胃体
body of stomach

左肾上腺
left suprarenal gland

左膈脚
left crus of diaphragm

左肾
left kidney

脾
spleen

竖脊肌
erector spinae

图 367　腹部水平断面
Horizontal section of the abdomen

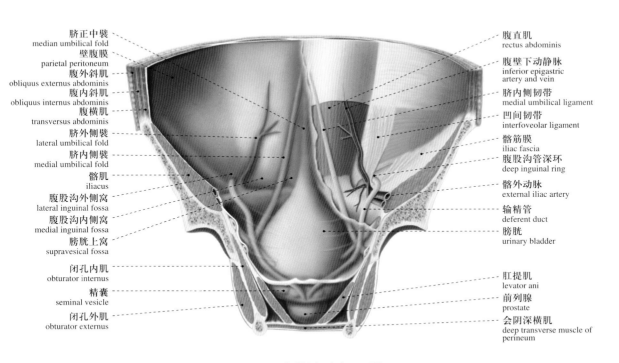

脐正中襞
median umbilical fold

壁腹膜
parietal peritoneum

腹外斜肌
obliquus externus abdominis

腹内斜肌
obliquus internus abdominis

腹横肌
transversus abdominis

脐外侧襞
lateral umbilical fold

脐内侧襞
medial umbilical fold

髂肌
iliacus

腹股沟外侧窝
lateral inguinal fossa

腹股沟内侧窝
medial inguinal fossa

膀胱上窝
supravesical fossa

闭孔内肌
obturator internus

精囊
seminal vesicle

闭孔外肌
obturator externus

腹直肌
rectus abdominis

腹壁下动静脉
inferior epigastric artery and vein

脐内侧韧带
medial umbilical ligament

凹间韧带
interfoveolar ligament

髂筋膜
iliac fascia

腹股沟管深环
deep inguinal ring

髂外动脉
external iliac artery

输精管
deferent duct

膀胱
urinary bladder

肛提肌
levator ani

前列腺
prostate

会阴深横肌
deep transverse muscle of perineum

图 368　腹前壁（内面观）
Anterior abdominal wall (interior aspect)

第一节

全身血管

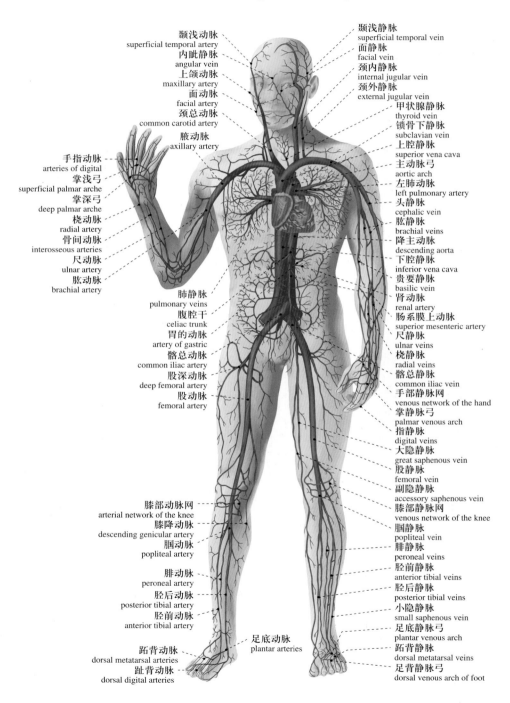

颞浅动脉
superficial temporal artery

内眦静脉
angular vein

上颌动脉
maxillary artery

面动脉
facial artery

颈总动脉
common carotid artery

腋动脉
axillary artery

手指动脉
arteries of digital

掌浅弓
superficial palmar arche

掌深弓
deep palmar arche

桡动脉
radial artery

骨间动脉
interosseous arteries

尺动脉
ulnar artery

肱动脉
brachial artery

肺静脉
pulmonary veins

腹腔干
celiac trunk

胃的动脉
artery of gastric

髂总动脉
common iliac artery

股深动脉
deep femoral artery

股动脉
femoral artery

膝部动脉网
arterial network of the knee

膝降动脉
descending genicular artery

腘动脉
popliteal artery

腓动脉
peroneal artery

胫后动脉
posterior tibial artery

胫前动脉
anterior tibial artery

跖背动脉
dorsal metatarsal arteries

趾背动脉
dorsal digital arteries

颞浅静脉
superficial temporal vein

面静脉
facial vein

颈内静脉
internal jugular vein

颈外静脉
external jugular vein

甲状腺静脉
thyroid vein

锁骨下静脉
subclavian vein

上腔静脉
superior vena cava

主动脉弓
aortic arch

左肺动脉
left pulmonary artery

头静脉
cephalic vein

肱静脉
brachial veins

降主动脉
descending aorta

下腔静脉
inferior vena cava

贵要静脉
basilic vein

肾动脉
renal artery

肠系膜上动脉
superior mesenteric artery

尺静脉
ulnar veins

桡静脉
radial veins

髂总静脉
common iliac vein

手部静脉网
venous network of the hand

掌静脉弓
palmar venous arch

指静脉
digital veins

大隐静脉
great saphenous vein

股静脉
femoral vein

副隐静脉
accessory saphenous vein

膝部静脉网
venous network of the knee

腘静脉
popliteal vein

腓静脉
peroneal veins

胫前静脉
anterior tibial veins

胫后静脉
posterior tibial veins

小隐静脉
small saphenous vein

足底静脉弓
plantar venous arch

跖背静脉
dorsal metatarsal veins

足背静脉弓
dorsal venous arch of foot

足底动脉
plantar arteries

图 369　血管分布（模式图）
Distrbution of blood vessels (diagram)

第二节

心

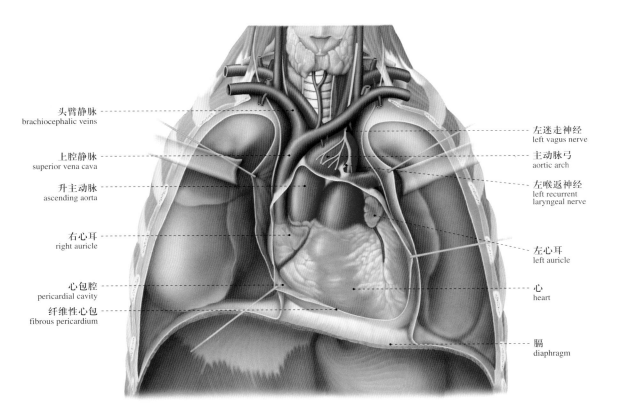

头臂静脉 brachiocephalic veins	左迷走神经 left vagus nerve
上腔静脉 superior vena cava	主动脉弓 aortic arch
升主动脉 ascending aorta	左喉返神经 left recurrent laryngeal nerve
右心耳 right auricle	左心耳 left auricle
心包腔 pericardial cavity	心 heart
纤维性心包 fibrous pericardium	膈 diaphragm

图 370　心脏的位置

Position of the heart

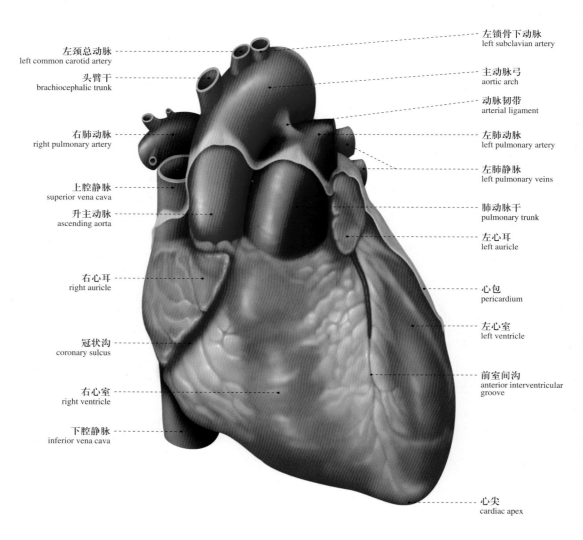

左颈总动脉
left common carotid artery

头臂干
brachiocephalic trunk

右肺动脉
right pulmonary artery

上腔静脉
superior vena cava

升主动脉
ascending aorta

右心耳
right auricle

冠状沟
coronary sulcus

右心室
right ventricle

下腔静脉
inferior vena cava

左锁骨下动脉
left subclavian artery

主动脉弓
aortic arch

动脉韧带
arterial ligament

左肺动脉
left pulmonary artery

左肺静脉
left pulmonary veins

肺动脉干
pulmonary trunk

左心耳
left auricle

心包
pericardium

左心室
left ventricle

前室间沟
anterior interventricular groove

心尖
cardiac apex

图 371 心脏的形状和结构（前面观）
Shape and structure of the heart (anterior aspect)

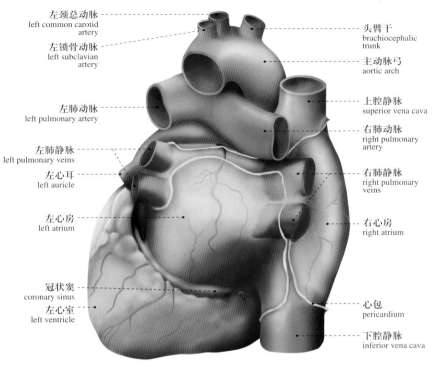

左颈总动脉
left common carotid artery

左锁骨下动脉
left subclavian artery

左肺动脉
left pulmonary artery

左肺静脉
left pulmonary veins

左心耳
left auricle

左心房
left atrium

冠状窦
coronary sinus

左心室
left ventricle

头臂干
brachiocephalic trunk

主动脉弓
aortic arch

上腔静脉
superior vena cava

右肺动脉
right pulmonary artery

右肺静脉
right pulmonary veins

右心房
right atrium

心包
pericardium

下腔静脉
inferior vena cava

图 372　心脏的形状和结构（后面观）

Shape and structure of the heart (posterior aspect)

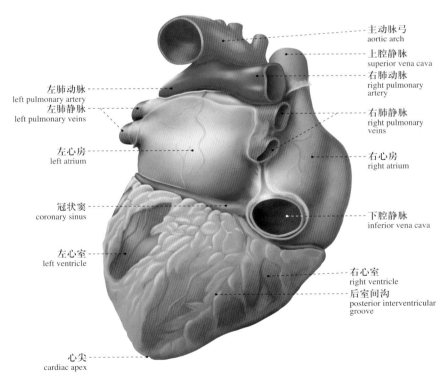

左肺动脉
left pulmonary artery

左肺静脉
left pulmonary veins

左心房
left atrium

冠状窦
coronary sinus

左心室
left ventricle

心尖
cardiac apex

主动脉弓
aortic arch

上腔静脉
superior vena cava

右肺动脉
right pulmonary artery

右肺静脉
right pulmonary veins

右心房
right atrium

下腔静脉
inferior vena cava

右心室
right ventricle

后室间沟
posterior interventricular groove

图 373　心脏的形状和结构（后下面观）

Shape and structure of the heart (posteroinferior aspect)

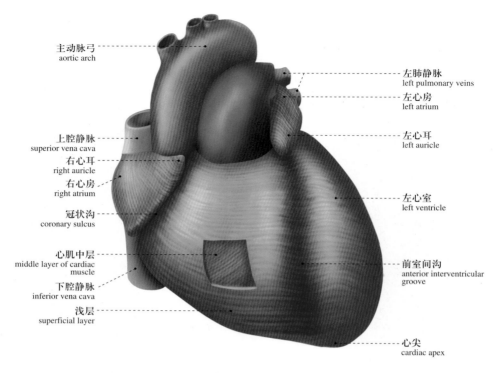

主动脉弓
aortic arch

左肺静脉
left pulmonary veins

左心房
left atrium

左心耳
left auricle

上腔静脉
superior vena cava

右心耳
right auricle

右心房
right atrium

左心室
left ventricle

冠状沟
coronary sulcus

心肌中层
middle layer of cardiac muscle

下腔静脉
inferior vena cava

前室间沟
anterior interventricular groove

浅层
superficial layer

心尖
cardiac apex

图 374　心脏的肌肉结构（前面观）
Muscular structure of the heart (anterior aspect)

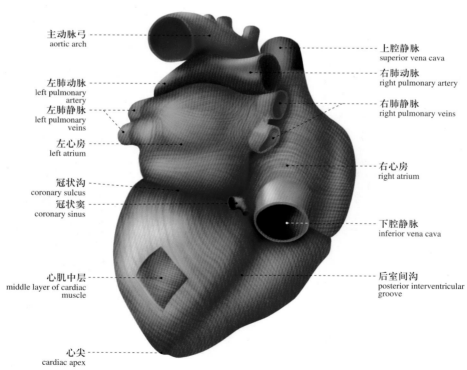

主动脉弓
aortic arch

左肺动脉
left pulmonary artery

左肺静脉
left pulmonary veins

左心房
left atrium

冠状沟
coronary sulcus

冠状窦
coronary sinus

心肌中层
middle layer of cardiac muscle

心尖
cardiac apex

上腔静脉
superior vena cava

右肺动脉
right pulmonary artery

右肺静脉
right pulmonary veins

右心房
right atrium

下腔静脉
inferior vena cava

后室间沟
posterior interventricular groove

图 375　心脏的肌肉结构（后下面观）
Muscular structure of the heart (posteroinferior aspect)

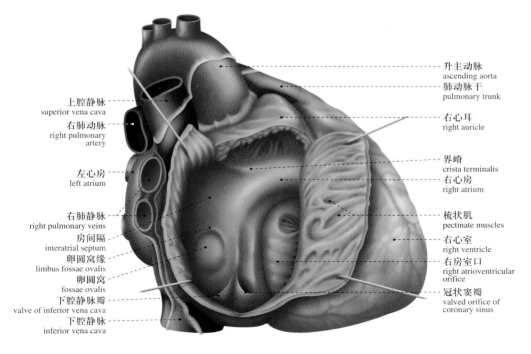

升主动脉
ascending aorta

肺动脉干
pulmonary trunk

右心耳
right auricle

界嵴
crista terminalis

右心房
right atrium

梳状肌
pectinate muscles

右心室
right ventricle

右房室口
right atrioventricular orifice

冠状窦瓣
valved orifice of coronary sinus

上腔静脉
superior vena cava

右肺动脉
right pulmonary artery

左心房
left atrium

右肺静脉
right pulmonary veins

房间隔
interatrial septum

卵圆窝缘
limbus fossae ovalis

卵圆窝
fossae ovalis

下腔静脉瓣
valve of inferior vena cava

下腔静脉
inferior vena cava

图 376　右心房的结构
Structure of right atrium

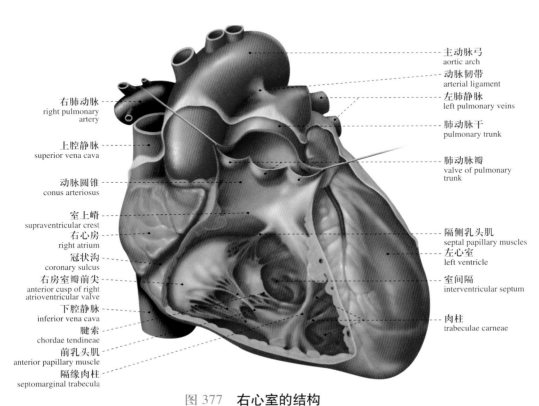

主动脉弓
aortic arch

动脉韧带
arterial ligament

左肺静脉
left pulmonary veins

肺动脉干
pulmonary trunk

肺动脉瓣
valve of pulmonary trunk

隔侧乳头肌
septal papillary muscles

左心室
left ventricle

室间隔
interventricular septum

肉柱
trabeculae carneae

右肺动脉
right pulmonary artery

上腔静脉
superior vena cava

动脉圆锥
conus arteriosus

室上嵴
supraventricular crest

右心房
right atrium

冠状沟
coronary sulcus

右房室瓣前尖
anterior cusp of right atrioventricular valve

下腔静脉
inferior vena cava

腱索
chordae tendineae

前乳头肌
anterior papillary muscle

隔缘肉柱
septomarginal trabecula

图 377　右心室的结构
Structure of right ventricular

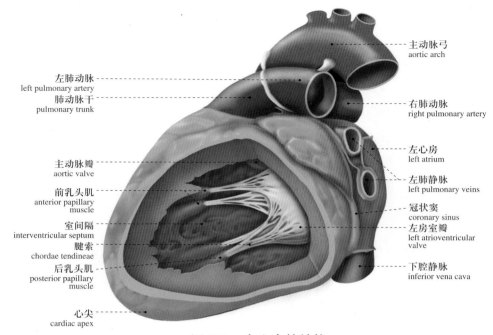

左肺动脉
left pulmonary artery

肺动脉干
pulmonary trunk

主动脉瓣
aortic valve

前乳头肌
anterior papillary muscle

室间隔
interventricular septum

腱索
chordae tendineae

后乳头肌
posterior papillary muscle

心尖
cardiac apex

主动脉弓
aortic arch

右肺动脉
right pulmonary artery

左心房
left atrium

左肺静脉
left pulmonary veins

冠状窦
coronary sinus

左房室瓣
left atrioventricular valve

下腔静脉
inferior vena cava

图 378　左心室的结构
Structure of left ventricular

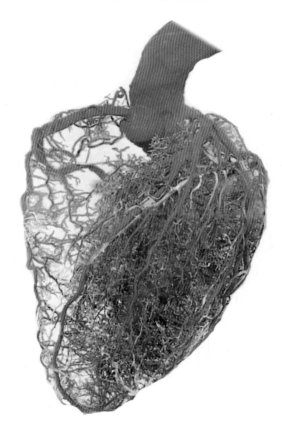

图 379　心脏血管铸型
Cast of the heart blood vessels

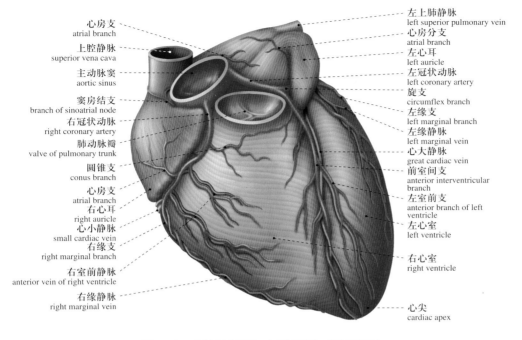

心房支
atrial branch

上腔静脉
superior vena cava

主动脉窦
aortic sinus

窦房结支
branch of sinoatrial node

右冠状动脉
right coronary artery

肺动脉瓣
valve of pulmonary trunk

圆锥支
conus branch

心房支
atrial branch

右心耳
right auricle

心小静脉
small cardiac vein

右缘支
right marginal branch

右室前静脉
anterior vein of right ventricle

右缘静脉
right marginal vein

左上肺静脉
left superior pulmonary vein

心房分支
atrial branch

左心耳
left auricle

左冠状动脉
left coronary artery

旋支
circumflex branch

左缘支
left marginal branch

左缘静脉
left marginal vein

心大静脉
great cardiac vein

前室间支
anterior interventricular branch

左室前支
anterior branch of left ventricle

左心室
left ventricle

右心室
right ventricle

心尖
cardiac apex

图 380　冠状动脉和心脏静脉（前面观）
Coronary arteries and cardiac veins (anterior aspect)

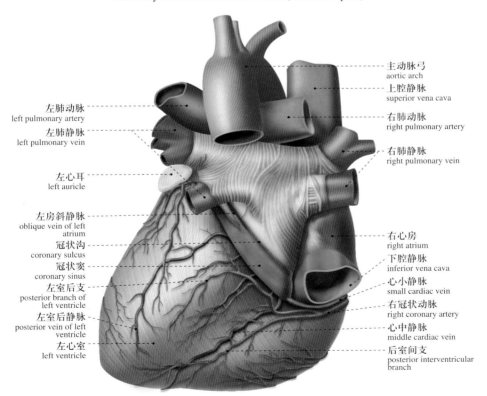

左肺动脉
left pulmonary artery

左肺静脉
left pulmonary vein

左心耳
left auricle

左房斜静脉
oblique vein of left atrium

冠状沟
coronary sulcus

冠状窦
coronary sinus

左室后支
posterior branch of left ventricle

左室后静脉
posterior vein of left ventricle

左心室
left ventricle

主动脉弓
aortic arch

上腔静脉
superior vena cava

右肺动脉
right pulmonary artery

右肺静脉
right pulmonary vein

右心房
right atrium

下腔静脉
inferior vena cava

心小静脉
small cardiac vein

右冠状动脉
right coronary artery

心中静脉
middle cardiac vein

后室间支
posterior interventricular branch

图 381　冠状动脉和心脏静脉（后面观）
Coronary arteries and cardiac veins (poster aspect)

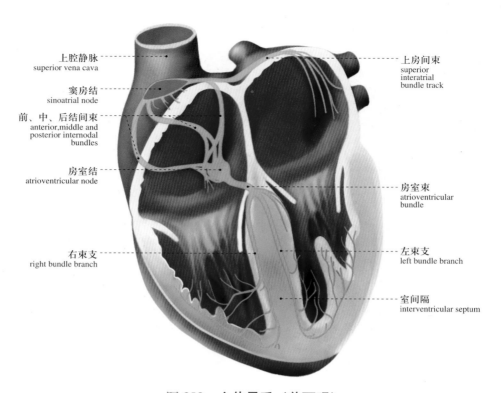

上腔静脉
superior vena cava

窦房结
sinoatrial node

前、中、后结间束
anterior,middle and
posterior internodal
bundles

房室结
atrioventricular node

右束支
right bundle branch

上房间束
superior
interatrial
bundle track

房室束
atrioventricular
bundle

左束支
left bundle branch

室间隔
interventricular septum

图 382　心传导系（前面观）
Conduction system of the heart (anterior aspect)

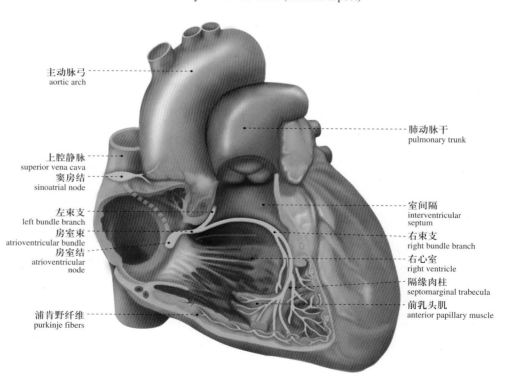

主动脉弓
aortic arch

上腔静脉
superior vena cava

窦房结
sinoatrial node

左束支
left bundle branch

房室束
atrioventricular bundle

房室结
atrioventricular
node

浦肯野纤维
purkinje fibers

肺动脉干
pulmonary trunk

室间隔
interventricular
septum

右束支
right bundle branch

右心室
right ventricle

隔缘肉柱
septomarginal trabecula

前乳头肌
anterior papillary muscle

图 383　心传导系（右侧面观）
Conduction system of the heart (right lateral aspect)

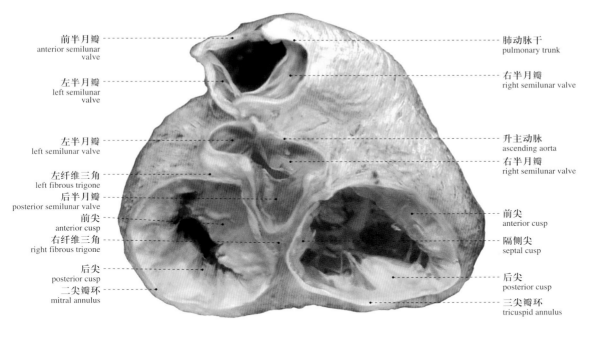

前半月瓣
anterior semilunar
valve

左半月瓣
left semilunar
valve

左半月瓣
left semilunar
valve

左纤维三角
left fibrous trigone

后半月瓣
posterior semilunar valve

前尖
anterior cusp

右纤维三角
right fibrous trigone

后尖
posterior cusp

二尖瓣环
mitral annulus

肺动脉干
pulmonary trunk

右半月瓣
right semilunar valve

升主动脉
ascending aorta

右半月瓣
right semilunar valve

前尖
anterior cusp

隔侧尖
septal cusp

后尖
posterior cusp

三尖瓣环
tricuspid annulus

图 384　心的瓣膜
Valves of the heart

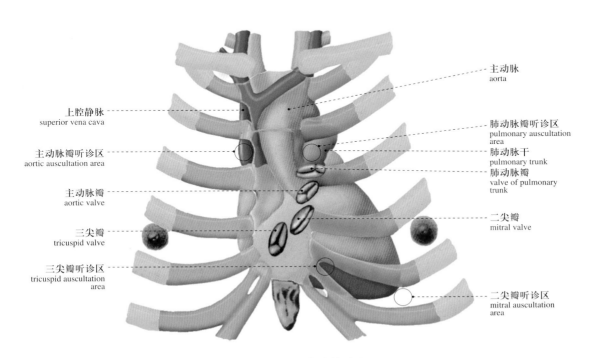

上腔静脉
superior vena cava

主动脉瓣听诊区
aortic auscultation area

主动脉瓣
aortic valve

三尖瓣
tricuspid valve

三尖瓣听诊区
tricuspid auscultation
area

主动脉
aorta

肺动脉瓣听诊区
pulmonary auscultation
area

肺动脉干
pulmonary trunk

肺动脉瓣
valve of pulmonary
trunk

二尖瓣
mitral valve

二尖瓣听诊区
mitral auscultation
area

图 385　心瓣膜的体表投影
Surface projection of the valves of the heart

第三节

动 脉

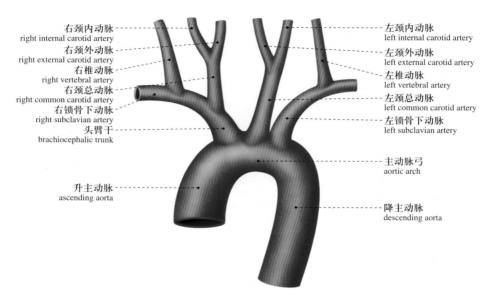

右颈内动脉
right internal carotid artery

右颈外动脉
right external carotid artery

右椎动脉
right vertebral artery

右颈总动脉
right common carotid artery

右锁骨下动脉
right subclavian artery

头臂干
brachiocephalic trunk

升主动脉
ascending aorta

左颈内动脉
left internal carotid artery

左颈外动脉
left external carotid artery

左椎动脉
left vertebral artery

左颈总动脉
left common carotid artery

左锁骨下动脉
left subclavian artery

主动脉弓
aortic arch

降主动脉
descending aorta

图 386　主动脉弓及其分支
Aortic arch and its branches

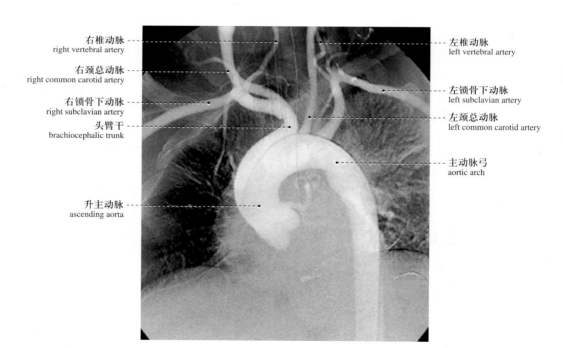

右椎动脉
right vertebral artery

右颈总动脉
right common carotid artery

右锁骨下动脉
right subclavian artery

头臂干
brachiocephalic trunk

升主动脉
ascending aorta

左椎动脉
left vertebral artery

左锁骨下动脉
left subclavian artery

左颈总动脉
left common carotid artery

主动脉弓
aortic arch

图 387　主动脉弓数字减影血管造影
DSA of the aortic arch

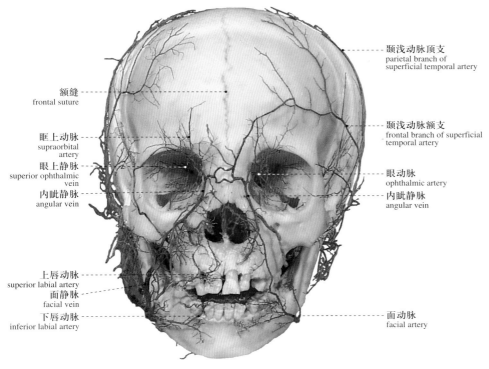

额缝
frontal suture

眶上动脉
supraorbital
artery

眼上静脉
superior ophthalmic
vein

内眦静脉
angular vein

上唇动脉
superior labial artery

面静脉
facial vein

下唇动脉
inferior labial artery

颞浅动脉顶支
parietal branch of
superficial temporal artery

颞浅动脉额支
frontal branch of superficial
temporal artery

眼动脉
ophthalmic artery

内眦静脉
angular vein

面动脉
facial artery

图 388　头部血管（前面观）
Blood vessels of the head (anterior aspect)

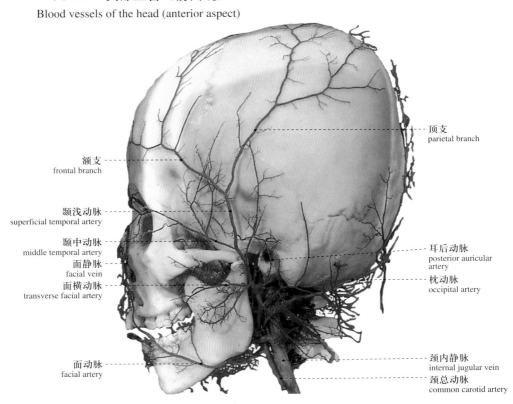

额支
frontal branch

颞浅动脉
superficial temporal artery

颞中动脉
middle temporal artery

面静脉
facial vein

面横动脉
transverse facial artery

面动脉
facial artery

顶支
parietal branch

耳后动脉
posterior auricular
artery

枕动脉
occipital artery

颈内静脉
internal jugular vein

颈总动脉
common carotid artery

图 389　头部血管（侧面观）
Blood vessels of the head (lateral aspect)

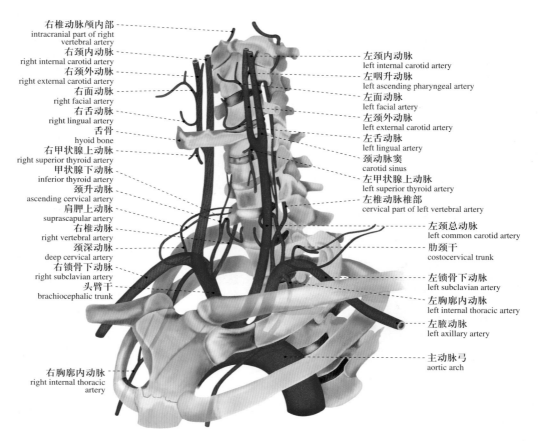

右椎动脉颅内部
intracranial part of right vertebral artery
右颈内动脉
right internal carotid artery
右颈外动脉
right external carotid artery
右面动脉
right facial artery
右舌动脉
right lingual artery
舌骨
hyoid bone
右甲状腺上动脉
right superior thyroid artery
甲状腺下动脉
inferior thyroid artery
颈升动脉
ascending cervical artery
肩胛上动脉
suprascapular artery
右椎动脉
right vertebral artery
颈深动脉
deep cervical artery
右锁骨下动脉
right subclavian artery
头臂干
brachiocephalic trunk

左颈内动脉
left internal carotid artery
左咽升动脉
left ascending pharyngeal artery
左面动脉
left facial artery
左颈外动脉
left external carotid artery
左舌动脉
left lingual artery
颈动脉窦
carotid sinus
左甲状腺上动脉
left superior thyroid artery
左椎动脉椎部
cervical part of left vertebral artery
左颈总动脉
left common carotid artery
肋颈干
costocervical trunk
左锁骨下动脉
left subclavian artery
左胸廓内动脉
left internal thoracic artery
左腋动脉
left axillary artery
主动脉弓
aortic arch

右胸廓内动脉
right internal thoracic artery

图 390　颈部动脉（左前斜位观）
Arteries of the neck (left anterior oblique aspect)

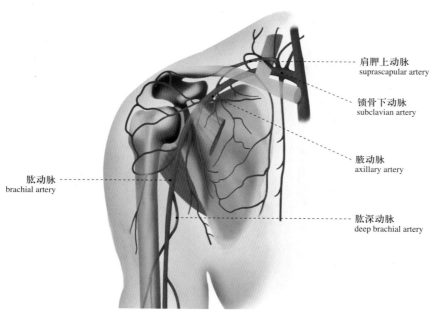

肩胛上动脉
suprascapular artery
锁骨下动脉
subclavian artery
腋动脉
axillary artery
肱动脉
brachial artery
肱深动脉
deep brachial artery

图 391　肩部动脉（前面观）
Shoulder arteries (anterior aspect)

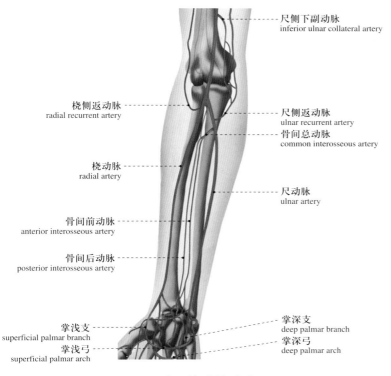

尺侧下副动脉
inferior ulnar collateral artery

桡侧返动脉
radial recurrent artery

尺侧返动脉
ulnar recurrent artery

骨间总动脉
common interosseous artery

桡动脉
radial artery

尺动脉
ulnar artery

骨间前动脉
anterior interosseous artery

骨间后动脉
posterior interosseous artery

掌浅支
superficial palmar branch

掌浅弓
superficial palmar arch

掌深支
deep palmar branch

掌深弓
deep palmar arch

图 392　肘及前臂的动脉
Arteries of the elbow and forearm

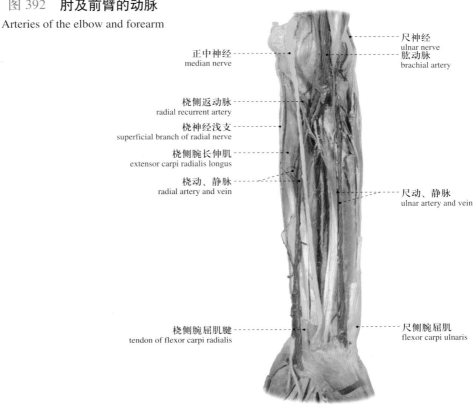

正中神经
median nerve

尺神经
ulnar nerve

肱动脉
brachial artery

桡侧返动脉
radial recurrent artery

桡神经浅支
superficial branch of radial nerve

桡侧腕长伸肌
extensor carpi radialis longus

桡动、静脉
radial artery and vein

尺动、静脉
ulnar artery and vein

桡侧腕屈肌腱
tendon of flexor carpi radialis

尺侧腕屈肌
flexor carpi ulnaris

图 393　前臂前区血管和神经
Blood vessels and nerves of the anterior antebrachial region

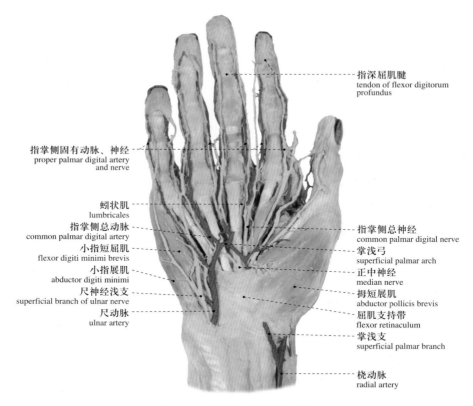

指深屈肌腱
tendon of flexor digitorum profundus

指掌侧固有动脉、神经
proper palmar digital artery and nerve

蚓状肌
lumbricales

指掌侧总动脉
common palmar digital artery

小指短屈肌
flexor digiti minimi brevis

小指展肌
abductor digiti minimi

尺神经浅支
superficial branch of ulnar nerve

尺动脉
ulnar artery

指掌侧总神经
common palmar digital nerve

掌浅弓
superficial palmar arch

正中神经
median nerve

拇短展肌
abductor pollicis brevis

屈肌支持带
flexor retinaculum

掌浅支
superficial palmar branch

桡动脉
radial artery

图 394　手掌面血管和神经

Blood vessels and nerves of the palmar aspect of the hand

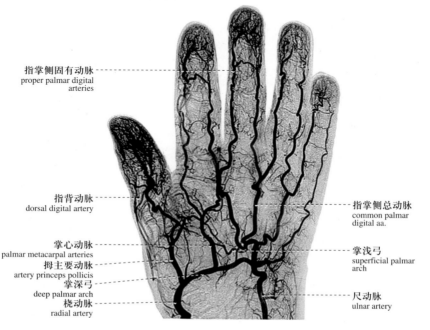

指掌侧固有动脉
proper palmar digital arteries

指背动脉
dorsal digital artery

掌心动脉
palmar metacarpal arteries

拇主要动脉
artery princeps pollicis

掌深弓
deep palmar arch

桡动脉
radial artery

指掌侧总动脉
common palmar digital aa.

掌浅弓
superficial palmar arch

尺动脉
ulnar artery

图 395　手部动脉数字减影血管造影

DSA of the hand arteries

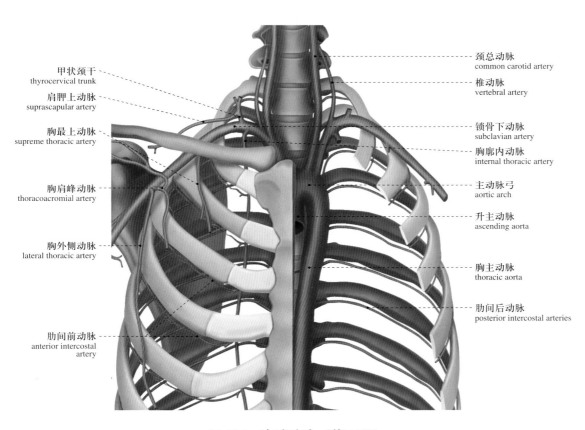

甲状颈干
thyrocervical trunk

肩胛上动脉
suprascapular artery

胸最上动脉
supreme thoracic artery

胸肩峰动脉
thoracoacromial artery

胸外侧动脉
lateral thoracic artery

肋间前动脉
anterior intercostal
artery

颈总动脉
common carotid artery

椎动脉
vertebral artery

锁骨下动脉
subclavian artery

胸廓内动脉
internal thoracic artery

主动脉弓
aortic arch

升主动脉
ascending aorta

胸主动脉
thoracic aorta

肋间后动脉
posterior intercostal arteries

图 396 胸壁动脉 （前面观）
Arteries of the chest wall (anterior aspect)

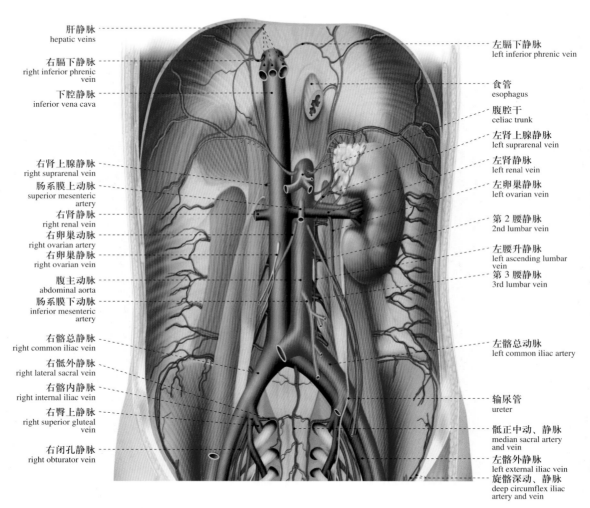

肝静脉
hepatic veins

右膈下静脉
right inferior phrenic vein

下腔静脉
inferior vena cava

右肾上腺静脉
right suprarenal vein

肠系膜上动脉
superior mesenteric artery

右肾静脉
right renal vein

右卵巢动脉
right ovarian artery

右卵巢静脉
right ovarian vein

腹主动脉
abdominal aorta

肠系膜下动脉
inferior mesenteric artery

右髂总静脉
right common iliac vein

右骶外静脉
right lateral sacral vein

右髂内静脉
right internal iliac vein

右臀上静脉
right superior gluteal vein

右闭孔静脉
right obturator vein

左膈下静脉
left inferior phrenic vein

食管
esophagus

腹腔干
celiac trunk

左肾上腺静脉
left suprarenal vein

左肾静脉
left renal vein

左卵巢静脉
left ovarian vein

第 2 腰静脉
2nd lumbar vein

左腰升静脉
left ascending lumbar vein

第 3 腰静脉
3rd lumbar vein

左髂总动脉
left common iliac artery

输尿管
ureter

骶正中动、静脉
median sacral artery and vein

左髂外静脉
left external iliac vein

旋髂深动、静脉
deep circumflex iliac artery and vein

图 397　腹后壁的血管（女）

Blood vessels of the posterior abdominal wall (female)

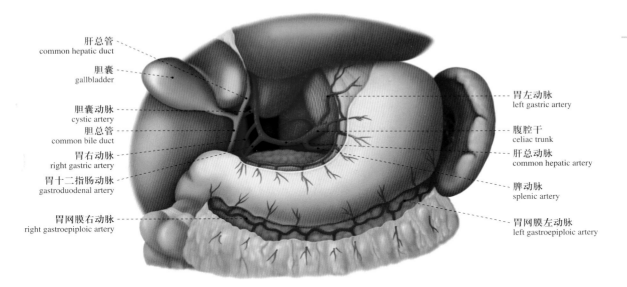

肝总管
common hepatic duct

胆囊
gallbladder

胆囊动脉
cystic artery

胆总管
common bile duct

胃右动脉
right gastric artery

胃十二指肠动脉
gastroduodenal artery

胃网膜右动脉
right gastroepiploic artery

胃左动脉
left gastric artery

腹腔干
celiac trunk

肝总动脉
common hepatic artery

脾动脉
splenic artery

胃网膜左动脉
left gastroepiploic artery

图 398　腹腔干及其分支（胃前面）

Celiac trunk and its branches (front of the stomach)

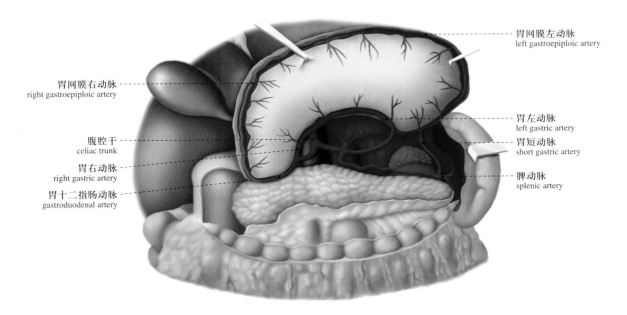

胃网膜右动脉
right gastroepiploic artery

腹腔干
celiac trunk

胃右动脉
right gastric artery

胃十二指肠动脉
gastroduodenal artery

胃网膜左动脉
left gastroepiploic artery

胃左动脉
left gastric artery

胃短动脉
short gastric artery

脾动脉
splenic artery

图 399　腹腔干及其分支（胃后面）

Celiac trunk and its branches (behind the stomach)

215

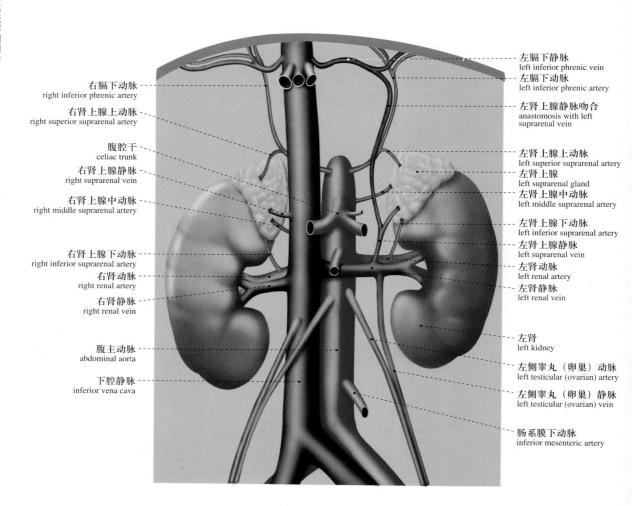

右膈下动脉
right inferior phrenic artery

右肾上腺上动脉
right superior suprarenal artery

腹腔干
celiac trunk

右肾上腺静脉
right suprarenal vein

右肾上腺中动脉
right middle suprarenal artery

右肾上腺下动脉
right inferior suprarenal artery

右肾动脉
right renal artery

右肾静脉
right renal vein

腹主动脉
abdominal aorta

下腔静脉
inferior vena cava

左膈下静脉
left inferior phrenic vein

左膈下动脉
left inferior phrenic artery

左肾上腺静脉吻合
anastomosis with left suprarenal vein

左肾上腺上动脉
left superior suprarenal artery

左肾上腺
left suprarenal gland

左肾上腺中动脉
left middle suprarenal artery

左肾上腺下动脉
left inferior suprarenal artery

左肾上腺静脉
left suprarenal vein

左肾动脉
left renal artery

左肾静脉
left renal vein

左肾
left kidney

左侧睾丸（卵巢）动脉
left testicular (ovarian) artery

左侧睾丸（卵巢）静脉
left testicular (ovarian) vein

肠系膜下动脉
inferior mesenteric artery

图 400　肾及肾上腺的动、静脉

Arteries and veins of the kidneys and suprarenal glands

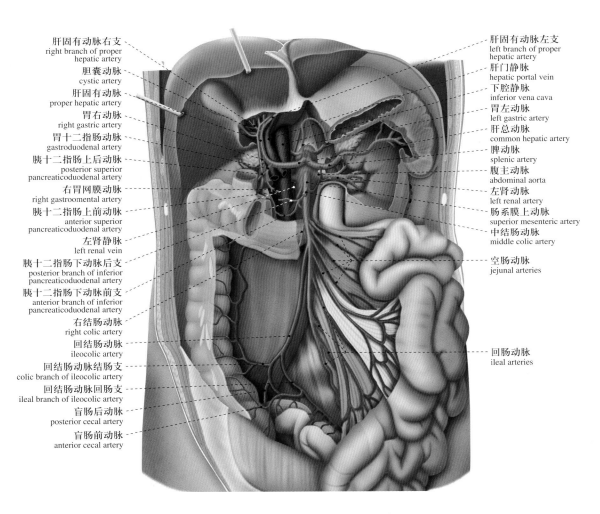

肝固有动脉右支
right branch of proper hepatic artery

胆囊动脉
cystic artery

肝固有动脉
proper hepatic artery

胃右动脉
right gastric artery

胃十二指肠动脉
gastroduodenal artery

胰十二指肠上后动脉
posterior superior pancreaticoduodenal artery

右胃网膜动脉
right gastroomental artery

胰十二指肠上前动脉
anterior superior pancreaticoduodenal artery

左肾静脉
left renal vein

胰十二指肠下动脉后支
posterior branch of inferior pancreaticoduodenal artery

胰十二指肠下动脉前支
anterior branch of inferior pancreaticoduodenal artery

右结肠动脉
right colic artery

回结肠动脉
ileocolic artery

回结肠动脉结肠支
colic branch of ileocolic artery

回结肠动脉回肠支
ileal branch of ileocolic artery

盲肠后动脉
posterior cecal artery

盲肠前动脉
anterior cecal artery

肝固有动脉左支
left branch of proper hepatic artery

肝门静脉
hepatic portal vein

下腔静脉
inferior vena cava

胃左动脉
left gastric artery

肝总动脉
common hepatic artery

脾动脉
splenic artery

腹主动脉
abdominal aorta

左肾动脉
left renal artery

肠系膜上动脉
superior mesenteric artery

中结肠动脉
middle colic artery

空肠动脉
jejunal arteries

回肠动脉
ileal arteries

图 401　肠系膜上动脉及其分支
Superior mesenteric artery and its branches

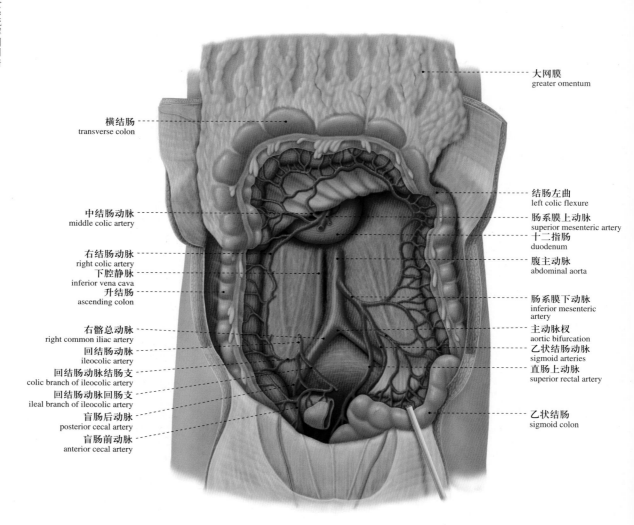

横结肠
transverse colon

中结肠动脉
middle colic artery

右结肠动脉
right colic artery

下腔静脉
inferior vena cava

升结肠
ascending colon

右髂总动脉
right common iliac artery

回结肠动脉
ileocolic artery

回结肠动脉结肠支
colic branch of ileocolic artery

回结肠动脉回肠支
ileal branch of ileocolic artery

盲肠后动脉
posterior cecal artery

盲肠前动脉
anterior cecal artery

大网膜
greater omentum

结肠左曲
left colic flexure

肠系膜上动脉
superior mesenteric artery

十二指肠
duodenum

腹主动脉
abdominal aorta

肠系膜下动脉
inferior mesenteric artery

主动脉杈
aortic bifurcation

乙状结肠动脉
sigmoid arteries

直肠上动脉
superior rectal artery

乙状结肠
sigmoid colon

图 402　肠系膜下动脉及其分支

Inferior mesenteric artery and its branches

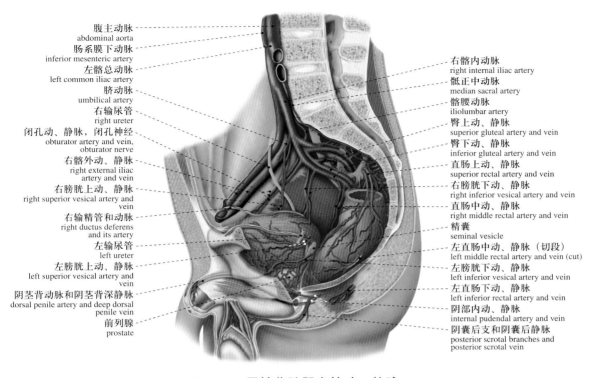

腹主动脉
abdominal aorta

肠系膜下动脉
inferior mesenteric artery

左髂总动脉
left common iliac artery

脐动脉
umbilical artery

右输尿管
right ureter

闭孔动、静脉，闭孔神经
obturator artery and vein,
obturator nerve

右髂外动、静脉
right external iliac
artery and vein

右膀胱上动、静脉
right superior vesical artery and
vein

右输精管和动脉
right ductus deferens
and its artery

左输尿管
left ureter

左膀胱上动、静脉
left superior vesical artery and
vein

阴茎背动脉和阴茎背深静脉
dorsal penile artery and deep dorsal
penile vein

前列腺
prostate

右髂内动脉
right internal iliac artery

骶正中动脉
median sacral artery

髂腰动脉
iliolumbar artery

臀上动、静脉
superior gluteal artery and vein

臀下动、静脉
inferior gluteal artery and vein

直肠上动、静脉
superior rectal artery and vein

右膀胱下动、静脉
right inferior vesical artery and vein

直肠中动、静脉
right middle rectal artery and vein

精囊
seminal vesicle

左直肠中动、静脉（切段）
left middle rectal artery and vein (cut)

左膀胱下动、静脉
left inferior vesical artery and vein

左直肠下动、静脉
left inferior rectal artery and vein

阴部内动、静脉
internal pudendal artery and vein

阴囊后支和阴囊后静脉
posterior scrotal branches and
posterior scrotal vein

图 403　男性盆腔器官的动、静脉

Arteries and veins of the pelvic organs in the male

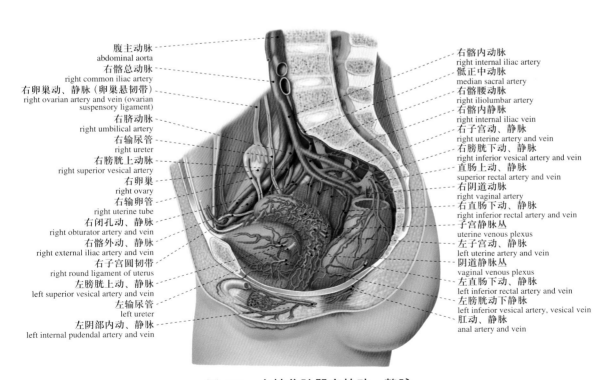

腹主动脉
abdominal aorta

右髂总动脉
right common iliac artery

右卵巢动、静脉（卵巢悬韧带）
right ovarian artery and vein (ovarian
suspensory ligament)

右脐动脉
right umbilical artery

右输尿管
right ureter

右膀胱上动脉
right superior vesical artery

右卵巢
right ovary

右输卵管
right uterine tube

右闭孔动、静脉
right obturator artery and vein

右髂外动、静脉
right external iliac artery and vein

右子宫圆韧带
right round ligament of uterus

左膀胱上动、静脉
left superior vesical artery and vein

左输尿管
left ureter

左阴部内动、静脉
left internal pudendal artery and vein

右髂内动脉
right internal iliac artery

骶正中动脉
median sacral artery

右髂腰动脉
right iliolumbar artery

右髂内静脉
right internal iliac vein

右子宫动、静脉
right uterine artery and vein

右膀胱下动、静脉
right inferior vesical artery and vein

直肠上动、静脉
superior rectal artery and vein

右阴道动脉
right vaginal artery

右直肠下动、静脉
right inferior rectal artery and vein

子宫静脉丛
uterine venous plexus

左子宫动、静脉
left uterine artery and vein

阴道静脉丛
vaginal venous plexus

左直肠下动、静脉
left inferior rectal artery and vein

左膀胱下静脉
left inferior vesical artery, vesical vein

肛动、静脉
anal artery and vein

图 404　女性盆腔器官的动、静脉

Arteries and veins of the pelvic organs in the female

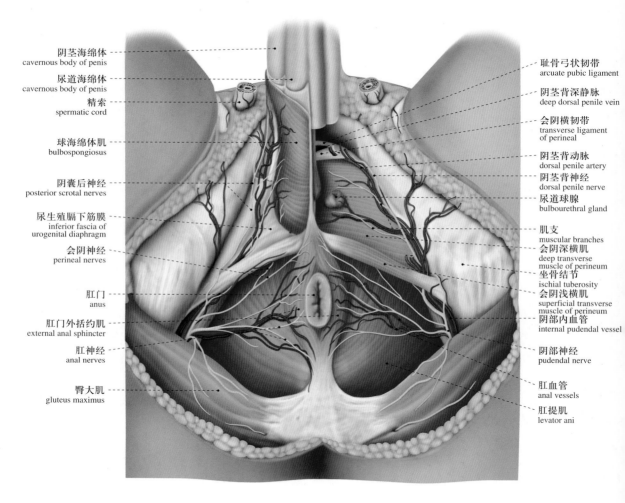

阴茎海绵体
cavernous body of penis

尿道海绵体
cavernous body of penis

精索
spermatic cord

球海绵体肌
bulbospongiosus

阴囊后神经
posterior scrotal nerves

尿生殖膈下筋膜
inferior fascia of
urogenital diaphragm

会阴神经
perineal nerves

肛门
anus

肛门外括约肌
external anal sphincter

肛神经
anal nerves

臀大肌
gluteus maximus

耻骨弓状韧带
arcuate pubic ligament

阴茎背深静脉
deep dorsal penile vein

会阴横韧带
transverse ligament
of perineal

阴茎背动脉
dorsal penile artery

阴茎背神经
dorsal penile nerve

尿道球腺
bulbourethral gland

肌支
muscular branches

会阴深横肌
deep transverse
muscle of perineum

坐骨结节
ischial tuberosity

会阴浅横肌
superficial transverse
muscle of perineum

阴部内血管
internal pudendal vessel

阴部神经
pudendal nerve

肛血管
anal vessels

肛提肌
levator ani

图 405　男性会阴部血管和神经
Blood vessels and nerves of the male perineum

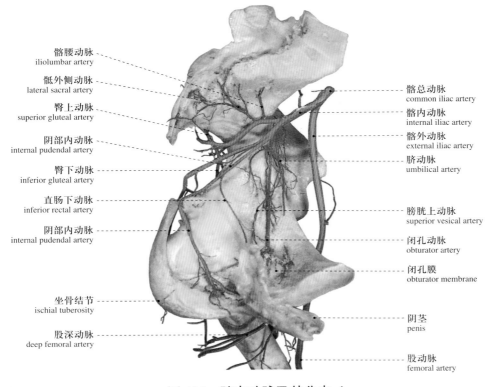

髂腰动脉
iliolumbar artery

骶外侧动脉
lateral sacral artery

臀上动脉
superior gluteal artery

阴部内动脉
internal pudendal artery

臀下动脉
inferior gluteal artery

直肠下动脉
inferior rectal artery

阴部内动脉
internal pudendal artery

坐骨结节
ischial tuberosity

股深动脉
deep femoral artery

髂总动脉
common iliac artery

髂内动脉
internal iliac artery

髂外动脉
external iliac artery

脐动脉
umbilical artery

膀胱上动脉
superior vesical artery

闭孔动脉
obturator artery

闭孔膜
obturator membrane

阴茎
penis

股动脉
femoral artery

图 406　髂内动脉及其分支 1
Internal iliac artery and its branches 1

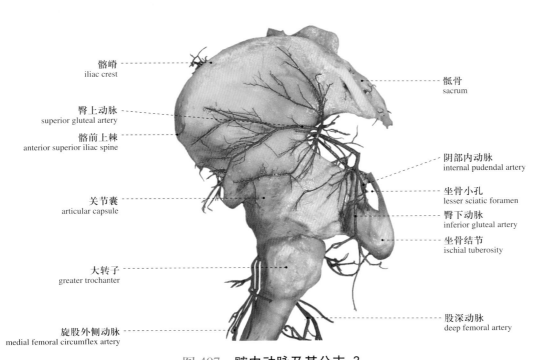

髂嵴
iliac crest

臀上动脉
superior gluteal artery

髂前上棘
anterior superior iliac spine

关节囊
articular capsule

大转子
greater trochanter

旋股外侧动脉
medial femoral circumflex artery

骶骨
sacrum

阴部内动脉
internal pudendal artery

坐骨小孔
lesser sciatic foramen

臀下动脉
inferior gluteal artery

坐骨结节
ischial tuberosity

股深动脉
deep femoral artery

图 407　髂内动脉及其分支 2
Internal iliac artery and its branches 2

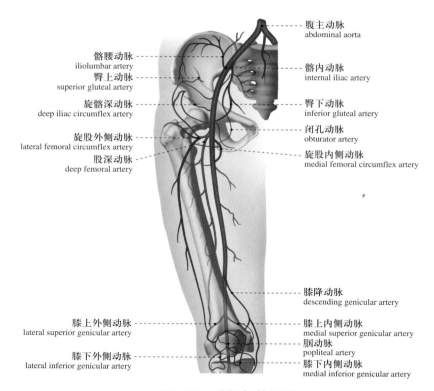

腹主动脉
abdominal aorta

髂腰动脉
iliolumbar artery

臀上动脉
superior gluteal artery

旋髂深动脉
deep iliac circumflex artery

旋股外侧动脉
lateral femoral circumflex artery

股深动脉
deep femoral artery

髂内动脉
internal iliac artery

臀下动脉
inferior gluteal artery

闭孔动脉
obturator artery

旋股内侧动脉
medial femoral circumflex artery

膝降动脉
descending genicular artery

膝上外侧动脉
lateral superior genicular artery

膝下外侧动脉
lateral inferior genicular artery

膝上内侧动脉
medial superior genicular artery

腘动脉
popliteal artery

膝下内侧动脉
medial inferior genicular artery

图 408　髋股部的动脉
Arteries of the hip and thigh

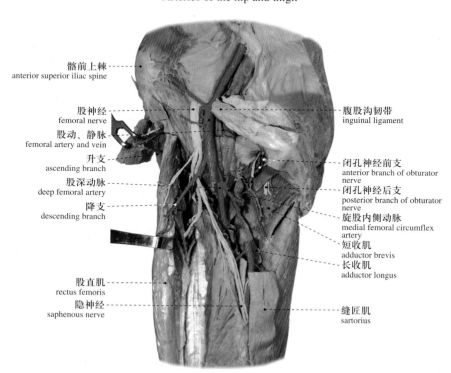

髂前上棘
anterior superior iliac spine

股神经
femoral nerve

股动、静脉
femoral artery and vein

升支
ascending branch

股深动脉
deep femoral artery

降支
descending branch

股直肌
rectus femoris

隐神经
saphenous nerve

腹股沟韧带
inguinal ligament

闭孔神经前支
anterior branch of obturator nerve

闭孔神经后支
posterior branch of obturator nerve

旋股内侧动脉
medial femoral circumflex artery

短收肌
adductor brevis

长收肌
adductor longus

缝匠肌
sartorius

图 409　闭孔区血管和神经
Blood vessels and nerves of the obturator region

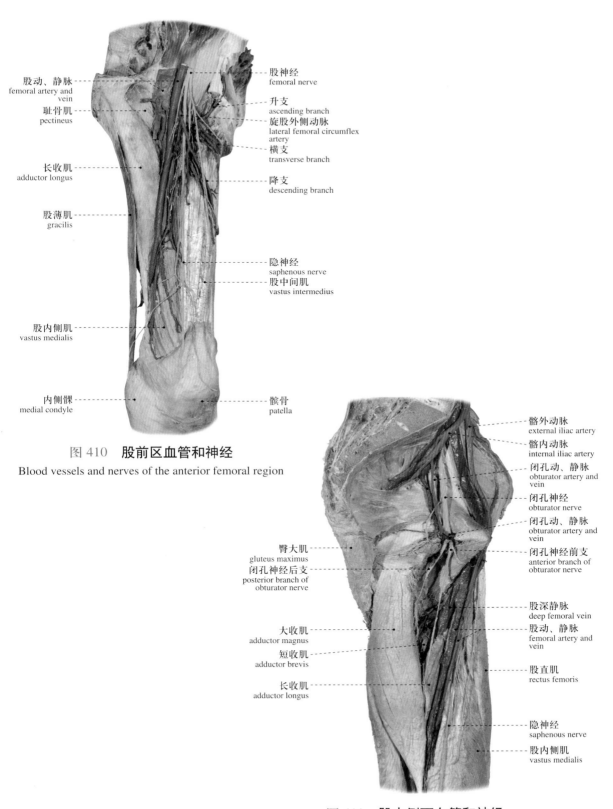

股动、静脉
femoral artery and vein

耻骨肌
pectineus

长收肌
adductor longus

股薄肌
gracilis

股内侧肌
vastus medialis

内侧髁
medial condyle

股神经
femoral nerve

升支
ascending branch

旋股外侧动脉
lateral femoral circumflex artery

横支
transverse branch

降支
descending branch

隐神经
saphenous nerve

股中间肌
vastus intermedius

髌骨
patella

图 410　股前区血管和神经

Blood vessels and nerves of the anterior femoral region

臀大肌
gluteus maximus

闭孔神经后支
posterior branch of obturator nerve

大收肌
adductor magnus

短收肌
adductor brevis

长收肌
adductor longus

髂外动脉
external iliac artery

髂内动脉
internal iliac artery

闭孔、静脉
obturator artery and vein

闭孔神经
obturator nerve

闭孔动、静脉
obturator artery and vein

闭孔神经前支
anterior branch of obturator nerve

股深静脉
deep femoral vein

股动、静脉
femoral artery and vein

股直肌
rectus femoris

隐神经
saphenous nerve

股内侧肌
vastus medialis

图 411　股内侧面血管和神经

Blood vessels and nerves of the medial femoral aspect

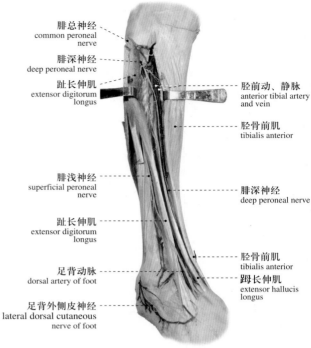

腓总神经
common peroneal nerve

腓深神经
deep peroneal nerve

趾长伸肌
extensor digitorum longus

胫前动、静脉
anterior tibial artery and vein

胫骨前肌
tibialis anterior

腓浅神经
superficial peroneal nerve

腓深神经
deep peroneal nerve

趾长伸肌
extensor digitorum longus

胫骨前肌
tibialis anterior

足背动脉
dorsal artery of foot

𧿹长伸肌
extensor hallucis longus

足背外侧皮神经
lateral dorsal cutaneous nerve of foot

图 413　小腿前区血管和神经

Blood vessels and nerves of the anterior crural region

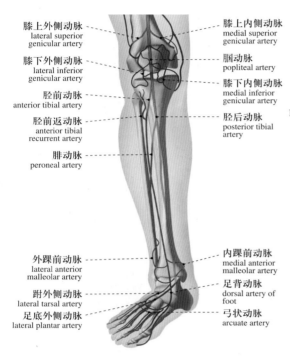

膝上外侧动脉
lateral superior genicular artery

膝上内侧动脉
medial superior genicular artery

膝下外侧动脉
lateral inferior genicular artery

腘动脉
popliteal artery

膝下内侧动脉
medial inferior genicular artery

胫前动脉
anterior tibial artery

胫前返动脉
anterior tibial recurrent artery

胫后动脉
posterior tibial artery

腓动脉
peroneal artery

外踝前动脉
lateral anterior malleolar artery

内踝前动脉
medial anterior malleolar artery

跗外侧动脉
lateral tarsal artery

足背动脉
dorsal artery of foot

足底外侧动脉
lateral plantar artery

弓状动脉
arcuate artery

图 412　膝及小腿的动脉

Arteries of the knee and leg

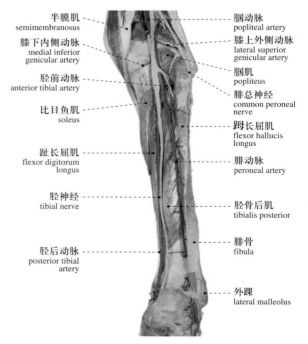

半膜肌
semimembranosus

腘动脉
popliteal artery

膝下内侧动脉
medial inferior genicular artery

膝上外侧动脉
lateral superior genicular artery

胫前动脉
anterior tibial artery

腘肌
popliteus

比目鱼肌
soleus

腓总神经
common peroneal nerve

趾长屈肌
flexor digitorum longus

𧿹长屈肌
flexor hallucis longus

胫神经
tibial nerve

腓动脉
peroneal artery

胫骨后肌
tibialis posterior

腓骨
fibula

胫后动脉
posterior tibial artery

外踝
lateral malleolus

图 414　小腿后区血管和神经

Blood vessels and nerves of the posterior crural region

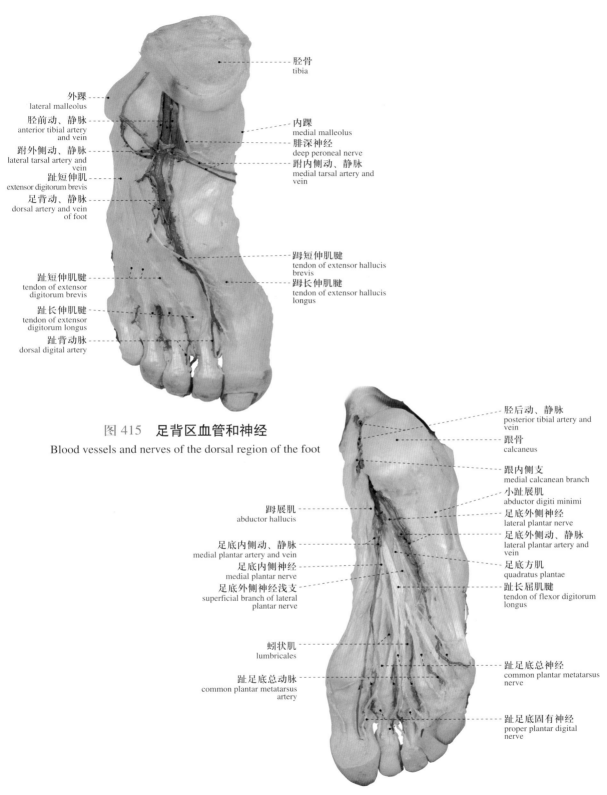

胫骨
tibia

外踝
lateral malleolus

胫前动、静脉
anterior tibial artery and vein

跗外侧动、静脉
lateral tarsal artery and vein

趾短伸肌
extensor digitorum brevis

足背动、静脉
dorsal artery and vein of foot

趾短伸肌腱
tendon of extensor digitorum brevis

趾长伸肌腱
tendon of extensor digitorum longus

趾背动脉
dorsal digital artery

内踝
medial malleolus

腓深神经
deep peroneal nerve

跗内侧动、静脉
medial tarsal artery and vein

跟短伸肌腱
tendon of extensor hallucis brevis

跟长伸肌腱
tendon of extensor hallucis longus

图 415　足背区血管和神经

Blood vessels and nerves of the dorsal region of the foot

胫后动、静脉
posterior tibial artery and vein

跟骨
calcaneus

跟内侧支
medial calcanean branch

小趾展肌
abductor digiti minimi

足底外侧神经
lateral plantar nerve

足底外侧动、静脉
lateral plantar artery and vein

足底方肌
quadratus plantae

趾长屈肌腱
tendon of flexor digitorum longus

跟展肌
abductor hallucis

足底内侧动、静脉
medial plantar artery and vein

足底内侧神经
medial plantar nerve

足底外侧神经浅支
superficial branch of lateral plantar nerve

蚓状肌
lumbricales

趾足底总动脉
common plantar metatarsus artery

趾足底总神经
common plantar metatarsus nerve

趾足底固有神经
proper plantar digital nerve

图 416　足底区血管和神经

Blood vessels and nerves of the plantar region of the foot

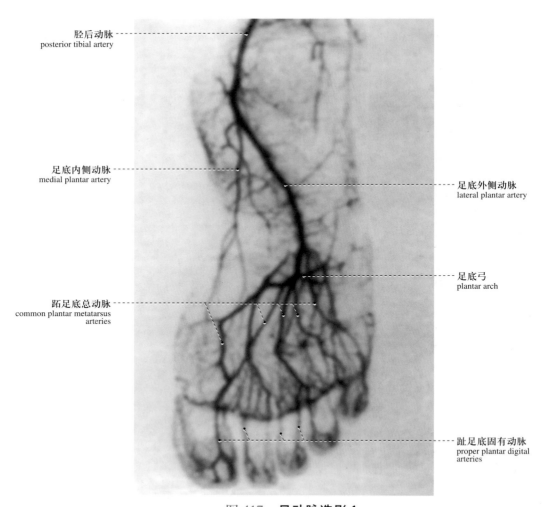

胫后动脉
posterior tibial artery

足底内侧动脉
medial plantar artery

足底外侧动脉
lateral plantar artery

足底弓
plantar arch

跖足底总动脉
common plantar metatarsus
arteries

趾足底固有动脉
proper plantar digital
arteries

图 417 足动脉造影 1
Angiography of the foot arteries 1

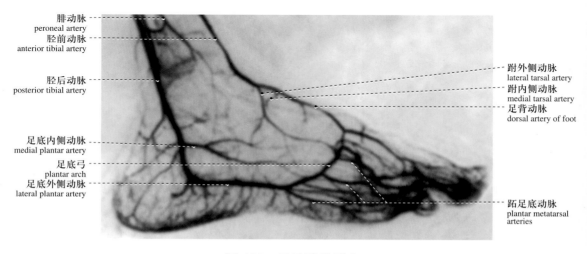

腓动脉
peroneal artery

胫前动脉
anterior tibial artery

胫后动脉
posterior tibial artery

足底内侧动脉
medial plantar artery

足底弓
plantar arch

足底外侧动脉
lateral plantar artery

跗外侧动脉
lateral tarsal artery

跗内侧动脉
medial tarsal artery

足背动脉
dorsal artery of foot

跖足底动脉
plantar metatarsal
arteries

图 418 足动脉造影 2
Angiography of the foot arteries 2

第四节

静 脉

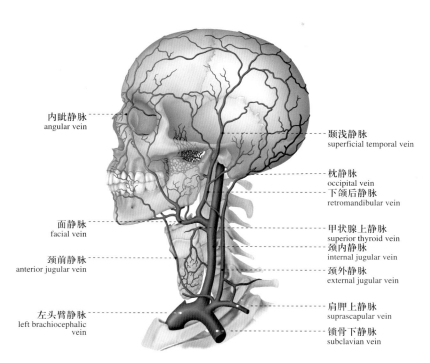

内眦静脉
angular vein

颞浅静脉
superficial temporal vein

枕静脉
occipital vein

下颌后静脉
retromandibular vein

面静脉
facial vein

甲状腺上静脉
superior thyroid vein

颈内静脉
internal jugular vein

颈前静脉
anterior jugular vein

颈外静脉
external jugular vein

左头臂静脉
left brachiocephalic
vein

肩胛上静脉
suprascapular vein

锁骨下静脉
subclavian vein

图 419　头部浅静脉（侧面观）
Superficial veins of the head (lateral aspect)

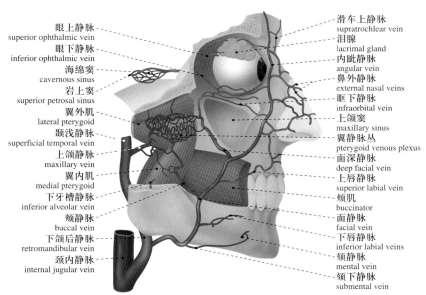

眼上静脉
superior ophthalmic vein

眼下静脉
inferior ophthalmic vein

海绵窦
cavernous sinus

岩上窦
superior petrosal sinus

翼外肌
lateral pterygoid

颞浅静脉
superficial temporal vein

上颌静脉
maxillary vein

翼内肌
medial pterygoid

下牙槽静脉
inferior alveolar vein

颊静脉
buccal vein

下颌后静脉
retromandibular vein

颈内静脉
internal jugular vein

滑车上静脉
supratrochlear vein

泪腺
lacrimal gland

内眦静脉
angular vein

鼻外静脉
external nasal veins

眶下静脉
infraorbital vein

上颌窦
maxillary sinus

翼静脉丛
pterygoid venous plexus

面深静脉
deep facial vein

上唇静脉
superior labial vein

颊肌
buccinator

面静脉
facial vein

下唇静脉
inferior labial veins

颏静脉
mental vein

颏下静脉
submental vein

图 420　头部深静脉（侧面观）
Deep veins of the head (lateral aspect)

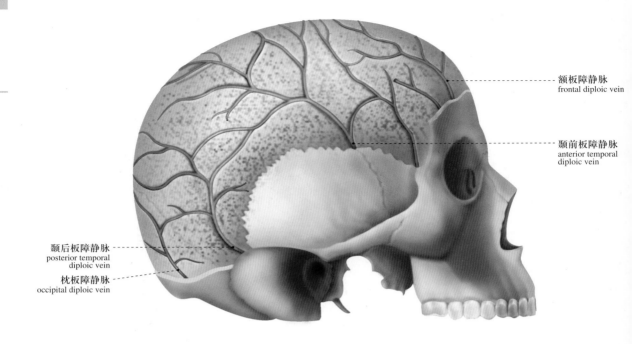

额板障静脉
frontal diploic vein

颞前板障静脉
anterior temporal
diploic vein

颞后板障静脉
posterior temporal
diploic vein

枕板障静脉
occipital diploic vein

图 421　**板障静脉**
Diploic veins

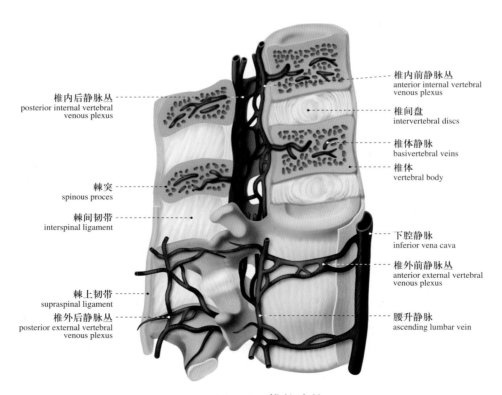

椎内后静脉丛
posterior internal vertebral
venous plexus

椎内前静脉丛
anterior internal vertebral
venous plexus

椎间盘
intervertebral discs

椎体静脉
basivertebral veins

椎体
vertebral body

棘突
spinous proces

棘间韧带
interspinal ligament

下腔静脉
inferior vena cava

椎外前静脉丛
anterior external vertebral
venous plexus

棘上韧带
supraspinal ligament

椎外后静脉丛
posterior external vertebral
venous plexus

腰升静脉
ascending lumbar vein

图 422　**椎静脉丛**
Vertebral venous plexus

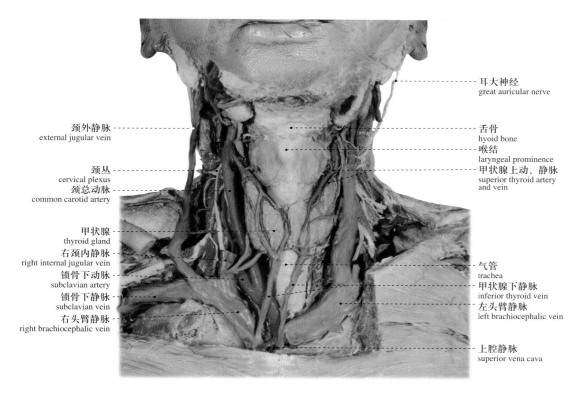

耳大神经
great auricular nerve

颈外静脉
external jugular vein

舌骨
hyoid bone

喉结
laryngeal prominence

颈丛
cervical plexus

颈总动脉
common carotid artery

甲状腺上动、静脉
superior thyroid artery and vein

甲状腺
thyroid gland

右颈内静脉
right internal jugular vein

锁骨下动脉
subclavian artery

锁骨下静脉
subclavian vein

右头臂静脉
right brachiocephalic vein

气管
trachea

甲状腺下静脉
inferior thyroid vein

左头臂静脉
left brachiocephalic vein

上腔静脉
superior vena cava

图 423　颈前区血管和神经

Blood vessels and nerves of anterior region of the neck

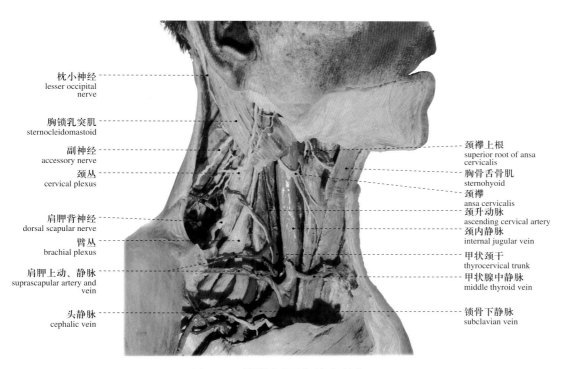

枕小神经
lesser occipital nerve

胸锁乳突肌
sternocleidomastoid

副神经
accessory nerve

颈丛
cervical plexus

肩胛背神经
dorsal scapular nerve

臂丛
brachial plexus

肩胛上动、静脉
suprascapular artery and vein

头静脉
cephalic vein

颈襻上根
superior root of ansa cervicalis

胸骨舌骨肌
sternohyoid

颈襻
ansa cervicalis

颈升动脉
ascending cervical artery

颈内静脉
internal jugular vein

甲状颈干
thyrocervical trunk

甲状腺中静脉
middle thyroid vein

锁骨下静脉
subclavian vein

图 424　颈外侧区血管和神经

Blood vessels and nerves of lateral region of the neck

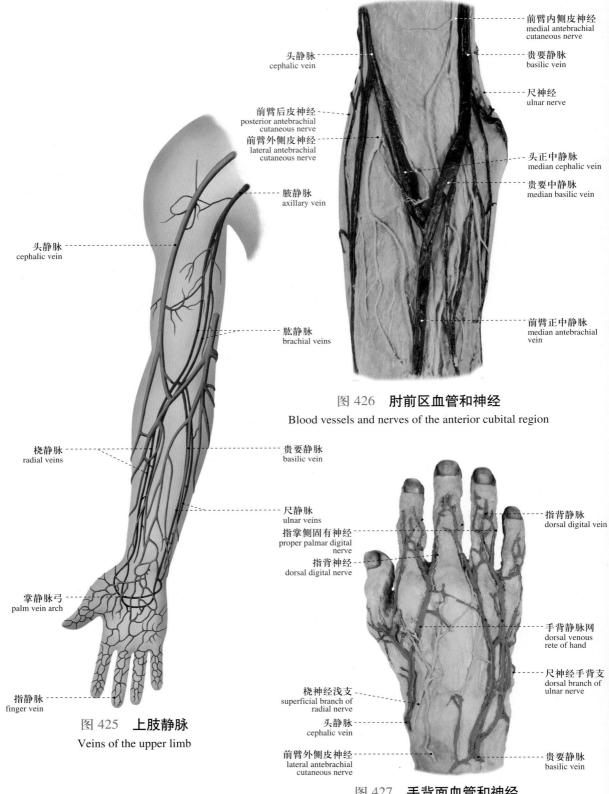

头静脉
cephalic vein

前臂内侧皮神经
medial antebrachial
cutaneous nerve

贵要静脉
basilic vein

尺神经
ulnar nerve

前臂后皮神经
posterior antebrachial
cutaneous nerve

前臂外侧皮神经
lateral antebrachial
cutaneous nerve

腋静脉
axillary vein

头正中静脉
median cephalic vein

贵要中静脉
median basilic vein

头静脉
cephalic vein

肱静脉
brachial veins

前臂正中静脉
median antebrachial
vein

图 426　肘前区血管和神经

Blood vessels and nerves of the anterior cubital region

桡静脉
radial veins

贵要静脉
basilic vein

尺静脉
ulnar veins

指掌侧固有神经
proper palmar digital
nerve

指背神经
dorsal digital nerve

指背静脉
dorsal digital vein

手背静脉网
dorsal venous
rete of hand

掌静脉弓
palm vein arch

尺神经手背支
dorsal branch of
ulnar nerve

桡神经浅支
superficial branch of
radial nerve

头静脉
cephalic vein

指静脉
finger vein

前臂外侧皮神经
lateral antebrachial
cutaneous nerve

贵要静脉
basilic vein

图 425　上肢静脉

Veins of the upper limb

图 427　手背面血管和神经

Blood vessels and nerves of the dorsal aspect of the hand

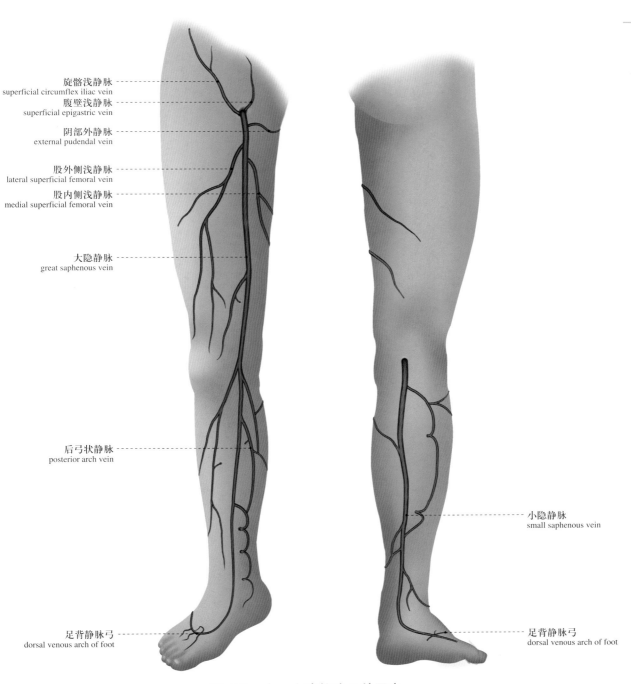

旋髂浅静脉
superficial circumflex iliac vein

腹壁浅静脉
superficial epigastric vein

阴部外静脉
external pudendal vein

股外侧浅静脉
lateral superficial femoral vein

股内侧浅静脉
medial superficial femoral vein

大隐静脉
great saphenous vein

后弓状静脉
posterior arch vein

小隐静脉
small saphenous vein

足背静脉弓
dorsal venous arch of foot

足背静脉弓
dorsal venous arch of foot

图 428　大、小隐静脉及其属支
Great and small saphenous veins and its tributaries

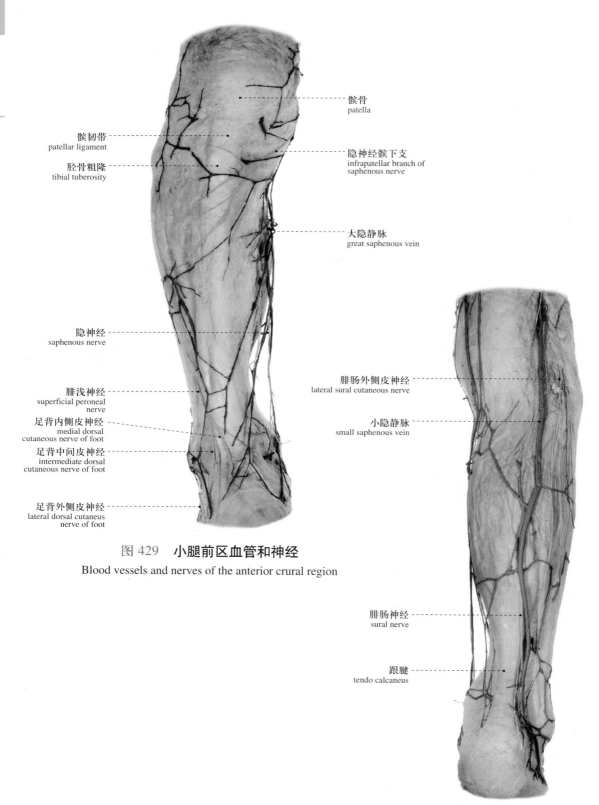

髌骨
patella

髌韧带
patellar ligament

隐神经髌下支
infrapatellar branch of
saphenous nerve

胫骨粗隆
tibial tuberosity

大隐静脉
great saphenous vein

隐神经
saphenous nerve

腓肠外侧皮神经
lateral sural cutaneous nerve

腓浅神经
superficial peroneal
nerve

小隐静脉
small saphenous vein

足背内侧皮神经
medial dorsal
cutaneous nerve of foot

足背中间皮神经
intermediate dorsal
cutaneous nerve of foot

足背外侧皮神经
lateral dorsal cutaneus
nerve of foot

图 429　小腿前区血管和神经
Blood vessels and nerves of the anterior crural region

腓肠神经
sural nerve

跟腱
tendo calcaneus

图 430　小腿后区血管和神经
Blood vessels and nerves of the posterior crural region

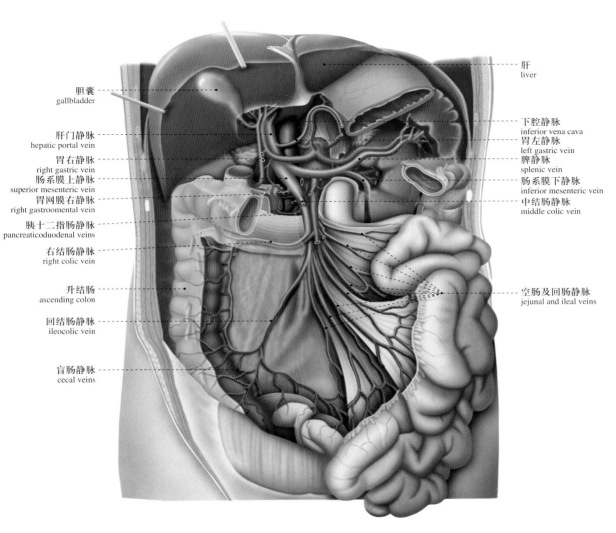

胆囊
gallbladder

肝门静脉
hepatic portal vein

胃右静脉
right gastric vein

肠系膜上静脉
superior mesenteric vein

胃网膜右静脉
right gastroomental vein

胰十二指肠静脉
pancreaticoduodenal veins

右结肠静脉
right colic vein

升结肠
ascending colon

回结肠静脉
ileocolic vein

盲肠静脉
cecal veins

肝
liver

下腔静脉
inferior vena cava

胃左静脉
left gastric vein

脾静脉
splenic vein

肠系膜下静脉
inferior mesenteric vein

中结肠静脉
middle colic vein

空肠及回肠静脉
jejunal and ileal veins

图 431　肠系膜上静脉及其属支
Superior mesenteric vein and its tributaries

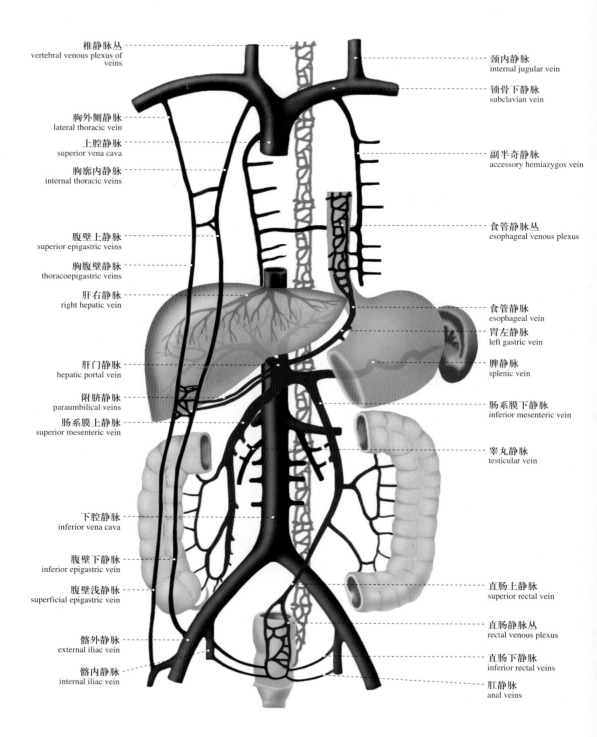

椎静脉丛
vertebral venous plexus of veins

胸外侧静脉
lateral thoracic vein

上腔静脉
superior vena cava

胸廓内静脉
internal thoracic veins

腹壁上静脉
superior epigastric veins

胸腹壁静脉
thoracoepigastric veins

肝右静脉
right hepatic vein

肝门静脉
hepatic portal vein

附脐静脉
paraumbilical veins

肠系膜上静脉
superior mesenteric vein

下腔静脉
inferior vena cava

腹壁下静脉
inferior epigastric vein

腹壁浅静脉
superficial epigastric vein

髂外静脉
external iliac vein

髂内静脉
internal iliac vein

颈内静脉
internal jugular vein

锁骨下静脉
subclavian vein

副半奇静脉
accessory hemiazygos vein

食管静脉丛
esophageal venous plexus

食管静脉
esophageal vein

胃左静脉
left gastric vein

脾静脉
splenic vein

肠系膜下静脉
inferior mesenteric vein

睾丸静脉
testicular vein

直肠上静脉
superior rectal vein

直肠静脉丛
rectal venous plexus

直肠下静脉
inferior rectal veins

肛静脉
anal veins

图 432　门腔静脉吻合（模式图）
Porta-caval venous communications (diagram)

第一节

总 论

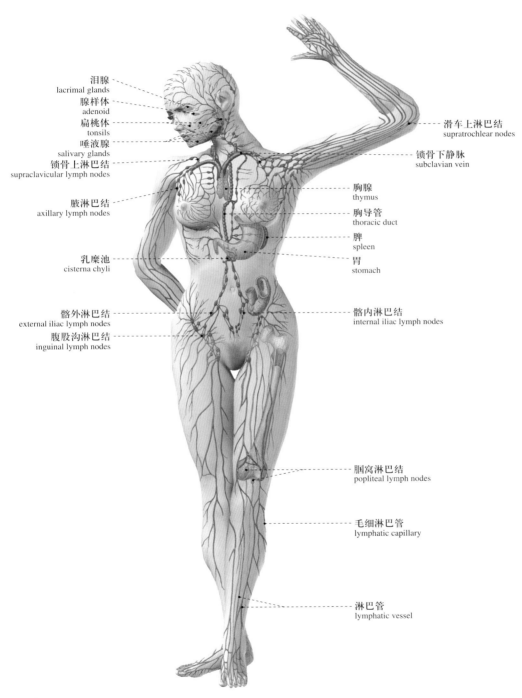

泪腺
lacrimal glands

腺样体
adenoid

扁桃体
tonsils

唾液腺
salivary glands

锁骨上淋巴结
supraclavicular lymph nodes

腋淋巴结
axillary lymph nodes

乳糜池
cisterna chyli

髂外淋巴结
external iliac lymph nodes

腹股沟淋巴结
inguinal lymph nodes

滑车上淋巴结
supratrochlear nodes

锁骨下静脉
subclavian vein

胸腺
thymus

胸导管
thoracic duct

脾
spleen

胃
stomach

髂内淋巴结
internal iliac lymph nodes

腘窝淋巴结
popliteal lymph nodes

毛细淋巴管
lymphatic capillary

淋巴管
lymphatic vessel

图 433 淋巴系统（模式图）
Lymph system (diagram)

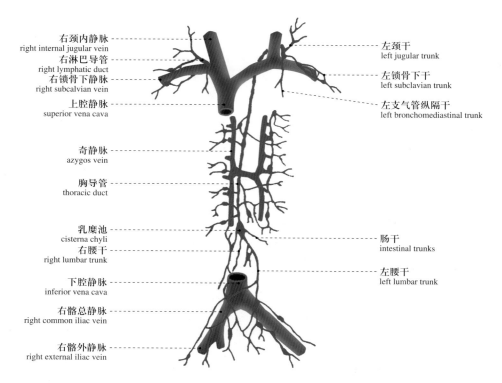

右颈内静脉
right internal jugular vein
右淋巴导管
right lymphatic duct
右锁骨下静脉
right subcalvian vein
上腔静脉
superior vena cava

奇静脉
azygos vein

胸导管
thoracic duct

乳糜池
cisterna chyli
右腰干
right lumbar trunk

下腔静脉
inferior vena cava

右髂总静脉
right common iliac vein

右髂外静脉
right external iliac vein

左颈干
left jugular trunk

左锁骨下干
left subclavian trunk

左支气管纵隔干
left bronchomediastinal trunk

肠干
intestinal trunks

左腰干
left lumbar trunk

图 434　淋巴干及淋巴导管
Lymphatic trunks and lymphatic ducts

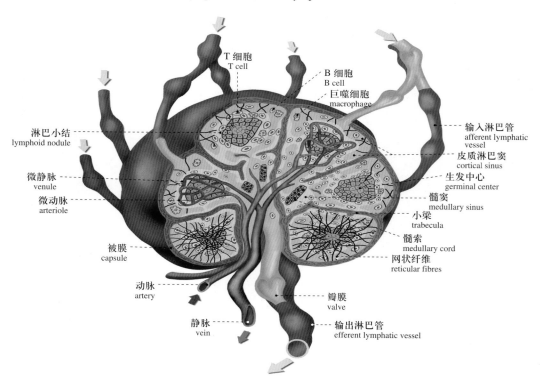

T 细胞
T cell

B 细胞
B cell
巨噬细胞
macrophage

淋巴小结
lymphoid nodule

微静脉
venule
微动脉
arteriole

被膜
capsule

动脉
artery

静脉
vein

输入淋巴管
afferent lymphatic vessel
皮质淋巴窦
cortical sinus
生发中心
germinal center
髓窦
medullary sinus
小梁
trabecula
髓索
medullary cord
网状纤维
reticular fibres

瓣膜
valve

输出淋巴管
efferent lymphatic vessel

图 435　淋巴结构造模式图
Diagram of construction of the lymph node

第二节

淋巴的位置和淋巴引流范围

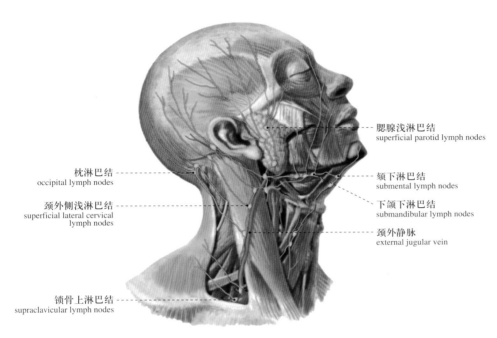

腮腺浅淋巴结
superficial parotid lymph nodes

枕淋巴结
occipital lymph nodes

颏下淋巴结
submental lymph nodes

颈外侧浅淋巴结
superficial lateral cervical
lymph nodes

下颌下淋巴结
submandibular lymph nodes

颈外静脉
external jugular vein

锁骨上淋巴结
supraclavicular lymph nodes

图 436　头颈部的淋巴管和淋巴结 1

Lymph vessels and the lymph nodes of the head and the neck 1

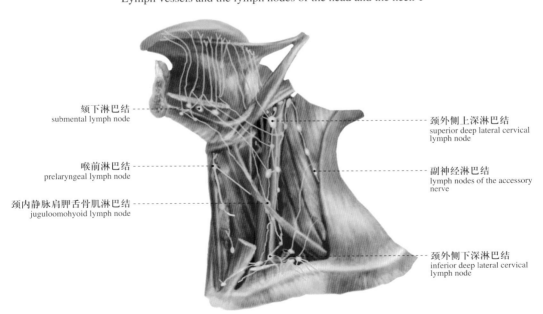

颏下淋巴结
submental lymph node

喉前淋巴结
prelaryngeal lymph node

颈内静脉肩胛舌骨肌淋巴结
juguloomohyoid lymph node

颈外侧上深淋巴结
superior deep lateral cervical
lymph node

副神经淋巴结
lymph nodes of the accessory
nerve

颈外侧下深淋巴结
inferior deep lateral cervical
lymph node

图 437　头颈部的淋巴管和淋巴结 2

Lymph vessels and the lymph nodes of the head and the neck 2

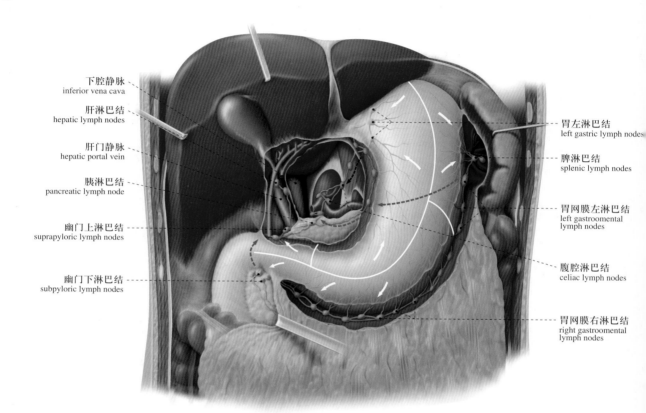

下腔静脉
inferior vena cava

肝淋巴结
hepatic lymph nodes

肝门静脉
hepatic portal vein

胰淋巴结
pancreatic lymph node

幽门上淋巴结
suprapyloric lymph nodes

幽门下淋巴结
subpyloric lymph nodes

胃左淋巴结
left gastric lymph nodes

脾淋巴结
splenic lymph nodes

胃网膜左淋巴结
left gastroomental
lymph nodes

腹腔淋巴结
celiac lymph nodes

胃网膜右淋巴结
right gastroomental
lymph nodes

图 438　胃的淋巴
Gastric lymphs

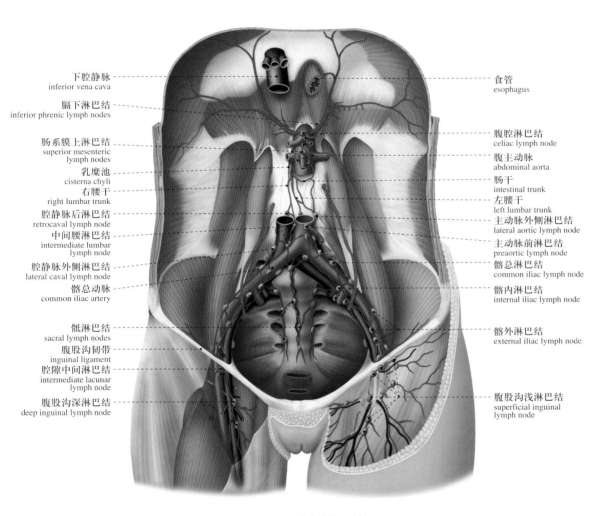

下腔静脉
inferior vena cava

膈下淋巴结
inferior phrenic lymph nodes

肠系膜上淋巴结
superior mesenteric
lymph nodes

乳糜池
cisterna chyli

右腰干
right lumbar trunk

腔静脉后淋巴结
retrocaval lymph node

中间腰淋巴结
intermediate lumbar
lymph node

腔静脉外侧淋巴结
lateral caval lymph node

髂总动脉
common iliac artery

骶淋巴结
sacral lymph nodes

腹股沟韧带
inguinal ligament

腔隙中间淋巴结
intermediate lacunar
lymph node

腹股沟深淋巴结
deep inguinal lymph node

食管
esophagus

腹腔淋巴结
celiac lymph node

腹主动脉
abdominal aorta

肠干
intestinal trunk

左腰干
left lumbar trunk

主动脉外侧淋巴结
lateral aortic lymph node

主动脉前淋巴结
preaortic lymph node

髂总淋巴结
common iliac lymph node

髂内淋巴结
internal iliac lymph node

髂外淋巴结
external iliac lymph node

腹股沟浅淋巴结
superficial inguinal
lymph node

图 439　盆部淋巴结
Pelvic lymph nodes

239

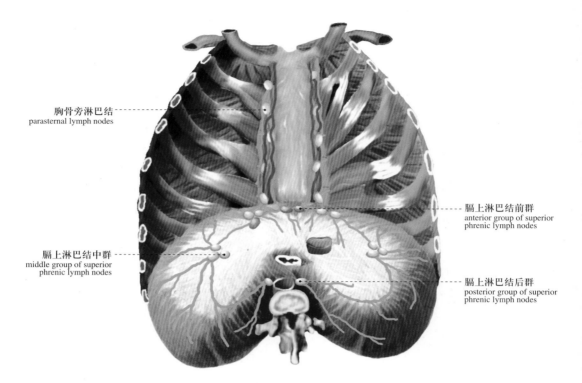

胸骨旁淋巴结
parasternal lymph nodes

膈上淋巴结前群
anterior group of superior
phrenic lymph nodes

膈上淋巴结中群
middle group of superior
phrenic lymph nodes

膈上淋巴结后群
posterior group of superior
phrenic lymph nodes

图 440　胸骨旁淋巴结和膈上淋巴结
Parasternal lymph nodes and superior phrenic lymph nodes

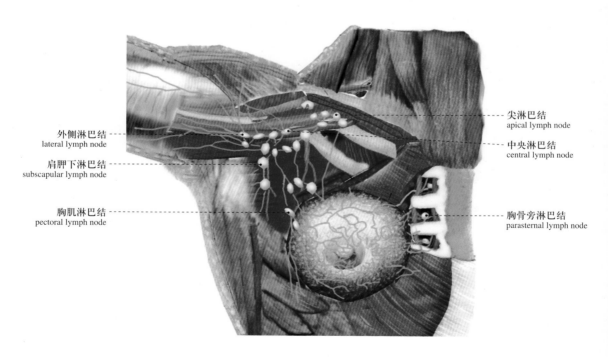

外侧淋巴结
lateral lymph node

肩胛下淋巴结
subscapular lymph node

胸肌淋巴结
pectoral lymph node

尖淋巴结
apical lymph node

中央淋巴结
central lymph node

胸骨旁淋巴结
parasternal lymph node

图 441　腋淋巴结和乳房淋巴管
Axillary lymph nodes and mamma lymph vessels

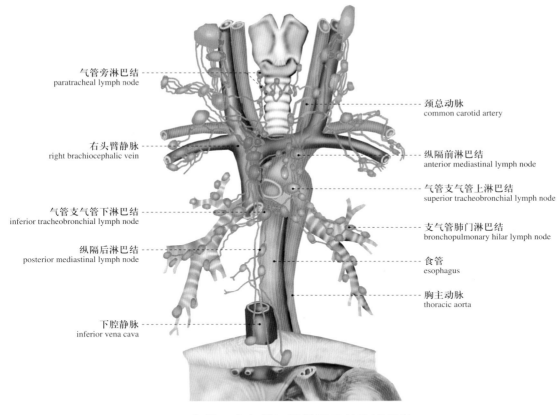

气管旁淋巴结
paratracheal lymph node

颈总动脉
common carotid artery

右头臂静脉
right brachiocephalic vein

纵隔前淋巴结
anterior mediastinal lymph node

气管支气管上淋巴结
superior tracheobronchial lymph node

气管支气管下淋巴结
inferior tracheobronchial lymph node

支气管肺门淋巴结
bronchopulmonary hilar lymph node

纵隔后淋巴结
posterior mediastinal lymph node

食管
esophagus

胸主动脉
thoracic aorta

下腔静脉
inferior vena cava

图 442　气管、支气管及肺的淋巴管和淋巴结
Lymph vessels and the lymph nodes of the trachea, the bronchi and the lungs

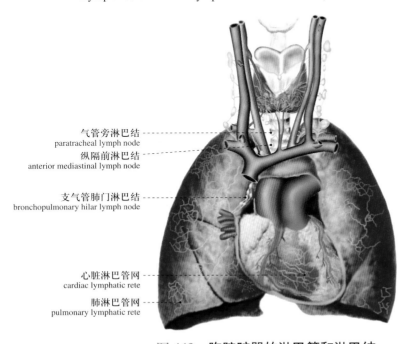

气管旁淋巴结
paratracheal lymph node

纵隔前淋巴结
anterior mediastinal lymph node

支气管肺门淋巴结
bronchopulmonary hilar lymph node

心脏淋巴管网
cardiac lymphatic rete

肺淋巴管网
pulmonary lymphatic rete

图 443　胸腔脏器的淋巴管和淋巴结
Lymph vessels and the lymph nodes of the thoracic viscerae

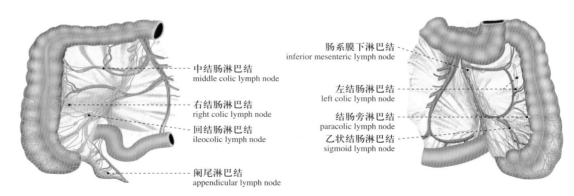

图 444 **大肠的淋巴管和淋巴结 1**
Lymph vessels and the lymph nodes of the large intestine 1

中结肠淋巴结
middle colic lymph node

右结肠淋巴结
right colic lymph node

回结肠淋巴结
ileocolic lymph node

阑尾淋巴结
appendicular lymph node

图 445 **大肠的淋巴管和淋巴结 2**
Lymph vessels and the lymph nodes of the large intestine 2

肠系膜下淋巴结
inferior mesenteric lymph node

左结肠淋巴结
left colic lymph node

结肠旁淋巴结
paracolic lymph node

乙状结肠淋巴结
sigmoid lymph node

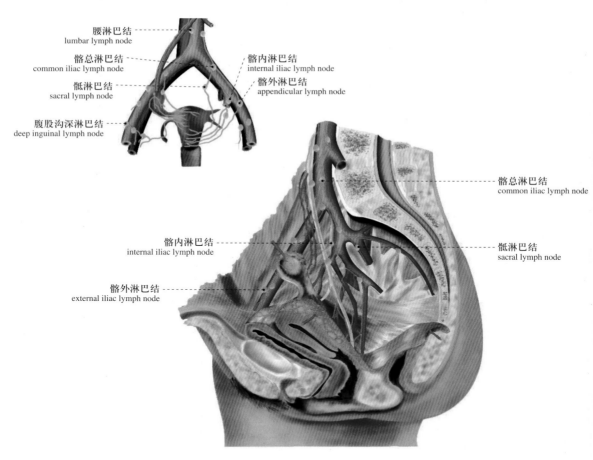

腰淋巴结
lumbar lymph node

髂总淋巴结
common iliac lymph node

骶淋巴结
sacral lymph node

腹股沟深淋巴结
deep inguinal lymph node

髂内淋巴结
internal iliac lymph node

髂外淋巴结
appendicular lymph node

髂总淋巴结
common iliac lymph node

骶淋巴结
sacral lymph node

髂内淋巴结
internal iliac lymph node

髂外淋巴结
external iliac lymph node

图 446 **女性盆部淋巴结**
Lymph nodes of the female pelvis

第三节

脾

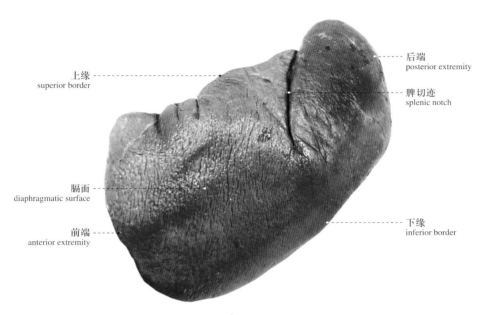

图 447　脾（膈面观）
Spleen (diaphragmatic aspect)

上缘
superior border

后端
posterior extremity

脾切迹
splenic notch

膈面
diaphragmatic surface

前端
anterior extremity

下缘
inferior border

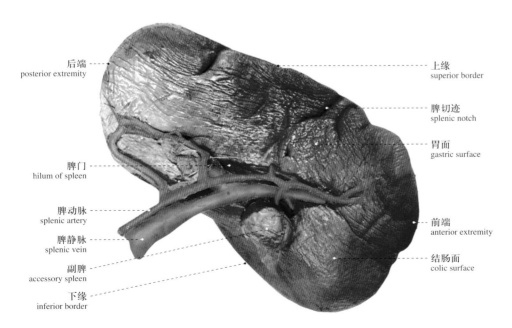

图 448　脾（脏面观）
Spleen (visceral aspect)

后端
posterior extremity

上缘
superior border

脾切迹
splenic notch

胃面
gastric surface

脾门
hilum of spleen

脾动脉
splenic artery

脾静脉
splenic vein

副脾
accessory spleen

下缘
inferior border

前端
anterior extremity

结肠面
colic surface

第一节

眼　球

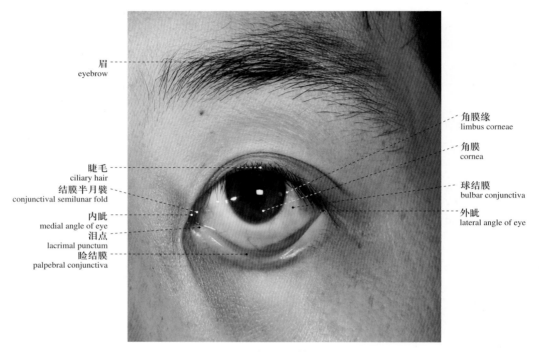

眉
eyebrow

角膜缘
limbus corneae

角膜
cornea

睫毛
ciliary hair

结膜半月襞
conjunctival semilunar fold

球结膜
bulbar conjunctiva

内眦
medial angle of eye

外眦
lateral angle of eye

泪点
lacrimal punctum

睑结膜
palpebral conjunctiva

图 449　左眼（前面观）

Left eye (anterior aspect)

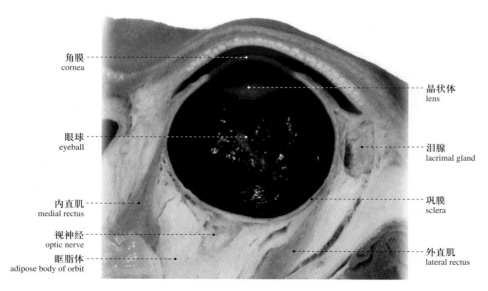

角膜
cornea

晶状体
lens

眼球
eyeball

泪腺
lacrimal gland

内直肌
medial rectus

巩膜
sclera

视神经
optic nerve

眶脂体
adipose body of orbit

外直肌
lateral rectus

图 450　眼水平断面

Horizontal section of the eye

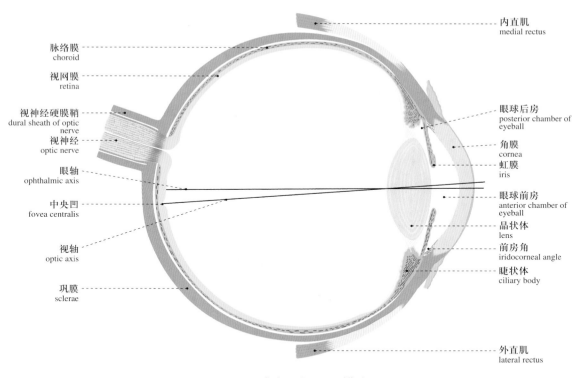

脉络膜
choroid

视网膜
retina

视神经硬膜鞘
dural sheath of optic nerve

视神经
optic nerve

眼轴
ophthalmic axis

中央凹
fovea centralis

视轴
optic axis

巩膜
sclerae

内直肌
medial rectus

眼球后房
posterior chamber of eyeball

角膜
cornea

虹膜
iris

眼球前房
anterior chamber of eyeball

晶状体
lens

前房角
iridocorneal angle

睫状体
ciliary body

外直肌
lateral rectus

图 451　眼球水平切面（模式图）

Horizontal section through the eyeball (diagram)

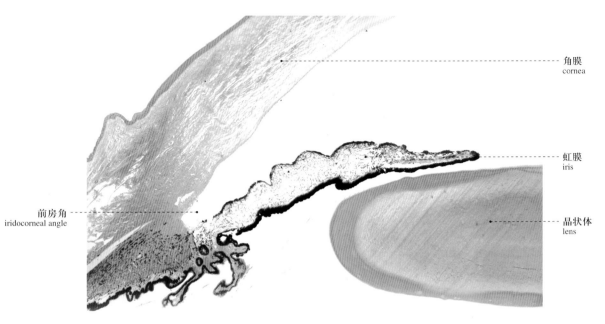

角膜
cornea

虹膜
iris

前房角
iridocorneal angle

晶状体
lens

图 452　眼球前部（人眼球，HE 染色，×40）

Anterior portion of the eyeball (human eyeball, HE staining, ×40)

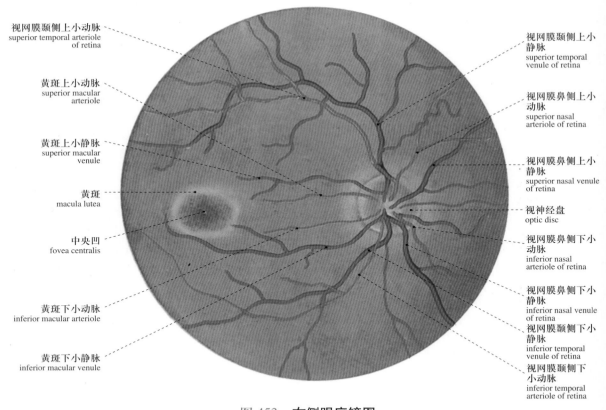

视网膜颞侧上小动脉
superior temporal arteriole
of retina

黄斑上小动脉
superior macular
arteriole

黄斑上小静脉
superior macular
venule

黄斑
macula lutea

中央凹
fovea centralis

黄斑下小动脉
inferior macular arteriole

黄斑下小静脉
inferior macular venule

视网膜颞侧上小
静脉
superior temporal
venule of retina

视网膜鼻侧上小
动脉
superior nasal
arteriole of retina

视网膜鼻侧上小
静脉
superior nasal venule
of retina

视神经盘
optic disc

视网膜鼻侧下小
动脉
inferior nasal
arteriole of retina

视网膜鼻侧下小
静脉
inferior nasal venule
of retina

视网膜颞侧下小
静脉
inferior temporal
venule of retina

视网膜颞侧下
小动脉
inferior temporal
arteriole of retina

图 453　右侧眼底镜图

Right ophthalmoscopic image of the fundus of the eyeball

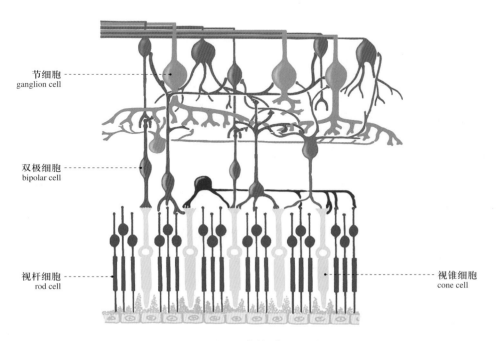

节细胞
ganglion cell

双极细胞
bipolar cell

视杆细胞
rod cell

视锥细胞
cone cell

图 454　视网膜的神经细胞

Nerve cells of the retina

眼 副 器

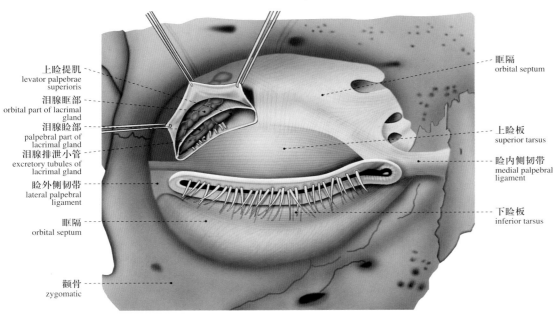

上睑提肌
levator palpebrae
superioris

泪腺眶部
orbital part of lacrimal
gland

泪腺睑部
palpebral part of
lacrimal gland

泪腺排泄小管
excretory tubules of
lacrimal gland

睑外侧韧带
lateral palpebral
ligament

眶隔
orbital septum

颧骨
zygomatic

眶隔
orbital septum

上睑板
superior tarsus

睑内侧韧带
medial palpebral
ligament

下睑板
inferior tarsus

图 455　泪腺（前面观）

Lacrimal gland (anterior aspect)

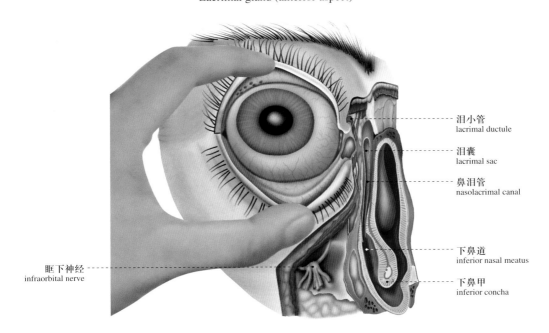

眶下神经
infraorbital nerve

泪小管
lacrimal ductule

泪囊
lacrimal sac

鼻泪管
nasolacrimal canal

下鼻道
inferior nasal meatus

下鼻甲
inferior concha

图 456　泪器（前面观）

Lacrimal apparatus (anterior aspect)

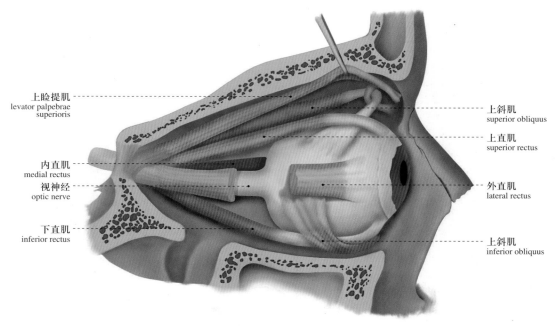

上睑提肌
levator palpebrae
superioris

上斜肌
superior obliquus

上直肌
superior rectus

内直肌
medial rectus

视神经
optic nerve

外直肌
lateral rectus

下直肌
inferior rectus

上斜肌
inferior obliquus

图 457　眼球外肌（外侧面观）

Ocular muscles (lateral aspect)

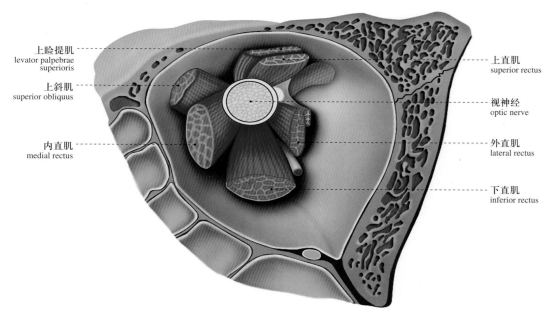

上睑提肌
levator palpebrae
superioris

上斜肌
superior obliquus

内直肌
medial rectus

上直肌
superior rectus

视神经
optic nerve

外直肌
lateral rectus

下直肌
inferior rectus

图 458　眼球外肌（前面观）

Ocular muscles (anterior aspect)

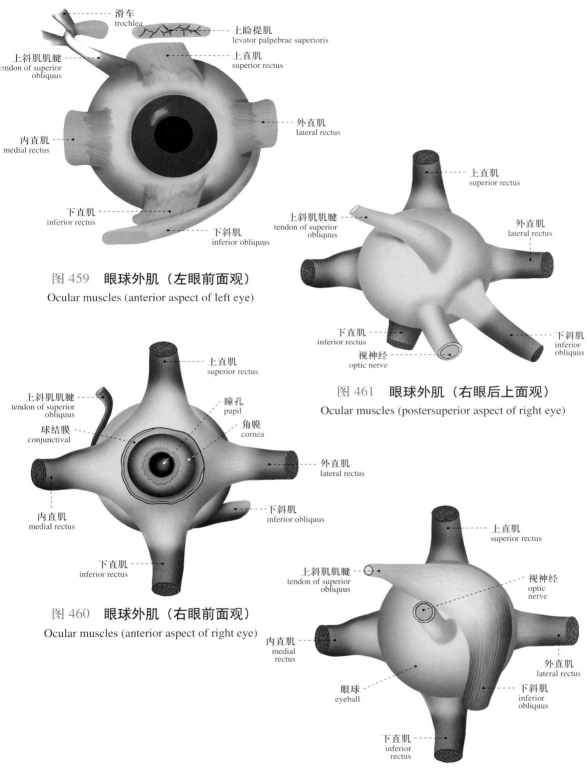

滑车
trochlea

上睑提肌
levator palpebrae superioris

上直肌
superior rectus

上斜肌肌腱
tendon of superior obliquus

内直肌
medial rectus

外直肌
lateral rectus

下直肌
inferior rectus

下斜肌
inferior obliquus

图 459　眼球外肌（左眼前面观）
Ocular muscles (anterior aspect of left eye)

上直肌
superior rectus

上斜肌肌腱
tendon of superior obliquus

外直肌
lateral rectus

下直肌
inferior rectus

视神经
optic nerve

下斜肌
inferior obliquus

图 461　眼球外肌（右眼后上面观）
Ocular muscles (postersuperior aspect of right eye)

上直肌
superior rectus

上斜肌肌腱
tendon of superior obliquus

瞳孔
pupil

角膜
cornea

球结膜
conjunctival

外直肌
lateral rectus

内直肌
medial rectus

下斜肌
inferior obliquus

下直肌
inferior rectus

图 460　眼球外肌（右眼前面观）
Ocular muscles (anterior aspect of right eye)

上直肌
superior rectus

上斜肌肌腱
tendon of superior obliquus

视神经
optic nerve

内直肌
medial rectus

外直肌
lateral rectus

眼球
eyeball

下斜肌
inferior obliquus

下直肌
inferior rectus

图 462　眼球外肌（右眼后面观）
Ocular muscles (posterior aspect of right eye)

第三节

眼的血管和神经

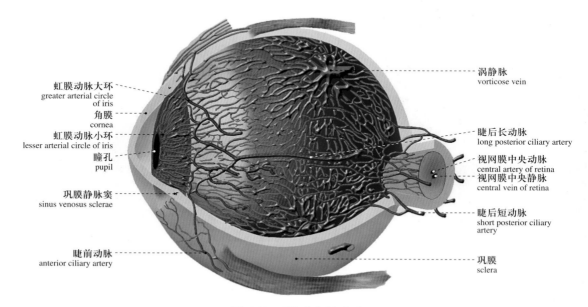

虹膜动脉大环
greater arterial circle of iris

角膜
cornea

虹膜动脉小环
lesser arterial circle of iris

瞳孔
pupil

巩膜静脉窦
sinus venosus sclerae

睫前动脉
anterior ciliary artery

涡静脉
vorticose vein

睫后长动脉
long posterior ciliary artery

视网膜中央动脉
central artery of retina

视网膜中央静脉
central vein of retina

睫后短动脉
short posterior ciliary artery

巩膜
sclera

图 463　眼球血管分布
Distribution of the blood vessels of the eyeball

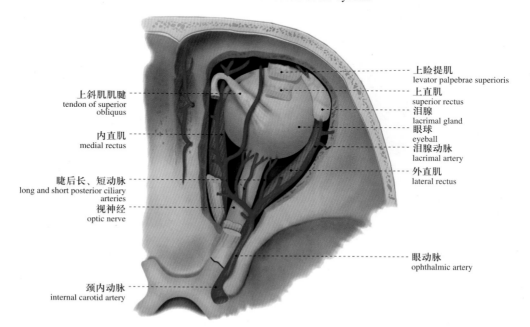

上斜肌肌腱
tendon of superior obliquus

内直肌
medial rectus

睫后长、短动脉
long and short posterior ciliary arteries

视神经
optic nerve

颈内动脉
internal carotid artery

上睑提肌
levator palpebrae superioris

上直肌
superior rectus

泪腺
lacrimal gland

眼球
eyeball

泪腺动脉
lacrimal artery

外直肌
lateral rectus

眼动脉
ophthalmic artery

图 464　右侧眶动脉（上面观）
Right orbital arteries (superior aspect)

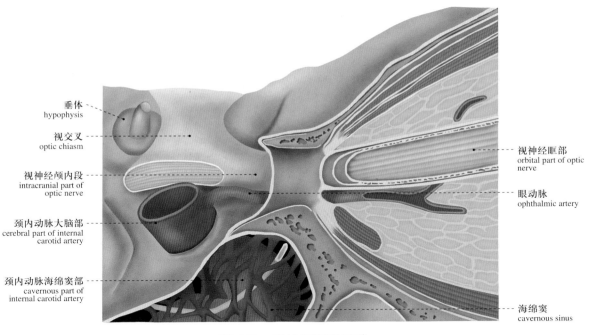

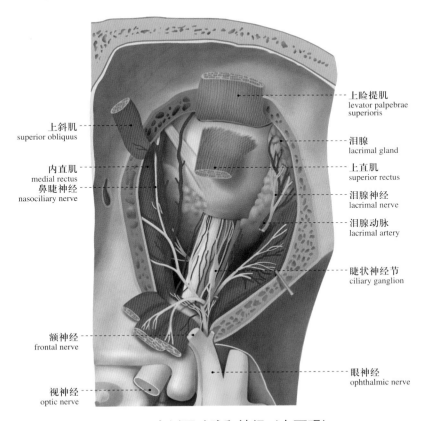

垂体
hypophysis

视交叉
optic chiasm

视神经颅内段
intracranial part of
optic nerve

颈内动脉大脑部
cerebral part of internal
carotid artery

颈内动脉海绵窦部
cavernous part of
internal carotid artery

视神经眶部
orbital part of optic
nerve

眼动脉
ophthalmic artery

海绵窦
cavernous sinus

图 465　视神经和眼动脉
Optic nerve and ophthalmic artery

上斜肌
superior obliquus

内直肌
medial rectus

鼻睫神经
nasociliary nerve

额神经
frontal nerve

视神经
optic nerve

上睑提肌
levator palpebrae
superioris

泪腺
lacrimal gland

上直肌
superior rectus

泪腺神经
lacrimal nerve

泪腺动脉
lacrimal artery

睫状神经节
ciliary ganglion

眼神经
ophthalmic nerve

图 466　右侧眶动脉和神经（上面观）
Right orbital arteries and nerves (superior aspect)

第一节

外 耳

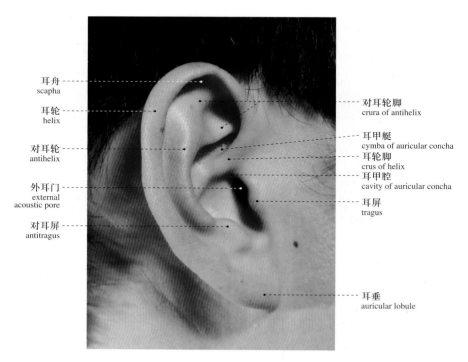

耳舟
scapha

耳轮
helix

对耳轮
antihelix

外耳门
external
acoustic pore

对耳屏
antitragus

对耳轮脚
crura of antihelix

耳甲艇
cymba of auricular concha

耳轮脚
crus of helix

耳甲腔
cavity of auricular concha

耳屏
tragus

耳垂
auricular lobule

图 467　**外耳**

External ear

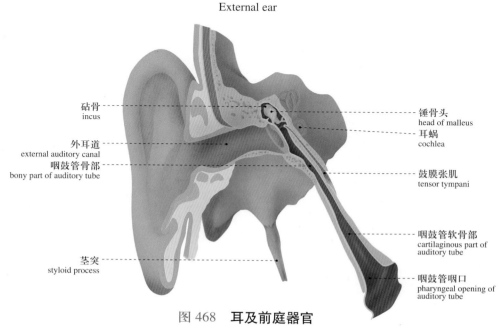

砧骨
incus

外耳道
external auditory canal

咽鼓管骨部
bony part of auditory tube

茎突
styloid process

锤骨头
head of malleus

耳蜗
cochlea

鼓膜张肌
tensor tympani

咽鼓管软骨部
cartilaginous part of
auditory tube

咽鼓管咽口
pharyngeal opening of
auditory tube

图 468　**耳及前庭器官**

Auditory and vestibular organs

第二节

中 耳

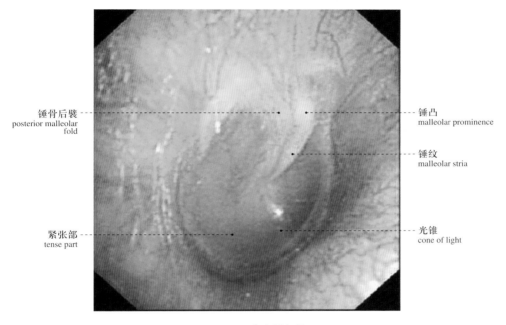

锤骨后襞
posterior malleolar
fold

锤凸
malleolar prominence

锤纹
malleolar stria

紧张部
tense part

光锥
cone of light

图 469　**右侧鼓膜**
Right tympanic membrane

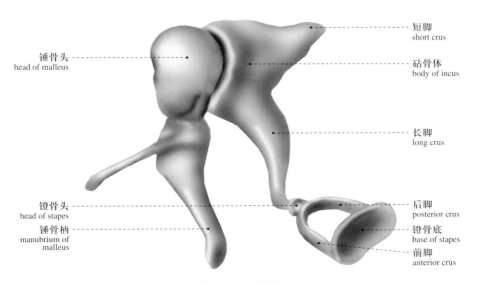

短脚
short crus

锤骨头
head of malleus

砧骨体
body of incus

长脚
long crus

镫骨头
head of stapes

后脚
posterior crus

锤骨柄
manubrium of
malleus

镫骨底
base of stapes

前脚
anterior crus

图 470　**听骨链**
Chain of the auditory ossicles

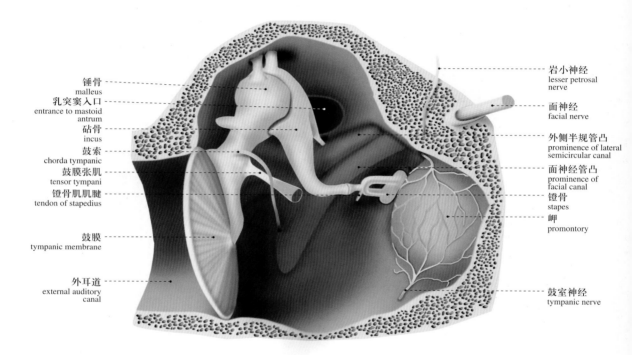

锤骨
malleus

乳突窦入口
entrance to mastoid antrum

砧骨
incus

鼓索
chorda tympanic

鼓膜张肌
tensor tympani

镫骨肌肌腱
tendon of stapedius

鼓膜
tympanic membrane

外耳道
external auditory canal

岩小神经
lesser petrosal nerve

面神经
facial nerve

外侧半规管凸
prominence of lateral semicircular canal

面神经管凸
prominence of facial canal

镫骨
stapes

岬
promontory

鼓室神经
tympanic nerve

图 471 鼓室壁
Walls of the tympanic cavity

第三节

内　耳

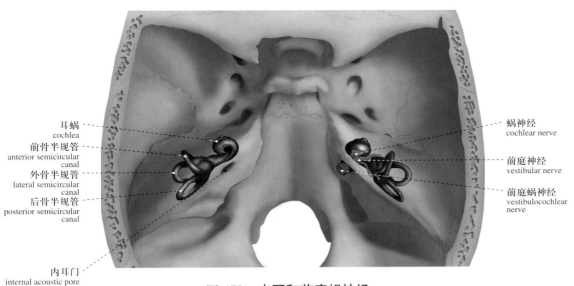

耳蜗
cochlea

前骨半规管
anterior semicircular canal

外骨半规管
lateral semicircular canal

后骨半规管
posterior semicircular canal

内耳门
internal acoustic pore

蜗神经
cochlear nerve

前庭神经
vestibular nerve

前庭蜗神经
vestibulocochlear nerve

图 472　内耳和前庭蜗神经
Internal ear and the vestibulocochlear nerve

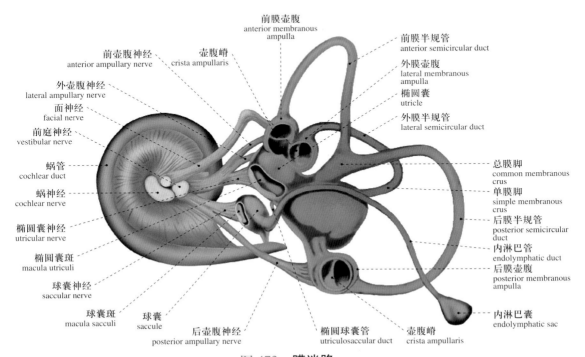

前膜壶腹
anterior membranous ampulla

壶腹嵴
crista ampullaris

前壶腹神经
anterior ampullary nerve

外壶腹神经
lateral ampullary nerve

面神经
facial nerve

前庭神经
vestibular nerve

蜗管
cochlear duct

蜗神经
cochlear nerve

椭圆囊神经
utricular nerve

椭圆囊斑
macula utriculi

球囊神经
saccular nerve

球囊斑
macula sacculi

球囊
saccule

后壶腹神经
posterior ampullary nerve

椭圆球囊管
utriculosaccular duct

壶腹嵴
crista ampullaris

前膜半规管
anterior semicircular duct

外膜壶腹
lateral membranous ampulla

椭圆囊
utricle

外膜半规管
lateral semicircular duct

总膜脚
common membranous crus

单膜脚
simple membranous crus

后膜半规管
posterior semicircular duct

内淋巴管
endolymphatic duct

后膜壶腹
posterior membranous ampulla

内淋巴囊
endolymphatic sac

图 473　膜迷路
Membranous labyrinth

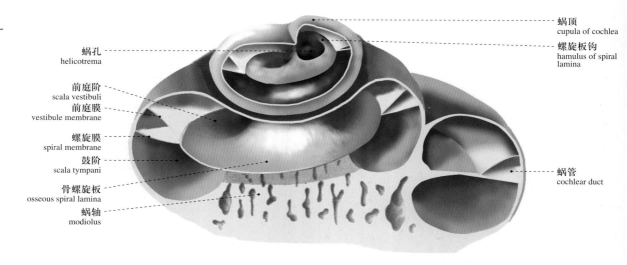

蜗顶
cupula of cochlea

螺旋板钩
hamulus of spiral lamina

蜗孔
helicotrema

前庭阶
scala vestibuli

前庭膜
vestibule membrane

螺旋膜
spiral membrane

鼓阶
scala tympani

骨螺旋板
osseous spiral lamina

蜗轴
modiolus

蜗管
cochlear duct

图 474　耳蜗切面
Section of the cochlea

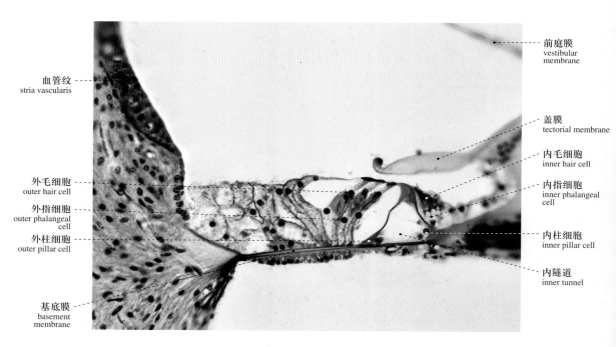

前庭膜
vestibular membrane

血管纹
stria vascularis

盖膜
tectorial membrane

内毛细胞
inner hair cell

外毛细胞
outer hair cell

内指细胞
inner phalangeal cell

外指细胞
outer phalangeal cell

外柱细胞
outer pillar cell

内柱细胞
inner pillar cell

内隧道
inner tunnel

基底膜
basement membrane

图 475　螺旋器（豚鼠内耳，镀银，×400）
Spiral organ (inner ear of the guinea pig, silver staining, ×400)

全身神经

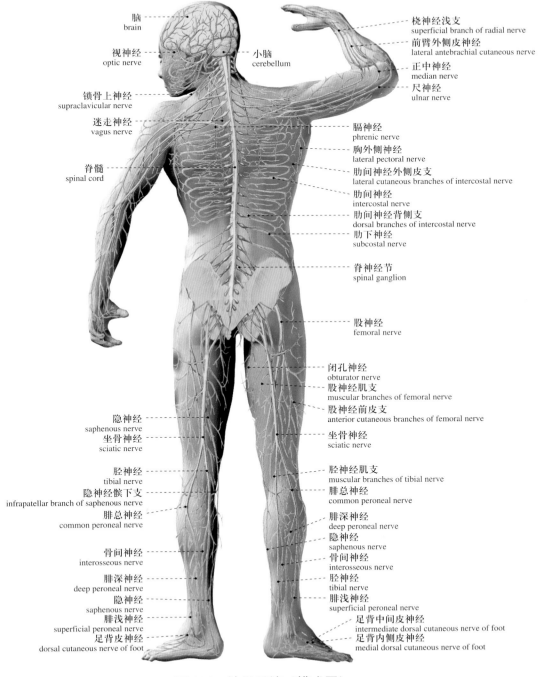

脑
brain

视神经
optic nerve

小脑
cerebellum

锁骨上神经
supraclavicular nerve

迷走神经
vagus nerve

脊髓
spinal cord

桡神经浅支
superficial branch of radial nerve

前臂外侧皮神经
lateral antebrachial cutaneous nerve

正中神经
median nerve

尺神经
ulnar nerve

膈神经
phrenic nerve

胸外侧神经
lateral pectoral nerve

肋间神经外侧皮支
lateral cutaneous branches of intercostal nerve

肋间神经
intercostal nerve

肋间神经背侧支
dorsal branches of intercostal nerve

肋下神经
subcostal nerve

脊神经节
spinal ganglion

股神经
femoral nerve

闭孔神经
obturator nerve

股神经肌支
muscular branches of femoral nerve

股神经前皮支
anterior cutaneous branches of femoral nerve

隐神经
saphenous nerve

坐骨神经
sciatic nerve

腔神经
tibial nerve

隐神经髌下支
infrapatellar branch of saphenous nerve

腓总神经
common peroneal nerve

骨间神经
interosseous nerve

腓深神经
deep peroneal nerve

隐神经
saphenous nerve

腓浅神经
superficial peroneal nerve

足背皮神经
dorsal cutaneous nerve of foot

坐骨神经
sciatic nerve

腔神经肌支
muscular branches of tibial nerve

腓总神经
common peroneal nerve

腓深神经
deep peroneal nerve

隐神经
saphenous nerve

骨间神经
interosseous nerve

腔神经
tibial nerve

腓浅神经
superficial peroneal nerve

足背中间皮神经
intermediate dorsal cutaneous nerve of foot

足背内侧皮神经
medial dorsal cutaneous nerve of foot

图 476 神经系统（模式图）
Nervous system (diagram)

第二节

神经元结构

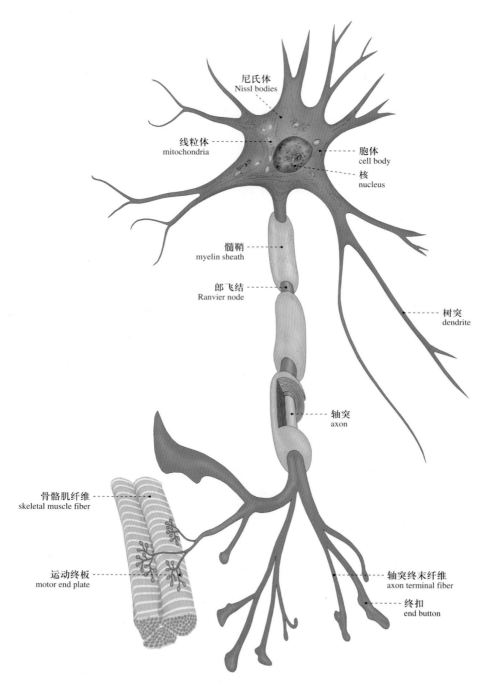

尼氏体
Nissl bodies

线粒体
mitochondria

胞体
cell body

核
nucleus

髓鞘
myelin sheath

郎飞结
Ranvier node

树突
dendrite

轴突
axon

骨骼肌纤维
skeletal muscle fiber

运动终板
motor end plate

轴突终末纤维
axon terminal fiber

终扣
end button

图 477　神经元的结构（模式图）
Neurons structure (diagram)

第一节

脊 髓

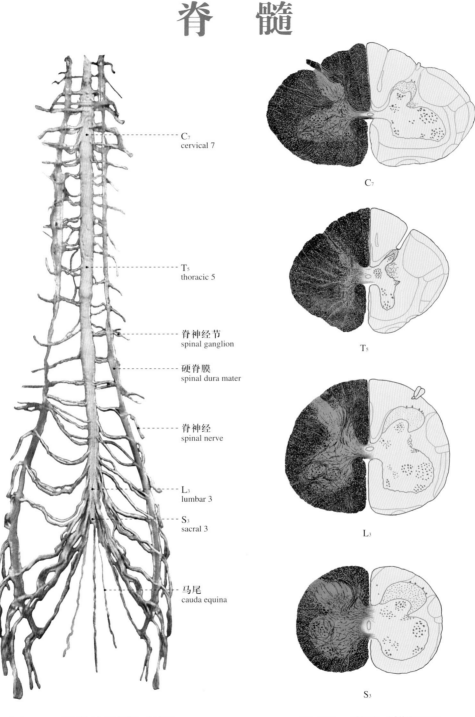

C₇
cervical 7

T₅
thoracic 5

脊 神 经 节
spinal ganglion

硬脊膜
spinal dura mater

脊 神 经
spinal nerve

L₃
lumbar 3

S₃
sacral 3

马尾
cauda equina

C₇

T₅

L₃

S₃

图 478　脊髓的外形和被膜

External morphology of the spinal cord and the meninges

图 479　脊髓（横切面）

Spinal cord (transverse section)

脑

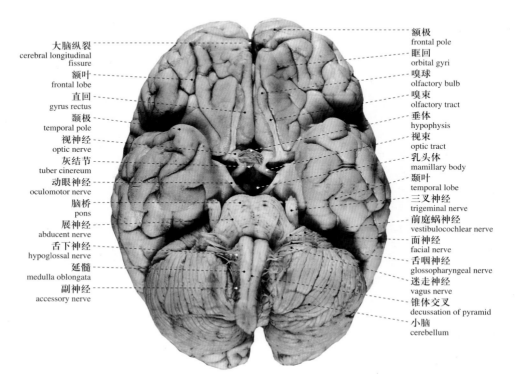

大脑纵裂 cerebral longitudinal fissure
额叶 frontal lobe
直回 gyrus rectus
颞极 temporal pole
视神经 optic nerve
灰结节 tuber cinereum
动眼神经 oculomotor nerve
脑桥 pons
展神经 abducent nerve
舌下神经 hypoglossal nerve
延髓 medulla oblongata
副神经 accessory nerve

额极 frontal pole
眶回 orbital gyri
嗅球 olfactory bulb
嗅束 olfactory tract
垂体 hypophysis
视束 optic tract
乳头体 mamillary body
颞叶 temporal lobe
三叉神经 trigeminal nerve
前庭蜗神经 vestibulocochlear nerve
面神经 facial nerve
舌咽神经 glossopharyngeal nerve
迷走神经 vagus nerve
锥体交叉 decussation of pyramid
小脑 cerebellum

图 480　大脑（下面观）
Cerebrum (inferior aspect)

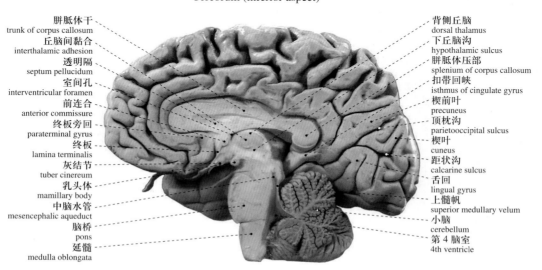

胼胝体干 trunk of corpus callosum
丘脑间黏合 interthalamic adhesion
透明隔 septum pellucidum
室间孔 interventricular foramen
前连合 anterior commissure
终板旁回 paraterminal gyrus
终板 lamina terminalis
灰结节 tuber cinereum
乳头体 mamillary body
中脑水管 mesencephalic aqueduct
脑桥 pons
延髓 medulla oblongata

背侧丘脑 dorsal thalamus
下丘脑沟 hypothalamic sulcus
胼胝体压部 splenium of corpus callosum
扣带回峡 isthmus of cingulate gyrus
楔前叶 precuneus
顶枕沟 parietooccipital sulcus
楔叶 cuneus
距状沟 calcarine sulcus
舌回 lingual gyrus
上髓帆 superior medullary velum
小脑 cerebellum
第 4 脑室 4th ventricle

图 481　大脑（正中矢状面）
Cerebrum (midsagittal section)

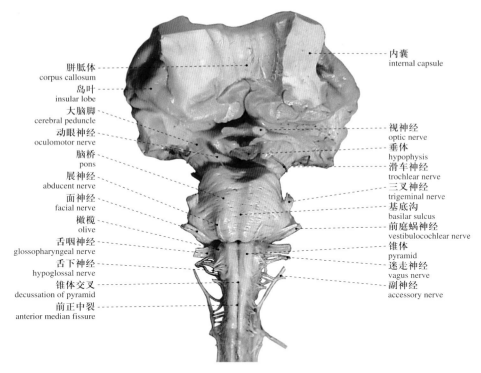

胼胝体
corpus callosum

岛叶
insular lobe

大脑脚
cerebral peduncle

动眼神经
oculomotor nerve

脑桥
pons

展神经
abducent nerve

面神经
facial nerve

橄榄
olive

舌咽神经
glossopharyngeal nerve

舌下神经
hypoglossal nerve

锥体交叉
decussation of pyramid

前正中裂
anterior median fissure

内囊
internal capsule

视神经
optic nerve

垂体
hypophysis

滑车神经
trochlear nerve

三叉神经
trigeminal nerve

基底沟
basilar sulcus

前庭蜗神经
vestibulocochlear nerve

锥体
pyramid

迷走神经
vagus nerve

副神经
accessory nerve

图 482　脑干（腹面观）
Brain stem (ventral aspect)

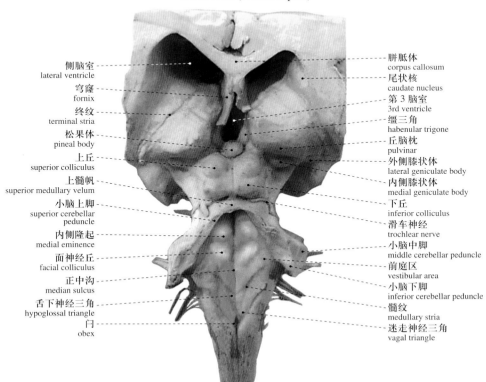

侧脑室
lateral ventricle

穹窿
fornix

终纹
terminal stria

松果体
pineal body

上丘
superior colliculus

上髓帆
superior medullary velum

小脑上脚
superior cerebellar peduncle

内侧隆起
medial eminence

面神经丘
facial colliculus

正中沟
median sulcus

舌下神经三角
hypoglossal triangle

闩
obex

胼胝体
corpus callosum

尾状核
caudate nucleus

第 3 脑室
3rd ventricle

缰三角
habenular trigone

丘脑枕
pulvinar

外侧膝状体
lateral geniculate body

内侧膝状体
medial geniculate body

下丘
inferior colliculus

滑车神经
trochlear nerve

小脑中脚
middle cerebellar peduncle

前庭区
vestibular area

小脑下脚
inferior cerebellar peduncle

髓纹
medullary stria

迷走神经三角
vagal triangle

图 483　脑干（背面观）
Brain stem (dorsal aspect)

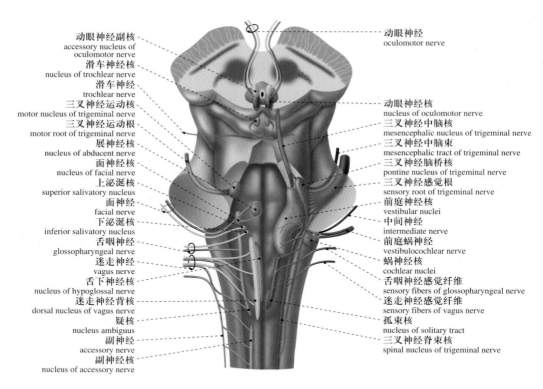

动眼神经副核
accessory nucleus of oculomotor nerve

滑车神经核
nucleus of trochlear nerve

滑车神经
trochlear nerve

三叉神经运动核
motor nucleus of trigeminal nerve

三叉神经运动根
motor root of trigeminal nerve

展神经核
nucleus of abducent nerve

面神经核
nucleus of facial nerve

上泌涎核
superior salivatory nucleus

面神经
facial nerve

下泌涎核
inferior salivatory nucleus

舌咽神经
glossopharyngeal nerve

迷走神经
vagus nerve

舌下神经核
nucleus of hypoglossal nerve

迷走神经背核
dorsal nucleus of vagus nerve

疑核
nucleus ambiguus

副神经
accessory nerve

副神经核
nucleus of accessory nerve

动眼神经
oculomotor nerve

动眼神经核
nucleus of oculomotor nerve

三叉神经中脑核
mesencephalic nucleus of trigeminal nerve

三叉神经中脑束
mesencephalic tract of trigeminal nerve

三叉神经脑桥核
pontine nucleus of trigeminal nerve

三叉神经感觉根
sensory root of trigeminal nerve

前庭神经核
vestibular nuclei

中间神经
intermediate nerve

前庭蜗神经
vestibulocochlear nerve

蜗神经核
cochlear nuclei

舌咽神经感觉纤维
sensory fibers of glossopharyngeal nerve

迷走神经感觉纤维
sensory fibers of vagus nerve

孤束核
nucleus of solitary tract

三叉神经脊束核
spinal nucleus of trigeminal nerve

图 484　脑神经核模式图（背面观）

Diagram of the nuclei of the cranial nerves (dorsal aspect)

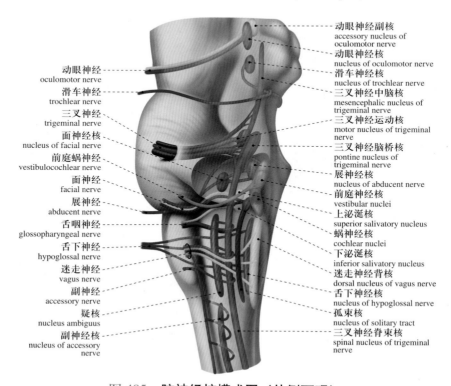

动眼神经
oculomotor nerve

滑车神经
trochlear nerve

三叉神经
trigeminal nerve

面神经核
nucleus of facial nerve

前庭蜗神经
vestibulocochlear nerve

面神经
facial nerve

展神经
abducent nerve

舌咽神经
glossopharyngeal nerve

舌下神经
hypoglossal nerve

迷走神经
vagus nerve

副神经
accessory nerve

疑核
nucleus ambiguus

副神经核
nucleus of accessory nerve

动眼神经副核
accessory nucleus of oculomotor nerve

动眼神经核
nucleus of oculomotor nerve

滑车神经核
nucleus of trochlear nerve

三叉神经中脑核
mesencephalic nucleus of trigeminal nerve

三叉神经运动核
motor nucleus of trigeminal nerve

三叉神经脑桥核
pontine nucleus of trigeminal nerve

展神经核
nucleus of abducent nerve

前庭神经核
vestibular nuclei

上泌涎核
superior salivatory nucleus

蜗神经核
cochlear nuclei

下泌涎核
inferior salivatory nucleus

迷走神经背核
dorsal nucleus of vagus nerve

舌下神经核
nucleus of hypoglossal nerve

孤束核
nucleus of solitary tract

三叉神经脊束核
spinal nucleus of trigeminal nerve

图 485　脑神经核模式图（外侧面观）

Diagram of the nuclei of the cranial nerves (lateral aspect)

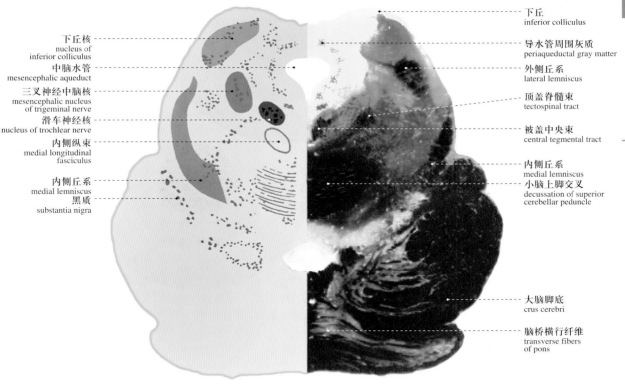

下丘
inferior colliculus

导水管周围灰质
periaqueductal gray matter

外侧丘系
lateral lemniscus

顶盖脊髓束
tectospinal tract

被盖中央束
central tegmental tract

内侧丘系
medial lemniscus

小脑上脚交叉
decussation of superior cerebellar peduncle

大脑脚底
crus cerebri

脑桥横行纤维
transverse fibers of pons

下丘核
nucleus of inferior colliculus

中脑水管
mesencephalic aqueduct

三叉神经中脑核
mesencephalic nucleus of trigeminal nerve

滑车神经核
nucleus of trochlear nerve

内侧纵束
medial longitudinal fasciculus

内侧丘系
medial lemniscus

黑质
substantia nigra

图 486　中脑横切面（经下丘）

Transverse section of the midbrain (through the inferior colliculus)

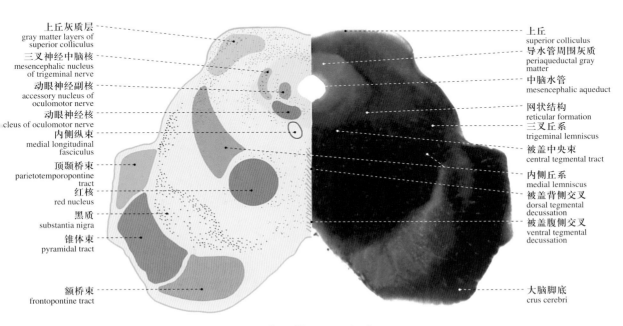

上丘
superior colliculus

导水管周围灰质
periaqueductal gray matter

中脑水管
mesencephalic aqueduct

网状结构
reticular formation

三叉丘系
trigeminal lemniscus

被盖中央束
central tegmental tract

内侧丘系
medial lemniscus

被盖背侧交叉
dorsal tegmental decussation

被盖腹侧交叉
ventral tegmental decussation

大脑脚底
crus cerebri

上丘灰质层
gray matter layers of superior colliculus

三叉神经中脑核
mesencephalic nucleus of trigeminal nerve

动眼神经副核
accessory nucleus of oculomotor nerve

动眼神经核
nucleus of oculomotor nerve

内侧纵束
medial longitudinal fasciculus

顶颞桥束
parietotemporopontine tract

红核
red nucleus

黑质
substantia nigra

锥体束
pyramidal tract

额桥束
frontopontine tract

图 487　中脑横切面（经上丘）

Transverse section of the midbrain (through the superior colliculus)

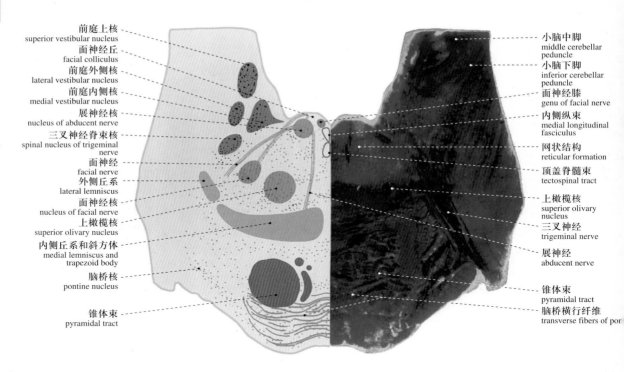

前庭上核
superior vestibular nucleus
面神经丘
facial colliculus
前庭外侧核
lateral vestibular nucleus
前庭内侧核
medial vestibular nucleus
展神经核
nucleus of abducent nerve
三叉神经脊束核
spinal nucleus of trigeminal nerve
面神经
facial nerve
外侧丘系
lateral lemniscus
面神经核
nucleus of facial nerve
上橄榄核
superior olivary nucleus
内侧丘系和斜方体
medial lemniscus and trapezoid body
脑桥核
pontine nucleus
锥体束
pyramidal tract

小脑中脚
middle cerebellar peduncle
小脑下脚
inferior cerebellar peduncle
面神经膝
genu of facial nerve
内侧纵束
medial longitudinal fasciculus
网状结构
reticular formation
顶盖脊髓束
tectospinal tract
上橄榄核
superior olivary nucleus
三叉神经
trigeminal nerve
展神经
abducent nerve
锥体束
pyramidal tract
脑桥横行纤维
transverse fibers of por

图 488　脑桥横切面（经面丘）
Transverse section of the pons (through the facial colliculus)

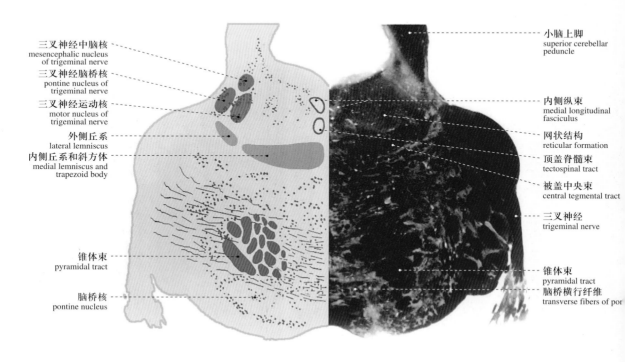

三叉神经中脑核
mesencephalic nucleus of trigeminal nerve
三叉神经脑桥核
pontine nucleus of trigeminal nerve
三叉神经运动核
motor nucleus of trigeminal nerve
外侧丘系
lateral lemniscus
内侧丘系和斜方体
medial lemniscus and trapezoid body
锥体束
pyramidal tract
脑桥核
pontine nucleus

小脑上脚
superior cerebellar peduncle
内侧纵束
medial longitudinal fasciculus
网状结构
reticular formation
顶盖脊髓束
tectospinal tract
被盖中央束
central tegmental tract
三叉神经
trigeminal nerve
锥体束
pyramidal tract
脑桥横行纤维
transverse fibers of por

图 489　脑桥中部横切面
Transverse section of the middle part of the pons

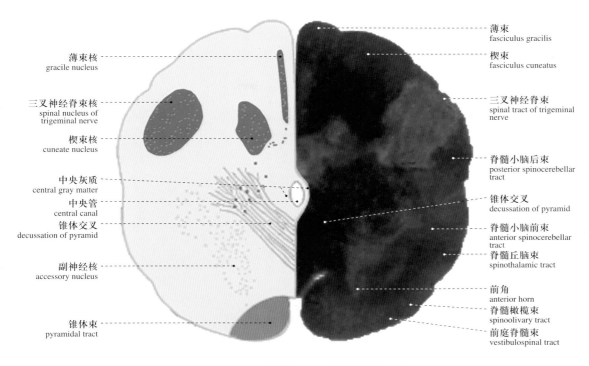

薄束
fasciculus gracilis

楔束
fasciculus cuneatus

三叉神经脊束
spinal tract of trigeminal nerve

脊髓小脑后束
posterior spinocerebellar tract

锥体交叉
decussation of pyramid

脊髓小脑前束
anterior spinocerebellar tract

脊髓丘脑束
spinothalamic tract

前角
anterior horn

脊髓橄榄束
spinoolivary tract

前庭脊髓束
vestibulospinal tract

薄束核
gracile nucleus

三叉神经脊束核
spinal nucleus of trigeminal nerve

楔束核
cuneate nucleus

中央灰质
central gray matter

中央管
central canal

锥体交叉
decussation of pyramid

副神经核
accessory nucleus

锥体束
pyramidal tract

图 490　延髓横切面（经锥体交叉）

Transverse section of the medulla oblongata (through the pyramidal decussation)

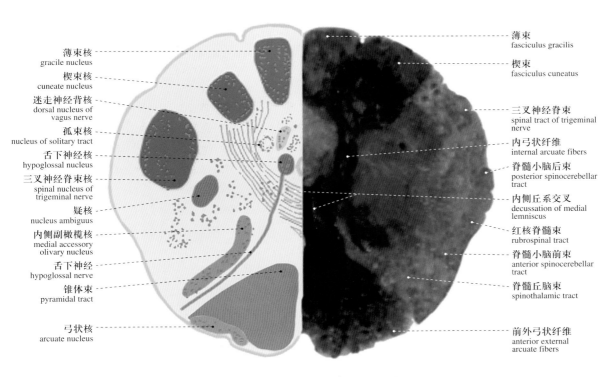

薄束核
gracile nucleus

楔束核
cuneate nucleus

迷走神经背核
dorsal nucleus of vagus nerve

孤束核
nucleus of solitary tract

舌下神经核
hypoglossal nucleus

三叉神经脊束核
spinal nucleus of trigeminal nerve

疑核
nucleus ambiguus

内侧副橄榄核
medial accessory olivary nucleus

舌下神经
hypoglossal nerve

锥体束
pyramidal tract

弓状核
arcuate nucleus

薄束
fasciculus gracilis

楔束
fasciculus cuneatus

三叉神经脊束
spinal tract of trigeminal nerve

内弓状纤维
internal arcuate fibers

脊髓小脑后束
posterior spinocerebellar tract

内侧丘系交叉
decussation of medial lemniscus

红核脊髓束
rubrospinal tract

脊髓小脑前束
anterior spinocerebellar tract

脊髓丘脑束
spinothalamic tract

前外弓状纤维
anterior external arcuate fibers

图 491　延髓横切面（经内侧丘系交叉）

Transverse section of the medulla oblongata (through the decussation of the medial lemniscus)

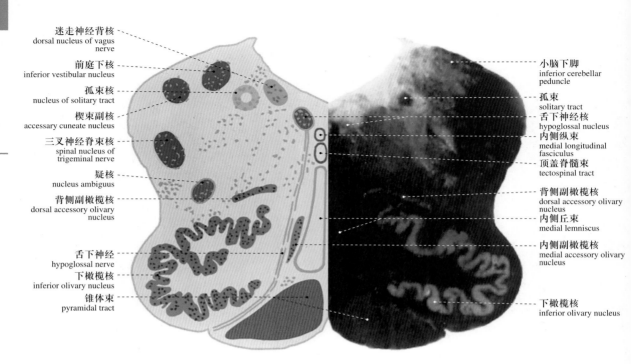

迷走神经背核
dorsal nucleus of vagus nerve

前庭下核
inferior vestibular nucleus

孤束核
nucleus of solitary tract

楔束副核
accessary cuneate nucleus

三叉神经脊束核
spinal nucleus of trigeminal nerve

疑核
nucleus ambiguus

背侧副橄榄核
dorsal accessory olivary nucleus

舌下神经
hypoglossal nerve

下橄榄核
inferior olivary nucleus

锥体束
pyramidal tract

小脑下脚
inferior cerebellar peduncle

孤束
solitary tract

舌下神经核
hypoglossal nucleus

内侧纵束
medial longitudinal fasciculus

顶盖脊髓束
tectospinal tract

背侧副橄榄核
dorsal accessory olivary nucleus

内侧丘束
medial lemniscus

内侧副橄榄核
medial accessory olivary nucleus

下橄榄核
inferior olivary nucleus

图 492　延髓横切面（经橄榄中部）

Transverse section of the medulla oblongata (through the middle portion of the olive)

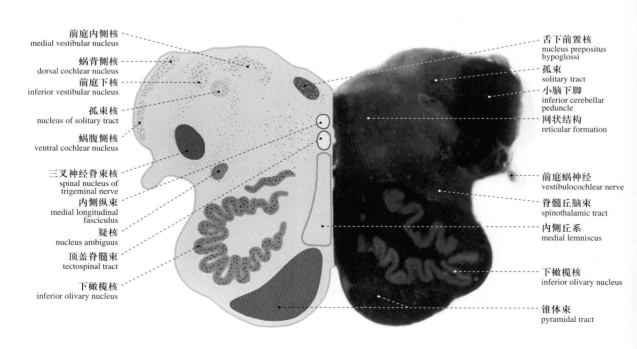

前庭内侧核
medial vestibular nucleus

蜗背侧核
dorsal cochlear nucleus

前庭下核
inferior vestibular nucleus

孤束核
nucleus of solitary tract

蜗腹侧核
ventral cochlear nucleus

三叉神经脊束核
spinal nucleus of trigeminal nerve

内侧纵束
medial longitudinal fasciculus

疑核
nucleus ambiguus

顶盖脊髓束
tectospinal tract

下橄榄核
inferior olivary nucleus

舌下前置核
nucleus prepositus hypoglossi

孤束
solitary tract

小脑下脚
inferior cerebellar peduncle

网状结构
reticular formation

前庭蜗神经
vestibulocochlear nerve

脊髓丘脑束
spinothalamic tract

内侧丘系
medial lemniscus

下橄榄核
inferior olivary nucleus

锥体束
pyramidal tract

图 493　延髓横切面（经橄榄上部）

Transverse section of the medulla oblongata (through the superior portion of the olive)

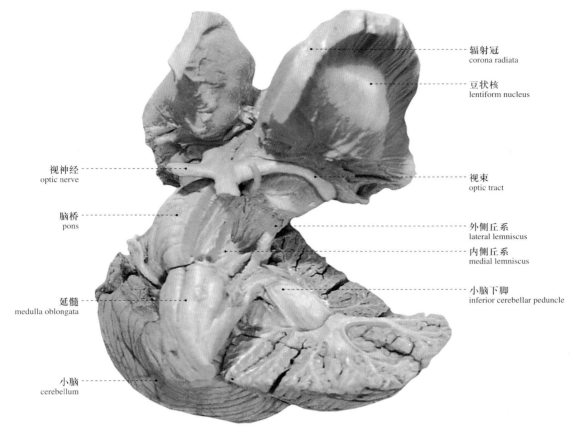

辐射冠
corona radiata

豆状核
lentiform nucleus

视神经
optic nerve

视束
optic tract

脑桥
pons

外侧丘系
lateral lemniscus

内侧丘系
medial lemniscus

延髓
medulla oblongata

小脑下脚
inferior cerebellar peduncle

小脑
cerebellum

图 494　内侧丘系和外侧丘系
Medial and lateral lemniscuses

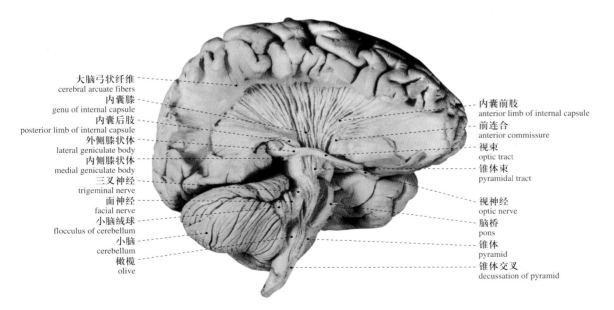

大脑弓状纤维
cerebral arcuate fibers

内囊膝
genu of internal capsule

内囊后肢
posterior limb of internal capsule

外侧膝状体
lateral geniculate body

内侧膝状体
medial geniculate body

三叉神经
trigeminal nerve

面神经
facial nerve

小脑绒球
flocculus of cerebellum

小脑
cerebellum

橄榄
olive

内囊前肢
anterior limb of internal capsule

前连合
anterior commissure

视束
optic tract

锥体束
pyramidal tract

视神经
optic nerve

脑桥
pons

锥体
pyramid

锥体交叉
decussation of pyramid

图 495　锥体束
Pyramidal tract

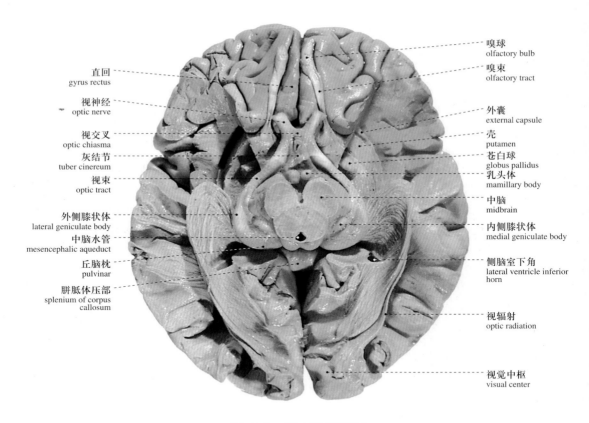

直回
gyrus rectus

视神经
optic nerve

视交叉
optic chiasma

灰结节
tuber cinereum

视束
optic tract

外侧膝状体
lateral geniculate body

中脑水管
mesencephalic aqueduct

丘脑枕
pulvinar

胼胝体压部
splenium of corpus callosum

嗅球
olfactory bulb

嗅束
olfactory tract

外囊
external capsule

壳
putamen

苍白球
globus pallidus

乳头体
mamillary body

中脑
midbrain

内侧膝状体
medial geniculate body

侧脑室下角
lateral ventricle inferior horn

视辐射
optic radiation

视觉中枢
visual center

图 496　视束及视辐射
Optic tract and the optic radiation

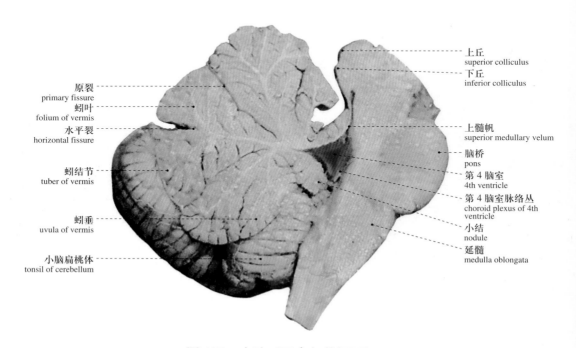

原裂
primary fissure

蚓叶
folium of vermis

水平裂
horizontal fissure

蚓结节
tuber of vermis

蚓垂
uvula of vermis

小脑扁桃体
tonsil of cerebellum

上丘
superior colliculus

下丘
inferior colliculus

上髓帆
superior medullary velum

脑桥
pons

第 4 脑室
4th ventricle

第 4 脑室脉络丛
choroid plexus of 4th ventricle

小结
nodule

延髓
medulla oblongata

图 497　小脑（正中矢状切面）
Cerebellum (median sagittal section)

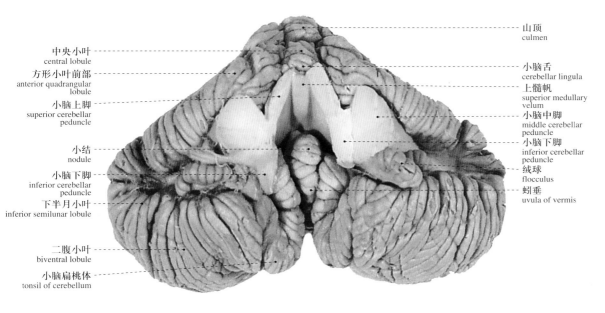

山顶
culmen

中央小叶
central lobule

方形小叶前部
anterior quadrangular lobule

小脑上脚
superior cerebellar peduncle

小结
nodule

小脑下脚
inferior cerebellar peduncle

下半月小叶
inferior semilunar lobule

二腹小叶
biventral lobule

小脑扁桃体
tonsil of cerebellum

小脑舌
cerebellar lingula

上髓帆
superior medullary velum

小脑中脚
middle cerebellar peduncle

小脑下脚
inferior cerebellar peduncle

绒球
flocculus

蚓垂
uvula of vermis

图 498　小脑（前面观）
Cerebellum (anterior aspect)

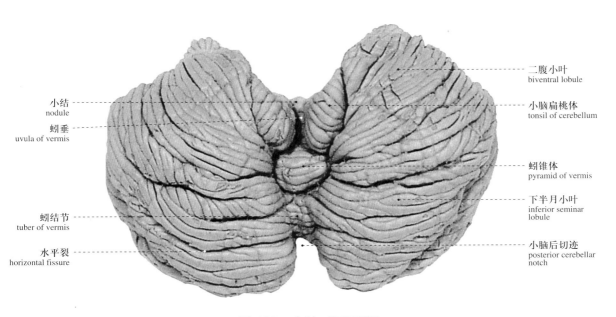

小结
nodule

蚓垂
uvula of vermis

蚓结节
tuber of vermis

水平裂
horizontal fissure

二腹小叶
biventral lobule

小脑扁桃体
tonsil of cerebellum

蚓锥体
pyramid of vermis

下半月小叶
inferior seminar lobule

小脑后切迹
posterior cerebellar notch

图 499　小脑（下面观）
Cerebellum (inferior aspect)

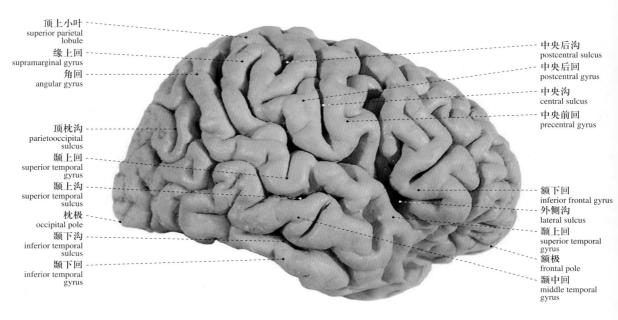

顶上小叶
superior parietal lobule

缘上回
supramarginal gyrus

角回
angular gyrus

顶枕沟
parietooccipital sulcus

颞上回
superior temporal gyrus

颞上沟
superior temporal sulcus

枕极
occipital pole

颞下沟
inferior temporal sulcus

颞下回
inferior temporal gyrus

中央后沟
postcentral sulcus

中央后回
postcentral gyrus

中央沟
central sulcus

中央前回
precentral gyrus

额下回
inferior frontal gyrus

外侧沟
lateral sulcus

颞上回
superior temporal gyrus

额极
frontal pole

颞中回
middle temporal gyrus

图 500　大脑（外侧面观）

Cerebrum (lateral aspect)

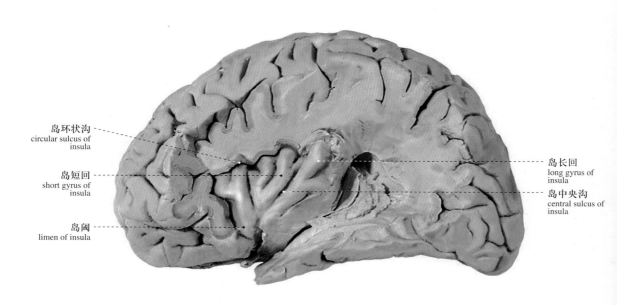

岛环状沟
circular sulcus of insula

岛短回
short gyrus of insula

岛阈
limen of insula

岛长回
long gyrus of insula

岛中央沟
central sulcus of insula

图 501　岛叶

Insular lobe

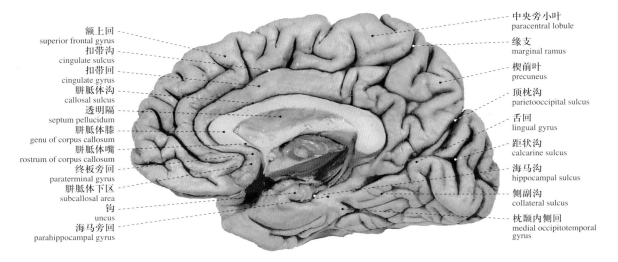

额上回
superior frontal gyrus

扣带沟
cingulate sulcus

扣带回
cingulate gyrus

胼胝体沟
callosal sulcus

透明隔
septum pellucidum

胼胝体膝
genu of corpus callosum

胼胝体嘴
rostrum of corpus callosum

终板旁回
paraterminal gyrus

胼胝体下区
subcallosal area

钩
uncus

海马旁回
parahippocampal gyrus

中央旁小叶
paracentral lobule

缘支
marginal ramus

楔前叶
precuneus

顶枕沟
parietooccipital sulcus

舌回
lingual gyrus

距状沟
calcarine sulcus

海马沟
hippocampal sulcus

侧副沟
collateral sulcus

枕颞内侧回
medial occipitotemporal gyrus

图 502 大脑（正中矢状面）
Cerebrum (midsagittal section)

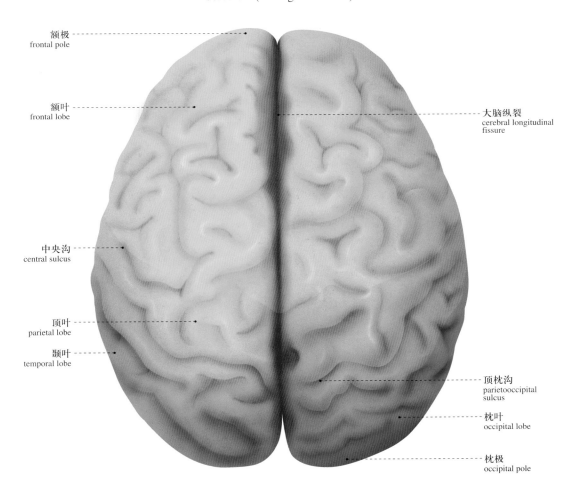

额极
frontal pole

额叶
frontal lobe

中央沟
central sulcus

顶叶
parietal lobe

颞叶
temporal lobe

大脑纵裂
cerebral longitudinal fissure

顶枕沟
parietooccipital sulcus

枕叶
occipital lobe

枕极
occipital pole

图 503 大脑分叶（上面观）
Division of the cerebrum into lobes (superior aspect)

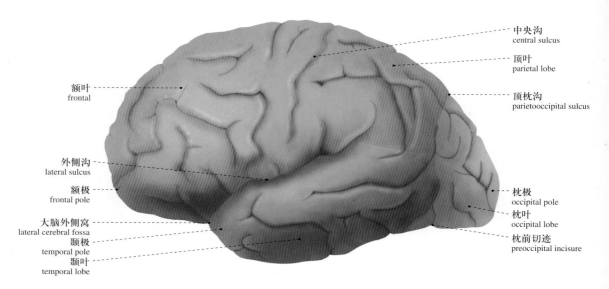

中央沟
central sulcus

顶叶
parietal lobe

顶枕沟
parietooccipital sulcus

额叶
frontal

外侧沟
lateral sulcus

额极
frontal pole

大脑外侧窝
lateral cerebral fossa

颞极
temporal pole

颞叶
temporal lobe

枕极
occipital pole

枕叶
occipital lobe

枕前切迹
preoccipital incisure

图 504　大脑分叶（外侧面观）
Division of the cerebrum into lobes (lateral aspect)

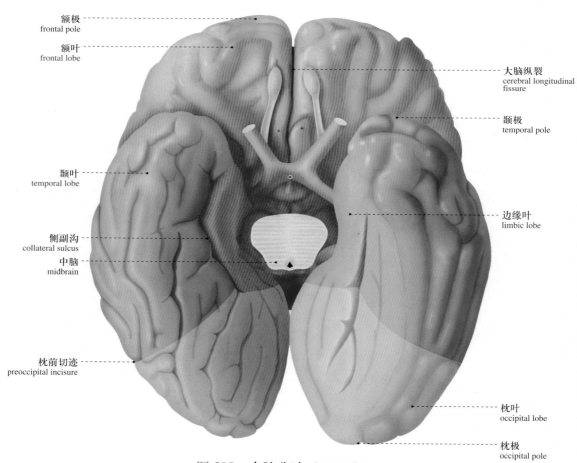

额极
frontal pole

额叶
frontal lobe

大脑纵裂
cerebral longitudinal fissure

颞极
temporal pole

颞叶
temporal lobe

侧副沟
collateral sulcus

中脑
midbrain

边缘叶
limbic lobe

枕前切迹
preoccipital incisure

枕叶
occipital lobe

枕极
occipital pole

图 505　大脑分叶（下面观）
Division of the cerebrum into lobes (inferior aspect)

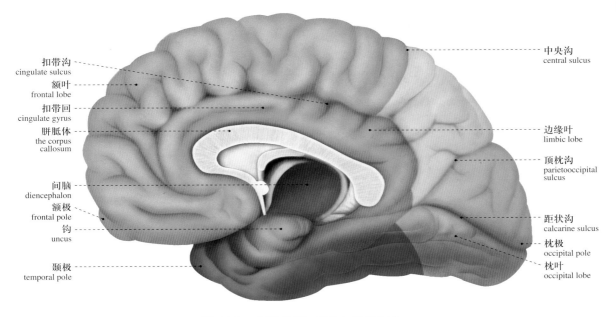

扣带沟
cingulate sulcus

额叶
frontal lobe

扣带回
cingulate gyrus

胼胝体
the corpus callosum

间脑
diencephalon

额极
frontal pole

钩
uncus

颞极
temporal pole

中央沟
central sulcus

边缘叶
limbic lobe

顶枕沟
parietooccipital sulcus

距状沟
calcarine sulcus

枕极
occipital pole

枕叶
occipital lobe

图 506　大脑分叶（正中矢状面）
Division of the cerebrum into lobes (midsagittal section aspect)

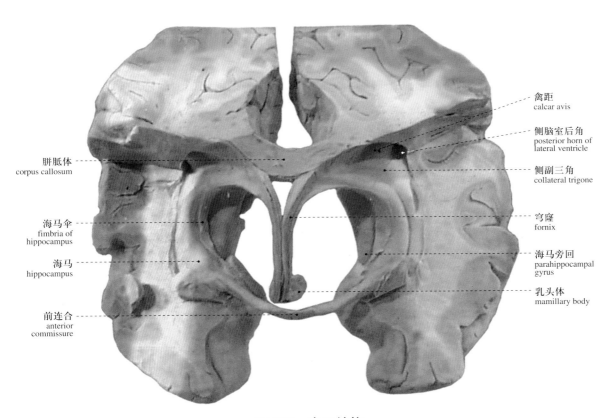

胼胝体
corpus callosum

海马伞
fimbria of hippocampus

海马
hippocampus

前连合
anterior commissure

禽距
calcar avis

侧脑室后角
posterior horn of lateral ventricle

侧副三角
collateral trigone

穹窿
fornix

海马旁回
parahippocampal gyrus

乳头体
mamillary body

图 507　海马结构
Hippocampal formation

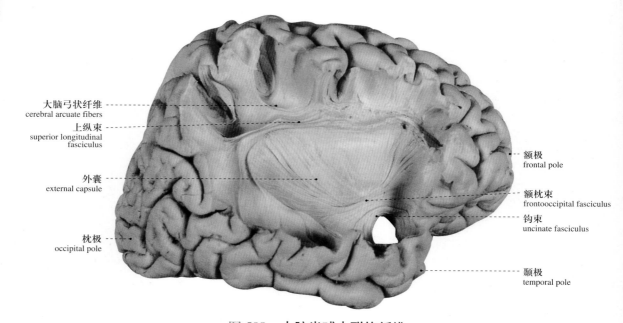

大脑弓状纤维
cerebral arcuate fibers

上纵束
superior longitudinal
fasciculus

外囊
external capsule

枕极
occipital pole

额极
frontal pole

额枕束
frontooccipital fasciculus

钩束
uncinate fasciculus

颞极
temporal pole

图 508　大脑半球内联络纤维
Association fibers in the cerebral hemisphere

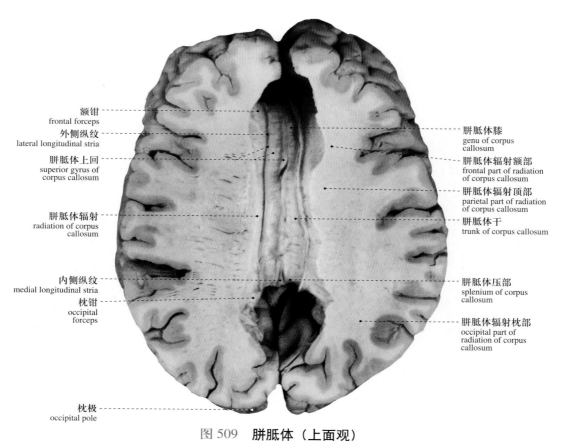

额钳
frontal forceps

外侧纵纹
lateral longitudinal stria

胼胝体上回
superior gyrus of
corpus callosum

胼胝体辐射
radiation of corpus
callosum

内侧纵纹
medial longitudinal stria

枕钳
occipital forceps

枕极
occipital pole

胼胝体膝
genu of corpus
callosum

胼胝体辐射额部
frontal part of radiation
of corpus callosum

胼胝体辐射顶部
parietal part of radiation
of corpus callosum

胼胝体干
trunk of corpus callosum

胼胝体压部
splenium of corpus
callosum

胼胝体辐射枕部
occipital part of
radiation of corpus
callosum

图 509　胼胝体（上面观）
Corpus callosum (superior aspect)

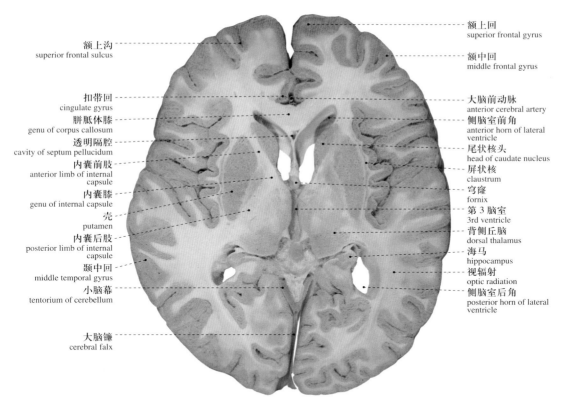

額上沟
superior frontal sulcus

扣带回
cingulate gyrus

胼胝体膝
genu of corpus callosum

透明隔腔
cavity of septum pellucidum

内囊前肢
anterior limb of internal capsule

内囊膝
genu of internal capsule

壳
putamen

内囊后肢
posterior limb of internal capsule

颞中回
middle temporal gyrus

小脑幕
tentorium of cerebellum

大脑镰
cerebral falx

额上回
superior frontal gyrus

额中回
middle frontal gyrus

大脑前动脉
anterior cerebral artery

侧脑室前角
anterior horn of lateral ventricle

尾状核头
head of caudate nucleus

屏状核
claustrum

穹窿
fornix

第 3 脑室
3rd ventricle

背侧丘脑
dorsal thalamus

海马
hippocampus

视辐射
optic radiation

侧脑室后角
posterior horn of lateral ventricle

图 510　脑水平断面
Horizontal section of the brain

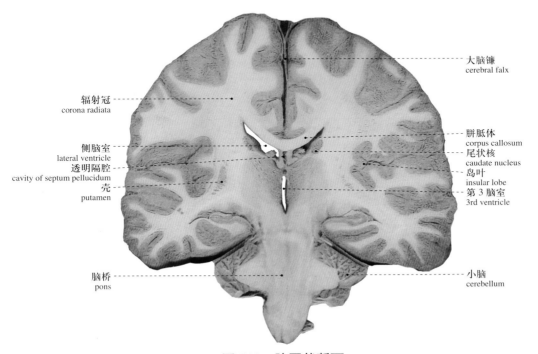

辐射冠
corona radiata

侧脑室
lateral ventricle

透明隔腔
cavity of septum pellucidum

壳
putamen

脑桥
pons

大脑镰
cerebral falx

胼胝体
corpus callosum

尾状核
caudate nucleus

岛叶
insular lobe

第 3 脑室
3rd ventricle

小脑
cerebellum

图 511　脑冠状断面
Frontal section of the brain

275

第一节

脊 神 经

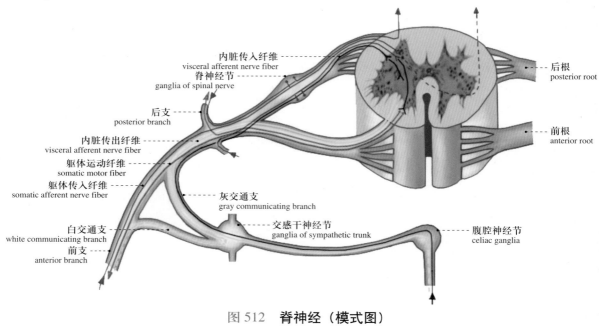

内脏传入纤维
visceral afferent nerve fiber
脊神经节
ganglia of spinal nerve
后支
posterior branch
内脏传出纤维
visceral efferent nerve fiber
躯体运动纤维
somatic motor fiber
躯体传入纤维
somatic afferent nerve fiber
白交通支
white communicating branch
前支
anterior branch
灰交通支
gray communicating branch
交感干神经节
ganglia of sympathetic trunk
后根
posterior root
前根
anterior root
腹腔神经节
celiac ganglia

图 512　脊神经（模式图）

Spinal nerve (diagram)

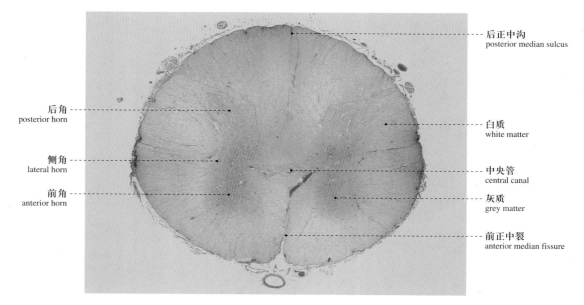

后角
posterior horn
侧角
lateral horn
前角
anterior horn
后正中沟
posterior median sulcus
白质
white matter
中央管
central canal
灰质
grey matter
前正中裂
anterior median fissure

图 513　脊髓（人脊髓，横切面，×40）

Spinal cord (human spinal cord, transverse section, ×40)

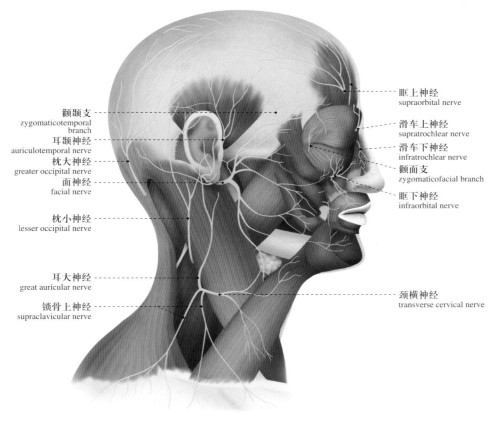

颞颧支
zygomaticotemporal branch

耳颞神经
auriculotemporal nerve

枕大神经
greater occipital nerve

面神经
facial nerve

枕小神经
lesser occipital nerve

耳大神经
great auricular nerve

锁骨上神经
supraclavicular nerve

眶上神经
supraorbital nerve

滑车上神经
supratrochlear nerve

滑车下神经
infratrochlear nerve

颧面支
zygomaticofacial branch

眶下神经
infraorbital nerve

颈横神经
transverse cervical nerve

图 514　头颈部感觉神经分布

Sensory nerve distribution of the head and neck

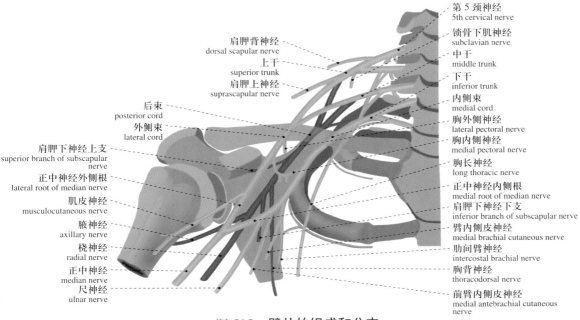

肩胛背神经
dorsal scapular nerve

上干
superior trunk

肩胛上神经
suprascapular nerve

后束
posterior cord

外侧束
lateral cord

肩胛下神经上支
superior branch of subscapular nerve

正中神经外侧根
lateral root of median nerve

肌皮神经
musculocutaneous nerve

腋神经
axillary nerve

桡神经
radial nerve

正中神经
median nerve

尺神经
ulnar nerve

第 5 颈神经
5th cervical nerve

锁骨下肌神经
subclavian nerve

中干
middle trunk

下干
inferior trunk

内侧束
medial cord

胸外侧神经
lateral pectoral nerve

胸内侧神经
medial pectoral nerve

胸长神经
long thoracic nerve

正中神经内侧根
medial root of median nerve

肩胛下神经下支
inferior branch of subscapular nerve

臂内侧皮神经
medial brachial cutaneous nerve

肋间臂神经
intercostal brachial nerve

胸背神经
thoracodorsal nerve

前臂内侧皮神经
medial antebrachial cutaneous nerve

图 515　臂丛的组成和分支

Constitution and branches of the brachial plexus

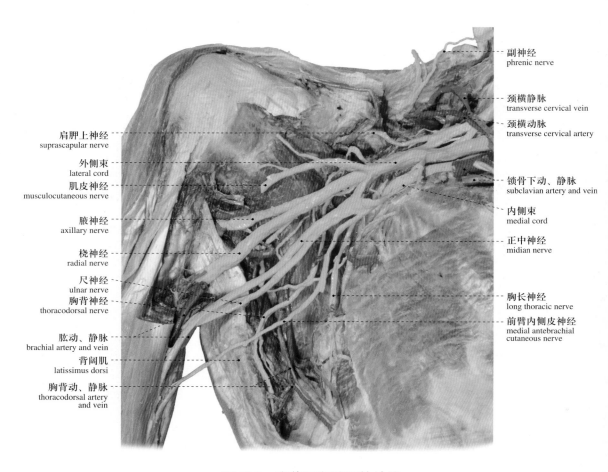

肩胛上神经
suprascapular nerve

外侧束
lateral cord

肌皮神经
musculocutaneous nerve

腋神经
axillary nerve

桡神经
radial nerve

尺神经
ulnar nerve

胸背神经
thoracodorsal nerve

肱动、静脉
brachial artery and vein

背阔肌
latissimus dorsi

胸背动、静脉
thoracodorsal artery
and vein

副神经
phrenic nerve

颈横静脉
transverse cervical vein

颈横动脉
transverse cervical artery

锁骨下动、静脉
subclavian artery and vein

内侧束
medial cord

正中神经
midian nerve

胸长神经
long thoracic nerve

前臂内侧皮神经
medial antebrachial
cutaneous nerve

图 516　肩前区和腋区的神经

Nerves of anterior region of the shoulder and the axillary region

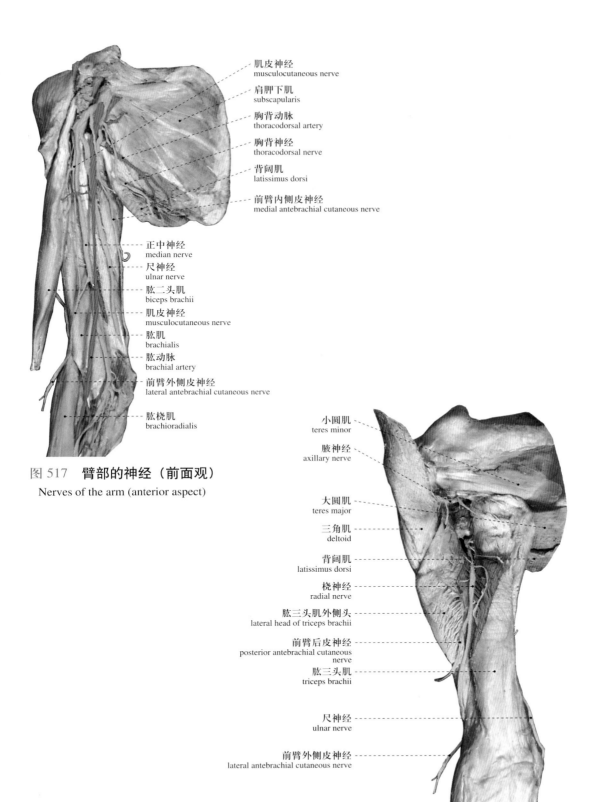

肌皮神经
musculocutaneous nerve

肩胛下肌
subscapularis

胸背动脉
thoracodorsal artery

胸背神经
thoracodorsal nerve

背阔肌
latissimus dorsi

前臂内侧皮神经
medial antebrachial cutaneous nerve

正中神经
median nerve

尺神经
ulnar nerve

肱二头肌
biceps brachii

肌皮神经
musculocutaneous nerve

肱肌
brachialis

肱动脉
brachial artery

前臂外侧皮神经
lateral antebrachial cutaneous nerve

肱桡肌
brachioradialis

图 517　臂部的神经（前面观）
Nerves of the arm (anterior aspect)

小圆肌
teres minor

腋神经
axillary nerve

大圆肌
teres major

三角肌
deltoid

背阔肌
latissimus dorsi

桡神经
radial nerve

肱三头肌外侧头
lateral head of triceps brachii

前臂后皮神经
posterior antebrachial cutaneous nerve

肱三头肌
triceps brachii

尺神经
ulnar nerve

前臂外侧皮神经
lateral antebrachial cutaneous nerve

图 518　臂部的神经（后面观）
Nerves of the arm (posterior aspect)

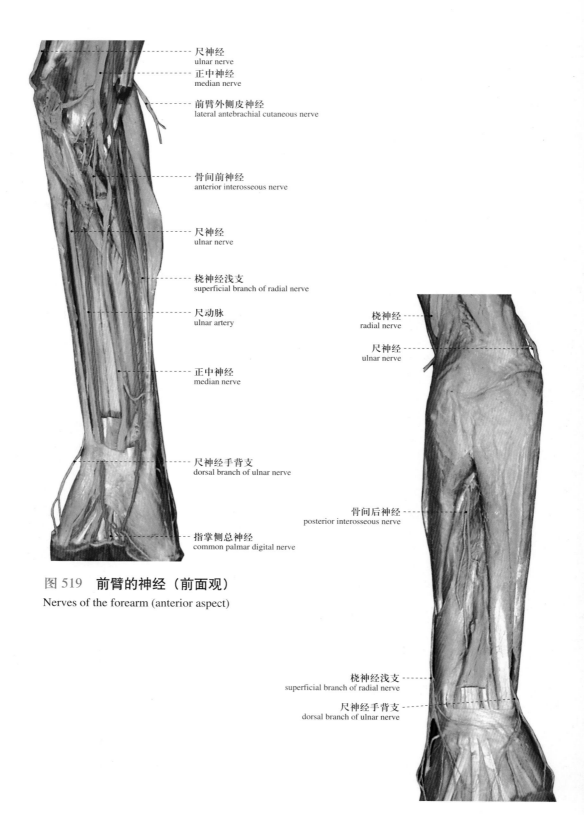

尺神经
ulnar nerve

正中神经
median nerve

前臂外侧皮神经
lateral antebrachial cutaneous nerve

骨间前神经
anterior interosseous nerve

尺神经
ulnar nerve

桡神经浅支
superficial branch of radial nerve

尺动脉
ulnar artery

正中神经
median nerve

尺神经手背支
dorsal branch of ulnar nerve

指掌侧总神经
common palmar digital nerve

图 519　前臂的神经（前面观）
Nerves of the forearm (anterior aspect)

桡神经
radial nerve

尺神经
ulnar nerve

骨间后神经
posterior interosseous nerve

桡神经浅支
superficial branch of radial nerve

尺神经手背支
dorsal branch of ulnar nerve

图 520　前臂的神经（后面观）
Nerves of the forearm (posterior aspect)

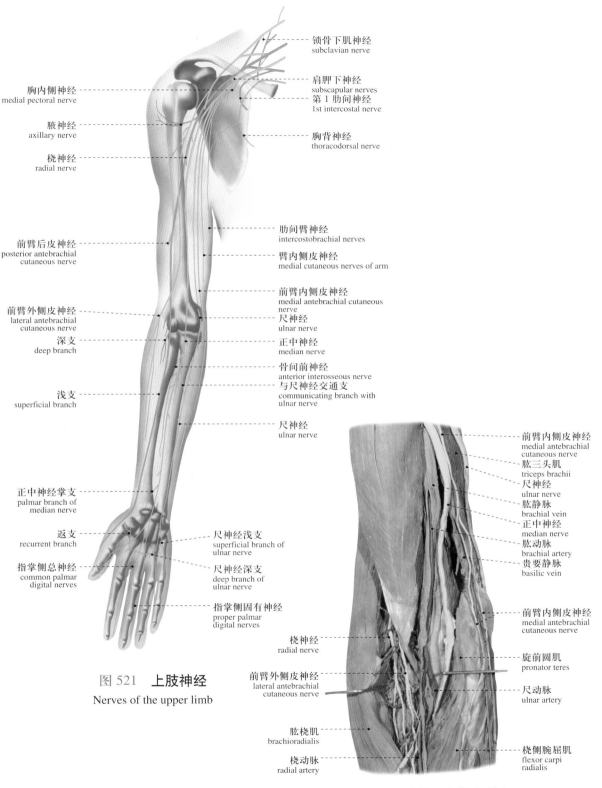

锁骨下肌神经
subclavian nerve

肩胛下神经
subscapular nerves

第 1 肋间神经
1st intercostal nerve

胸背神经
thoracodorsal nerve

胸内侧神经
medial pectoral nerve

腋神经
axillary nerve

桡神经
radial nerve

肋间臂神经
intercostobrachial nerves

臂内侧皮神经
medial cutaneous nerves of arm

前臂后皮神经
posterior antebrachial
cutaneous nerve

前臂内侧皮神经
medial antebrachial cutaneous
nerve

前臂外侧皮神经
lateral antebrachial
cutaneous nerve

尺神经
ulnar nerve

深支
deep branch

正中神经
median nerve

骨间前神经
anterior interosseous nerve

与尺神经交通支
communicating branch with
ulnar nerve

浅支
superficial branch

尺神经
ulnar nerve

正中神经掌支
palmar branch of
median nerve

返支
recurrent branch

指掌侧总神经
common palmar
digital nerves

尺神经浅支
superficial branch of
ulnar nerve

尺神经深支
deep branch of
ulnar nerve

指掌侧固有神经
proper palmar
digital nerves

图 521　上肢神经
Nerves of the upper limb

前臂内侧皮神经
medial antebrachial
cutaneous nerve

肱三头肌
triceps brachii

尺神经
ulnar nerve

肱静脉
brachial vein

正中神经
median nerve

肱动脉
brachial artery

贵要静脉
basilic vein

前臂内侧皮神经
medial antebrachial
cutaneous nerve

旋前圆肌
pronator teres

尺动脉
ulnar artery

桡侧腕屈肌
flexor carpi
radialis

桡神经
radial nerve

前臂外侧皮神经
lateral antebrachial
cutaneous nerve

肱桡肌
brachioradialis

桡动脉
radial artery

图 522　肘前区血管和神经
Blood vessels and nerves of the anterior cubital region

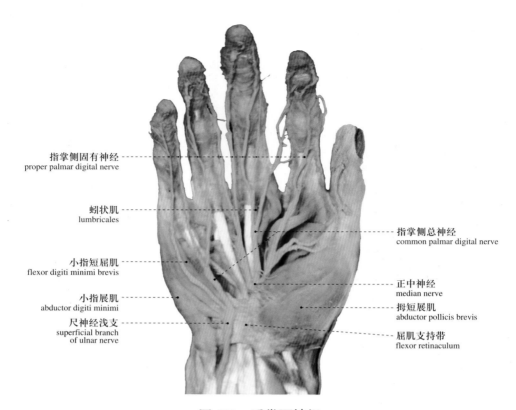

指掌侧固有神经
proper palmar digital nerve

蚓状肌
lumbricales

小指短屈肌
flexor digiti minimi brevis

小指展肌
abductor digiti minimi

尺神经浅支
superficial branch
of ulnar nerve

指掌侧总神经
common palmar digital nerve

正中神经
median nerve

拇短展肌
abductor pollicis brevis

屈肌支持带
flexor retinaculum

图 523　手掌面神经

Nerves of the palmar aspect of the hand

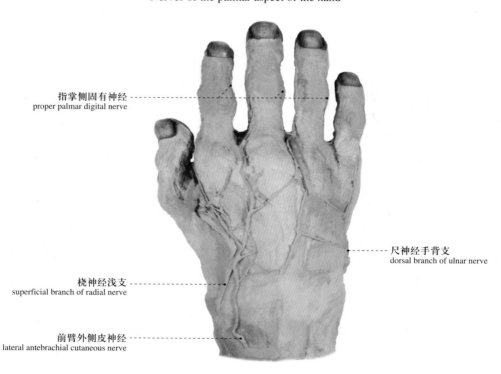

指掌侧固有神经
proper palmar digital nerve

尺神经手背支
dorsal branch of ulnar nerve

桡神经浅支
superficial branch of radial nerve

前臂外侧皮神经
lateral antebrachial cutaneous nerve

图 524　手背面神经

Nerves of the dorsal aspect of the hand

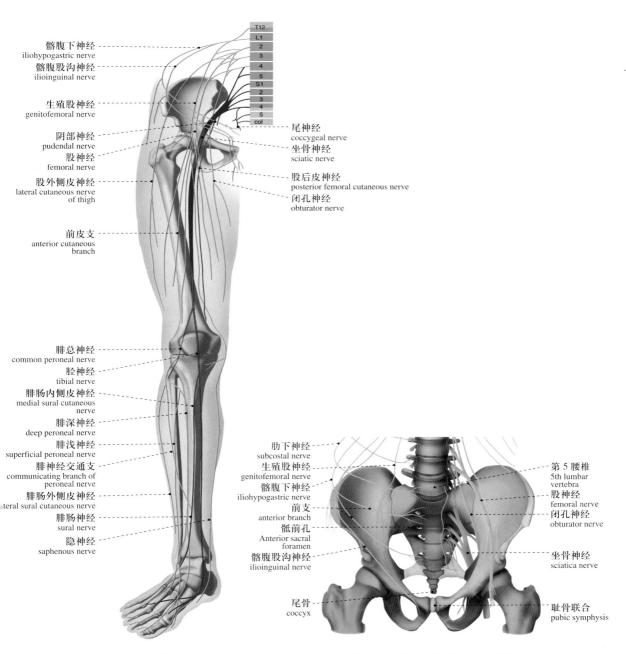

髂腹下神经
iliohypogastric nerve

髂腹股沟神经
ilioinguinal nerve

生殖股神经
genitofemoral nerve

阴部神经
pudendal nerve

股神经
femoral nerve

股外侧皮神经
lateral cutaneous nerve
of thigh

前皮支
anterior cutaneous
branch

腓总神经
common peroneal nerve

胫神经
tibial nerve

腓肠内侧皮神经
medial sural cutaneous
nerve

腓深神经
deep peroneal nerve

腓浅神经
superficial peroneal nerve

腓神经交通支
communicating branch of
peroneal nerve

腓肠外侧皮神经
lateral sural cutaneous nerve

腓肠神经
sural nerve

隐神经
saphenous nerve

T12
L1
2
3
4
5
S1
2
3
4
5
col

尾神经
coccygeal nerve

坐骨神经
sciatic nerve

股后皮神经
posterior femoral cutaneous nerve

闭孔神经
obturator nerve

图 525　下肢的神经（模式图）
Nerves of the lower limb (diagram)

肋下神经
subcostal nerve

生殖股神经
genitofemoral nerve

髂腹下神经
iliohypogastric nerve

前支
anterior branch

骶前孔
Anterior sacral
foramen

髂腹股沟神经
ilioinguinal nerve

尾骨
coccyx

第 5 腰椎
5th lumbar
vertebra

股神经
femoral nerve

闭孔神经
obturator nerve

坐骨神经
sciatica nerve

耻骨联合
pubic symphysis

图 526　盆腔的神经（模式图）
Pelvic nerves (diagram)

283

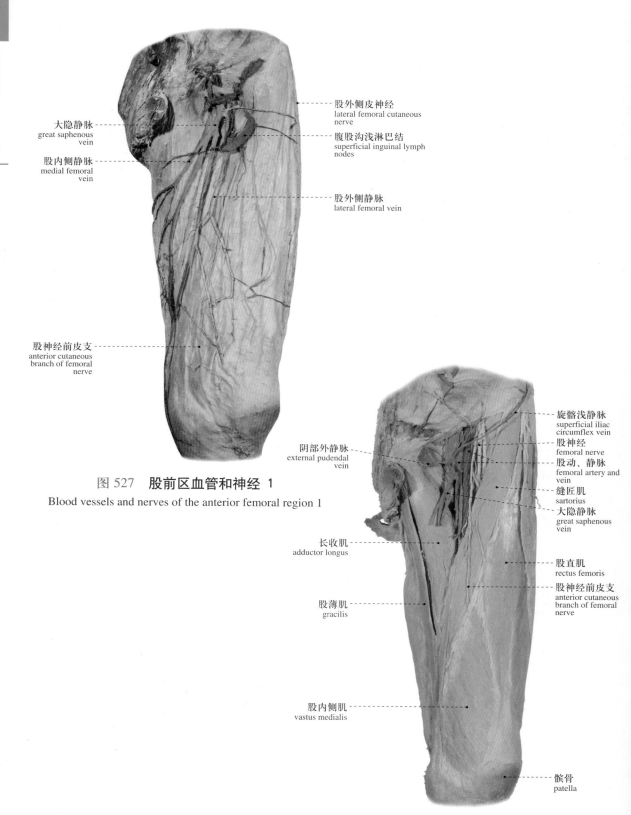

股外侧皮神经
lateral femoral cutaneous nerve

大隐静脉
great saphenous vein

腹股沟浅淋巴结
superficial inguinal lymph nodes

股内侧静脉
medial femoral vein

股外侧静脉
lateral femoral vein

股神经前皮支
anterior cutaneous branch of femoral nerve

图 527　股前区血管和神经 1
Blood vessels and nerves of the anterior femoral region 1

阴部外静脉
external pudendal vein

长收肌
adductor longus

股薄肌
gracilis

股内侧肌
vastus medialis

旋髂浅静脉
superficial iliac circumflex vein

股神经
femoral nerve

股动、静脉
femoral artery and vein

缝匠肌
sartorius

大隐静脉
great saphenous vein

股直肌
rectus femoris

股神经前皮支
anterior cutaneous branch of femoral nerve

髌骨
patella

图 528　股前区血管和神经 2
Blood vessels and nerves of the anterior femoral region 2

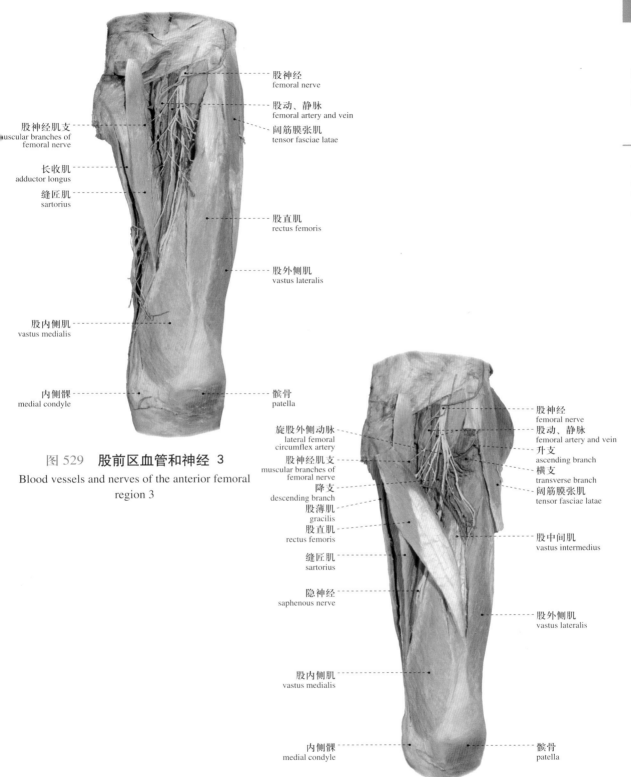

股神经
femoral nerve

股动、静脉
femoral artery and vein

阔筋膜张肌
tensor fasciae latae

股神经肌支
muscular branches of
femoral nerve

长收肌
adductor longus

缝匠肌
sartorius

股直肌
rectus femoris

股外侧肌
vastus lateralis

股内侧肌
vastus medialis

内侧髁
medial condyle

髌骨
patella

图 529　股前区血管和神经 3
Blood vessels and nerves of the anterior femoral
region 3

旋股外侧动脉
lateral femoral
circumflex artery

股神经肌支
muscular branches of
femoral nerve

降支
descending branch

股薄肌
gracilis

股直肌
rectus femoris

缝匠肌
sartorius

隐神经
saphenous nerve

股内侧肌
vastus medialis

内侧髁
medial condyle

股神经
femoral nerve

股动、静脉
femoral artery and vein

升支
ascending branch

横支
transverse branch

阔筋膜张肌
tensor fasciae latae

股中间肌
vastus intermedius

股外侧肌
vastus lateralis

髌骨
patella

图 530　股前区血管和神经 4
Blood vessels and nerves of the anterior femoral region 4

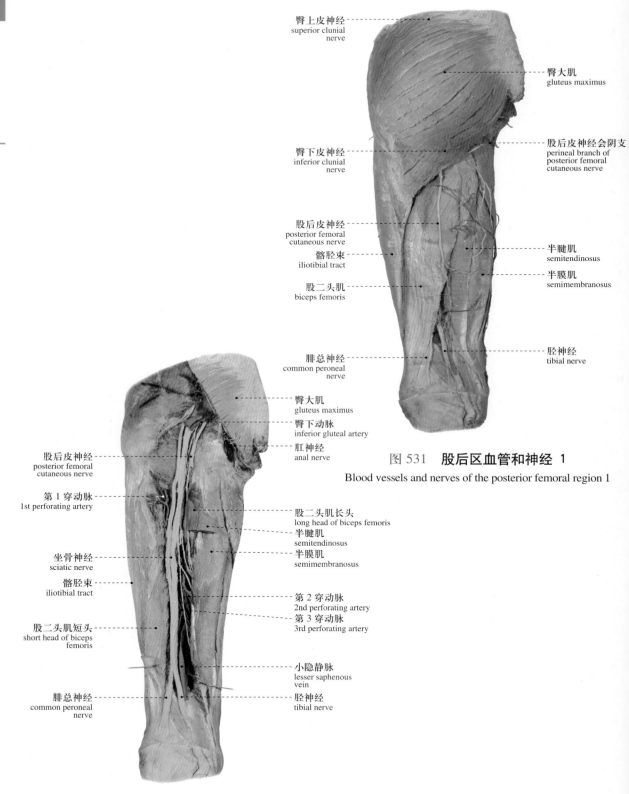

臀上皮神经
superior clunial nerve

臀大肌
gluteus maximus

股后皮神经会阴支
perineal branch of posterior femoral cutaneous nerve

臀下皮神经
inferior clunial nerve

股后皮神经
posterior femoral cutaneous nerve

髂胫束
iliotibial tract

股二头肌
biceps femoris

半腱肌
semitendinosus

半膜肌
semimembranosus

腓总神经
common peroneal nerve

胫神经
tibial nerve

图 531　股后区血管和神经 1
Blood vessels and nerves of the posterior femoral region 1

臀大肌
gluteus maximus

臀下动脉
inferior gluteal artery

肛神经
anal nerve

股后皮神经
posterior femoral cutaneous nerve

第 1 穿动脉
1st perforating artery

股二头肌长头
long head of biceps femoris

半腱肌
semitendinosus

半膜肌
semimembranosus

坐骨神经
sciatic nerve

髂胫束
iliotibial tract

第 2 穿动脉
2nd perforating artery

第 3 穿动脉
3rd perforating artery

股二头肌短头
short head of biceps femoris

小隐静脉
lesser saphenous vein

腓总神经
common peroneal nerve

胫神经
tibial nerve

图 532　股后区血管和神经 2
Blood vessels and nerves of the posterior femoral region 2

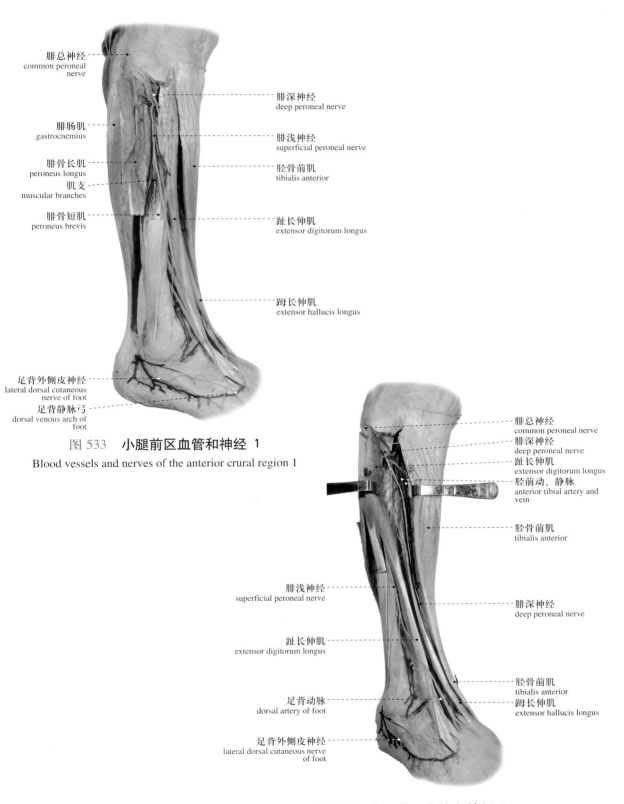

腓总神经
common peroneal nerve

腓肠肌
gastrocnemius

腓骨长肌
peroneus longus

肌支
muscular branches

腓骨短肌
peroneus brevis

足背外侧皮神经
lateral dorsal cutaneous nerve of foot

足背静脉弓
dorsal venous arch of foot

腓深神经
deep peroneal nerve

腓浅神经
superficial peroneal nerve

胫骨前肌
tibialis anterior

趾长伸肌
extensor digitorum longus

蹞长伸肌
extensor hallucis longus

图 533　小腿前区血管和神经　1
Blood vessels and nerves of the anterior crural region 1

腓总神经
common peroneal nerve

腓深神经
deep peroneal nerve

趾长伸肌
extensor digitorum longus

胫前动、静脉
anterior tibial artery and vein

胫骨前肌
tibialis anterior

腓深神经
deep peroneal nerve

腓浅神经
superficial peroneal nerve

趾长伸肌
extensor digitorum longus

胫骨前肌
tibialis anterior

足背动脉
dorsal artery of foot

蹞长伸肌
extensor hallucis longus

足背外侧皮神经
lateral dorsal cutaneous nerve of foot

图 534　小腿前区血管和神经　2
Blood vessels and nerves of the anterior crural region 2

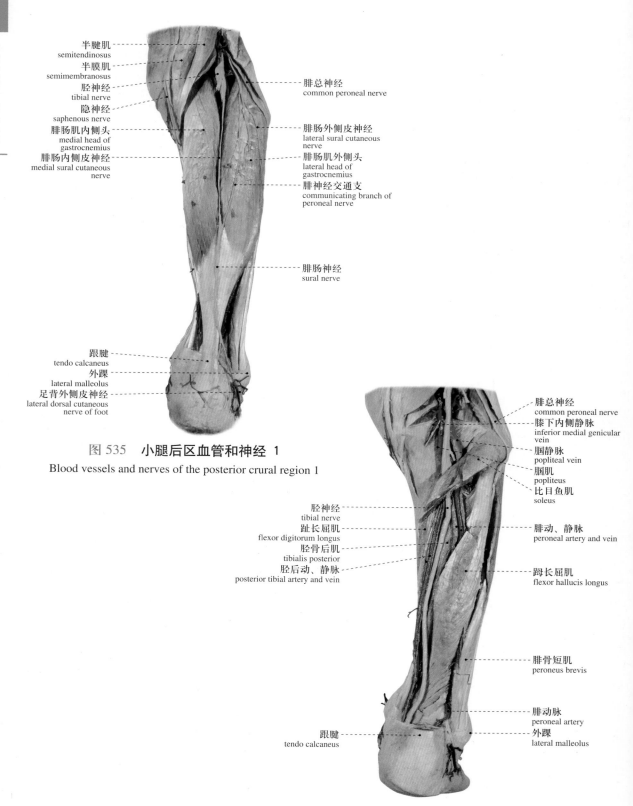

半腱肌
semitendinosus

半膜肌
semimembranosus

腓总神经
common peroneal nerve

胫神经
tibial nerve

隐神经
saphenous nerve

腓肠外侧皮神经
lateral sural cutaneous nerve

腓肠肌内侧头
medial head of gastrocnemius

腓肠肌外侧头
lateral head of gastrocnemius

腓肠内侧皮神经
medial sural cutaneous nerve

腓神经交通支
communicating branch of peroneal nerve

腓肠神经
sural nerve

跟腱
tendo calcaneus

外踝
lateral malleolus

足背外侧皮神经
lateral dorsal cutaneous nerve of foot

图 535　小腿后区血管和神经 1
Blood vessels and nerves of the posterior crural region 1

腓总神经
common peroneal nerve

膝下内侧静脉
inferior medial genicular vein

腘静脉
popliteal vein

腘肌
popliteus

比目鱼肌
soleus

腓动、静脉
peroneal artery and vein

胫神经
tibial nerve

趾长屈肌
flexor digitorum longus

胫骨后肌
tibialis posterior

胫后动、静脉
posterior tibial artery and vein

蹬长屈肌
flexor hallucis longus

腓骨短肌
peroneus brevis

腓动脉
peroneal artery

外踝
lateral malleolus

跟腱
tendo calcaneus

图 536　小腿后区血管和神经 2
Blood vessels and nerves of the posterior crural region 2

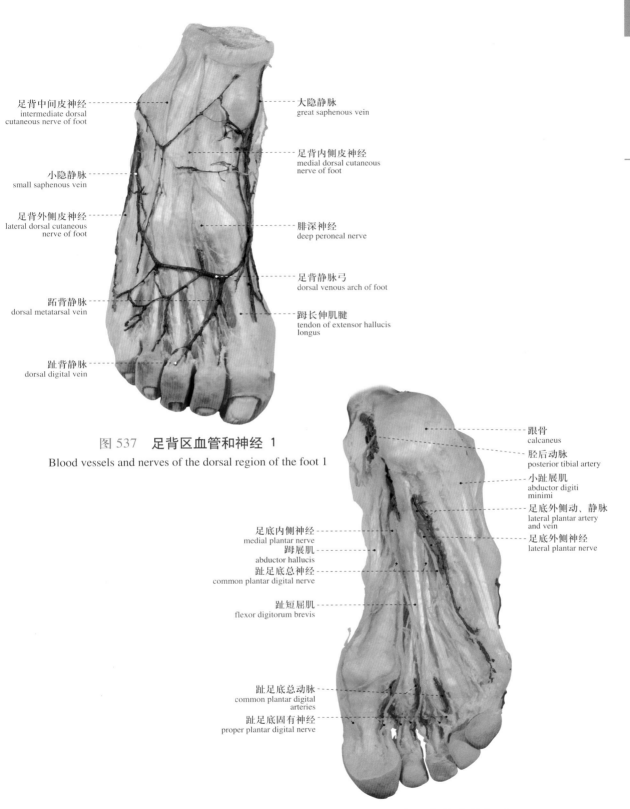

足背中间皮神经
intermediate dorsal
cutaneous nerve of foot

大隐静脉
great saphenous vein

小隐静脉
small saphenous vein

足背内侧皮神经
medial dorsal cutaneous
nerve of foot

足背外侧皮神经
lateral dorsal cutaneous
nerve of foot

腓深神经
deep peroneal nerve

跖背静脉
dorsal metatarsal vein

足背静脉弓
dorsal venous arch of foot

趾背静脉
dorsal digital vein

𧿹长伸肌腱
tendon of extensor hallucis
longus

图 537 足背区血管和神经 1

Blood vessels and nerves of the dorsal region of the foot 1

跟骨
calcaneus

胫后动脉
posterior tibial artery

小趾展肌
abductor digiti
minimi

足底外侧动、静脉
lateral plantar artery
and vein

足底内侧神经
medial plantar nerve

𧿹展肌
abductor hallucis

趾足底总神经
common plantar digital nerve

足底外侧神经
lateral plantar nerve

趾短屈肌
flexor digitorum brevis

趾足底总动脉
common plantar digital
arteries

趾足底固有神经
proper plantar digital nerve

图 538 足底区血管和神经 2

Blood vessels and nerves of the plantar region of the foot 2

脑 神 经

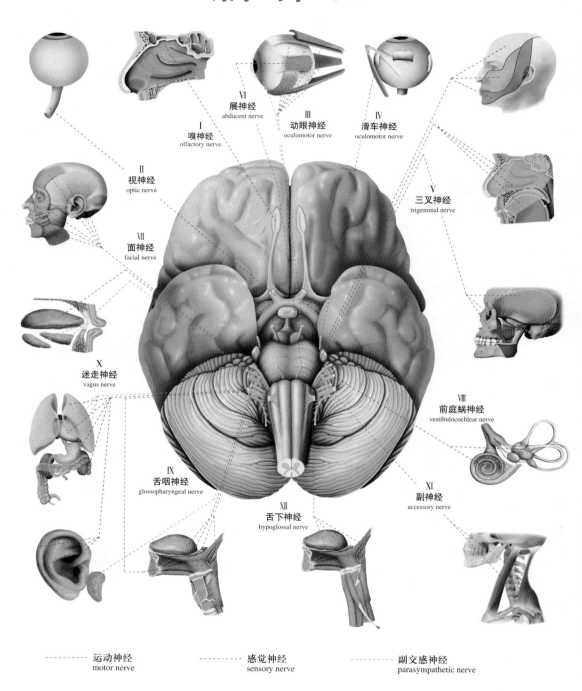

VI
展神经
abducent nerve

III
动眼神经
oculomotor nerve

IV
滑车神经
oculomotor nerve

I
嗅神经
olfactory nerve

V
三叉神经
trigeminal nerve

II
视神经
optic nerve

VII
面神经
facial nerve

X
迷走神经
vagus nerve

VIII
前庭蜗神经
vestibulocochlear nerve

IX
舌咽神经
glossopharyngeal nerve

XI
副神经
accessory nerve

XII
舌下神经
hypoglossal nerve

- - - - - 运动神经
motor nerve

- - - - - 感觉神经
sensory nerve

- - - - - 副交感神经
parasympathetic nerve

图 539　脑神经（模式图）

Cranial nerves (diagram)

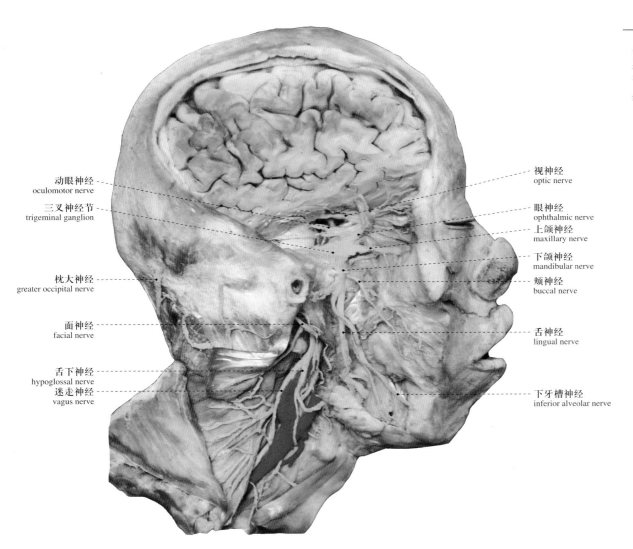

动眼神经
oculomotor nerve

三叉神经节
trigeminal ganglion

枕大神经
greater occipital nerve

面神经
facial nerve

舌下神经
hypoglossal nerve

迷走神经
vagus nerve

视神经
optic nerve

眼神经
ophthalmic nerve

上颌神经
maxillary nerve

下颌神经
mandibular nerve

颊神经
buccal nerve

舌神经
lingual nerve

下牙槽神经
inferior alveolar nerve

图 540　脑神经（侧面观）

Cranial nerve (lateral aspect)

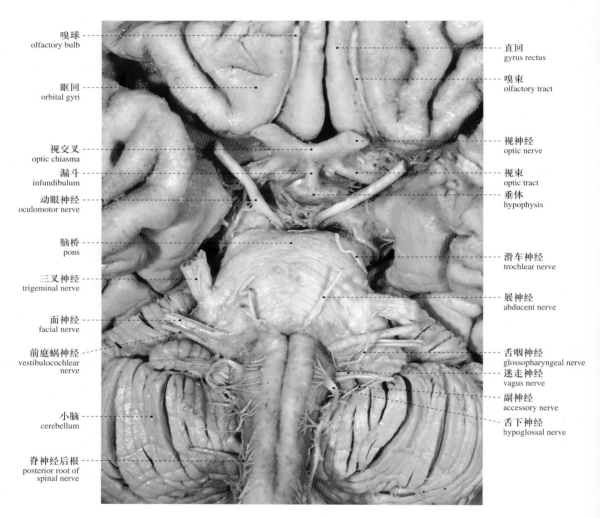

嗅球
olfactory bulb

眶回
orbital gyri

视交叉
optic chiasma

漏斗
infundibulum

动眼神经
oculomotor nerve

脑桥
pons

三叉神经
trigeminal nerve

面神经
facial nerve

前庭蜗神经
vestibulocochlear
nerve

小脑
cerebellum

脊神经后根
posterior root of
spinal nerve

直回
gyrus rectus

嗅束
olfactory tract

视神经
optic nerve

视束
optic tract

垂体
hypophysis

滑车神经
trochlear nerve

展神经
abducent nerve

舌咽神经
glossopharyngeal nerve

迷走神经
vagus nerve

副神经
accessory nerve

舌下神经
hypoglossal nerve

图 541　脑神经（底面）
Cranial nerves (basal surface)

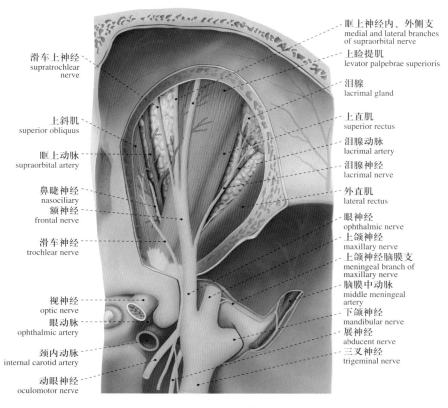

滑车上神经
supratrochlear
nerve

上斜肌
superior obliquus

眶上动脉
supraorbital artery

鼻睫神经
nasociliary
额神经
frontal nerve

滑车神经
trochlear nerve

视神经
optic nerve

眼动脉
ophthalmic artery

颈内动脉
internal carotid artery

动眼神经
oculomotor nerve

眶上神经内、外侧支
medial and lateral branches
of supraorbital nerve

上睑提肌
levator palpebrae superioris

泪腺
lacrimal gland

上直肌
superior rectus

泪腺动脉
lacrimal artery

泪腺神经
lacrimal nerve

外直肌
lateral rectus

眼神经
ophthalmic nerve
上颌神经
maxillary nerve
上颌神经脑膜支
meningeal branch of
maxillary nerve
脑膜中动脉
middle meningeal
artery
下颌神经
mandibular nerve
展神经
abducent nerve
三叉神经
trigeminal nerve

图 542　右侧眶动脉和神经（上面观）
Right orbital arteries and nerves (superior aspect)

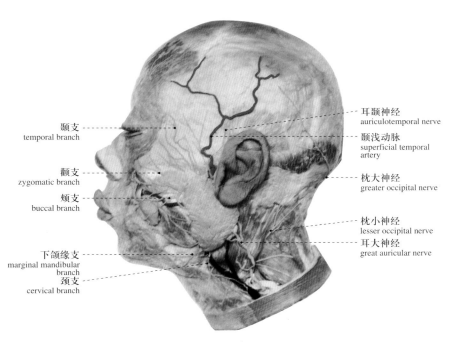

颞支
temporal branch

颧支
zygomatic branch

颊支
buccal branch

下颌缘支
marginal mandibular
branch
颈支
cervical branch

耳颞神经
auriculotemporal nerve

颞浅动脉
superficial temporal
artery

枕大神经
greater occipital nerve

枕小神经
lesser occipital nerve
耳大神经
great auricular nerve

图 543　面神经
Facial nerve

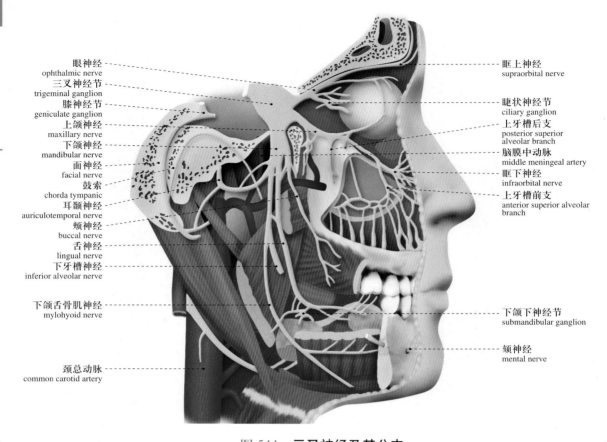

眼神经
ophthalmic nerve
三叉神经节
trigeminal ganglion
膝神经节
geniculate ganglion
上颌神经
maxillary nerve
下颌神经
mandibular nerve
面神经
facial nerve
鼓索
chorda tympanic
耳颞神经
auriculotemporal nerve
颊神经
buccal nerve
舌神经
lingual nerve
下牙槽神经
inferior alveolar nerve
下颌舌骨肌神经
mylohyoid nerve
颈总动脉
common carotid artery

眶上神经
supraorbital nerve
睫状神经节
ciliary ganglion
上牙槽后支
posterior superior alveolar branch
脑膜中动脉
middle meningeal artery
眶下神经
infraorbital nerve
上牙槽前支
anterior superior alveolar branch
下颌下神经节
submandibular ganglion
颏神经
mental nerve

图 544　三叉神经及其分支
Trigeminal nerve and its branches

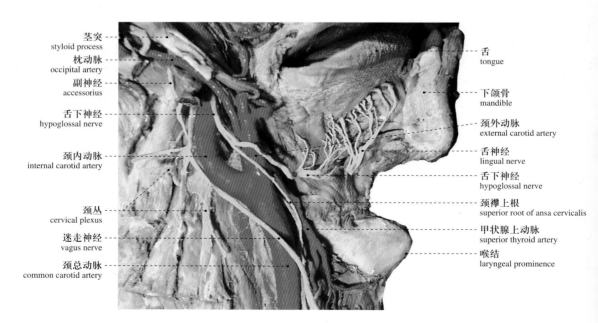

茎突
styloid process
枕动脉
occipital artery
副神经
accessorius
舌下神经
hypoglossal nerve
颈内动脉
internal carotid artery
颈丛
cervical plexus
迷走神经
vagus nerve
颈总动脉
common carotid artery

舌
tongue
下颌骨
mandible
颈外动脉
external carotid artery
舌神经
lingual nerve
舌下神经
hypoglossal nerve
颈襻上根
superior root of ansa cervicalis
甲状腺上动脉
superior thyroid artery
喉结
laryngeal prominence

图 545　舌下神经
Hypoglossal nerve

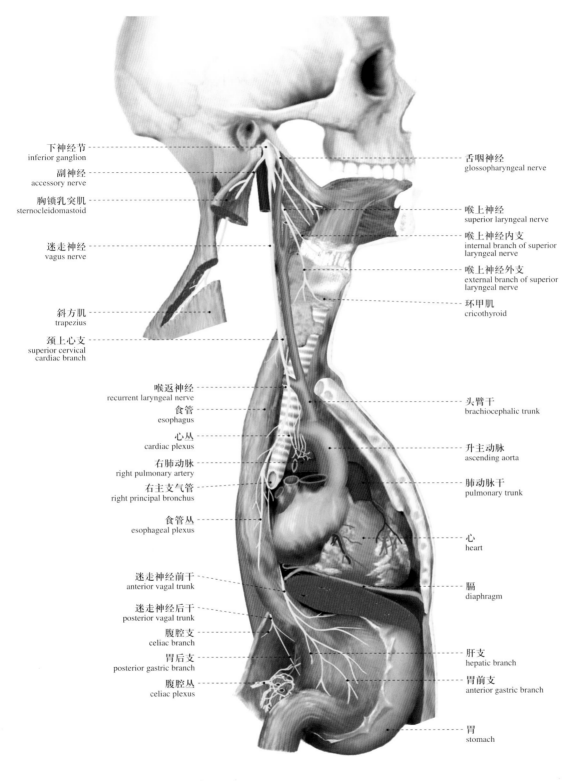

下神经节
inferior ganglion

副神经
accessory nerve

胸锁乳突肌
sternocleidomastoid

迷走神经
vagus nerve

斜方肌
trapezius

颈上心支
superior cervical
cardiac branch

喉返神经
recurrent laryngeal nerve

食管
esophagus

心丛
cardiac plexus

右肺动脉
right pulmonary artery

右主支气管
right principal bronchus

食管丛
esophageal plexus

迷走神经前干
anterior vagal trunk

迷走神经后干
posterior vagal trunk

腹腔支
celiac branch

胃后支
posterior gastric branch

腹腔丛
celiac plexus

舌咽神经
glossopharyngeal nerve

喉上神经
superior laryngeal nerve

喉上神经内支
internal branch of superior
laryngeal nerve

喉上神经外支
external branch of superior
laryngeal nerve

环甲肌
cricothyroid

头臂干
brachiocephalic trunk

升主动脉
ascending aorta

肺动脉干
pulmonary trunk

心
heart

膈
diaphragm

肝支
hepatic branch

胃前支
anterior gastric branch

胃
stomach

图 546　舌咽、迷走、副神经的走行和分布
Course and the distribution of the glossopharyngeal, the vagus and the accessory nerves

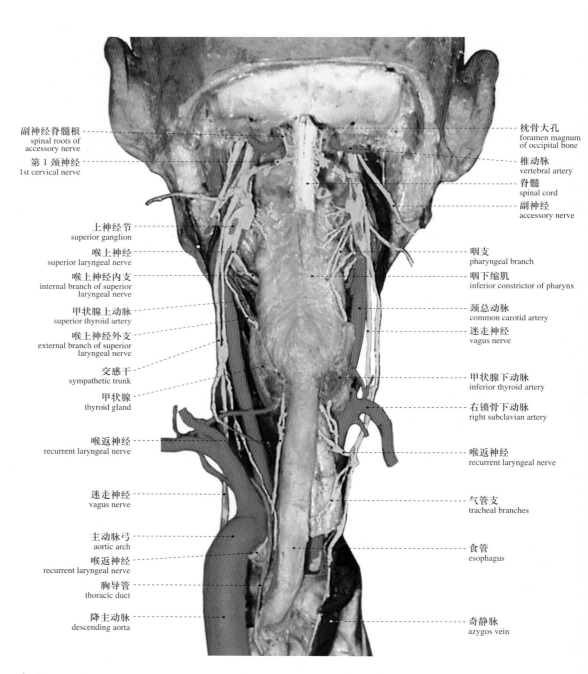

副神经脊髓根
spinal roots of accessory nerve

第 1 颈神经
1st cervical nerve

上神经节
superior ganglion

喉上神经
superior laryngeal nerve

喉上神经内支
internal branch of superior laryngeal nerve

甲状腺上动脉
superior thyroid artery

喉上神经外支
external branch of superior laryngeal nerve

交感干
sympathetic trunk

甲状腺
thyroid gland

喉返神经
recurrent laryngeal nerve

迷走神经
vagus nerve

主动脉弓
aortic arch

喉返神经
recurrent laryngeal nerve

胸导管
thoracic duct

降主动脉
descending aorta

枕骨大孔
foramen magnum of occipital bone

椎动脉
vertebral artery

脊髓
spinal cord

副神经
accessory nerve

咽支
pharyngeal branch

咽下缩肌
inferior constrictor of pharynx

颈总动脉
common carotid artery

迷走神经
vagus nerve

甲状腺下动脉
inferior thyroid artery

右锁骨下动脉
right subclavian artery

喉返神经
recurrent laryngeal nerve

气管支
tracheal branches

食管
esophagus

奇静脉
azygos vein

图 547　迷走神经的分支（后面观）
Branches of the vagus nerve (posterior aspect)

第三节

内脏神经系统

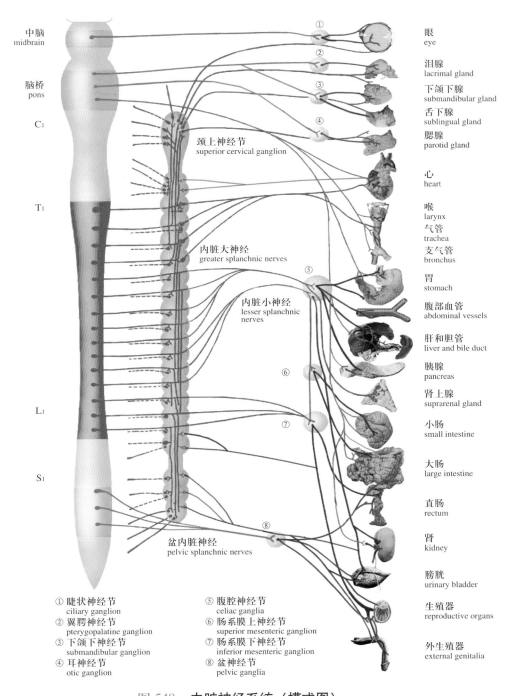

中脑
midbrain

脑桥
pons

C_1

T_1

L_1

S_1

颈上神经节
superior cervical ganglion

内脏大神经
greater splanchnic nerves

内脏小神经
lesser splanchnic nerves

盆内脏神经
pelvic splanchnic nerves

眼
eye

泪腺
lacrimal gland

下颌下腺
submandibular gland

舌下腺
sublingual gland

腮腺
parotid gland

心
heart

喉
larynx

气管
trachea

支气管
bronchus

胃
stomach

腹部血管
abdominal vessels

肝和胆管
liver and bile duct

胰腺
pancreas

肾上腺
suprarenal gland

小肠
small intestine

大肠
large intestine

直肠
rectum

肾
kidney

膀胱
urinary bladder

生殖器
reproductive organs

外生殖器
external genitalia

① 睫状神经节
ciliary ganglion
② 翼腭神经节
pterygopalatine ganglion
③ 下颌下神经节
submandibular ganglion
④ 耳神经节
otic ganglion

⑤ 腹腔神经节
celiac ganglia
⑥ 肠系膜上神经节
superior mesenteric ganglion
⑦ 肠系膜下神经节
inferior mesenteric ganglion
⑧ 盆神经节
pelvic ganglia

图 548　内脏神经系统（模式图）
Visceral nervous system (diagram)

297

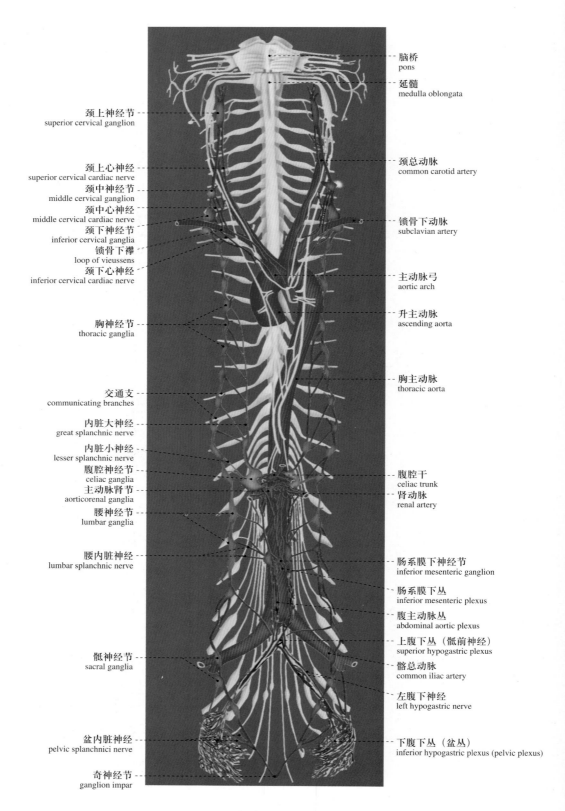

颈上神经节
superior cervical ganglion

颈上心神经
superior cervical cardiac nerve

颈中神经节
middle cervical ganglion

颈中心神经
middle cervical cardiac nerve

颈下神经节
inferior cervical ganglia

锁骨下襻
loop of vieussens

颈下心神经
inferior cervical cardiac nerve

胸神经节
thoracic ganglia

交通支
communicating branches

内脏大神经
great splanchnic nerve

内脏小神经
lesser splanchnic nerve

腹腔神经节
celiac ganglia

主动脉肾节
aorticorenal ganglia

腰神经节
lumbar ganglia

腰内脏神经
lumbar splanchnic nerve

骶神经节
sacral ganglia

盆内脏神经
pelvic splanchnici nerve

奇神经节
ganglion impar

脑桥
pons

延髓
medulla oblongata

颈总动脉
common carotid artery

锁骨下动脉
subclavian artery

主动脉弓
aortic arch

升主动脉
ascending aorta

胸主动脉
thoracic aorta

腹腔干
celiac trunk

肾动脉
renal artery

肠系膜下神经节
inferior mesenteric ganglion

肠系膜下丛
inferior mesenteric plexus

腹主动脉丛
abdominal aortic plexus

上腹下丛（骶前神经）
superior hypogastric plexus

髂总动脉
common iliac artery

左腹下神经
left hypogastric nerve

下腹下丛（盆丛）
inferior hypogastric plexus (pelvic plexus)

图 549　交感神经系统（模式图）
Sympathetic nervous system (diagram)

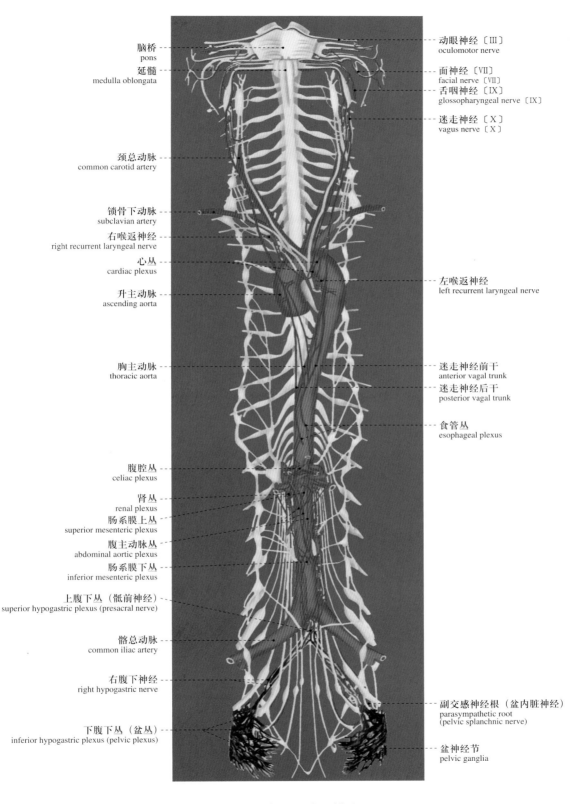

脑桥
pons

延髓
medulla oblongata

颈总动脉
common carotid artery

锁骨下动脉
subclavian artery

右喉返神经
right recurrent laryngeal nerve

心丛
cardiac plexus

升主动脉
ascending aorta

胸主动脉
thoracic aorta

腹腔丛
celiac plexus

肾丛
renal plexus

肠系膜上丛
superior mesenteric plexus

腹主动脉丛
abdominal aortic plexus

肠系膜下丛
inferior mesenteric plexus

上腹下丛（骶前神经）
superior hypogastric plexus (presacral nerve)

髂总动脉
common iliac artery

右腹下神经
right hypogastric nerve

下腹下丛（盆丛）
inferior hypogastric plexus (pelvic plexus)

动眼神经〔Ⅲ〕
oculomotor nerve

面神经〔Ⅶ〕
facial nerve〔Ⅶ〕

舌咽神经〔Ⅸ〕
glossopharyngeal nerve〔Ⅸ〕

迷走神经〔Ⅹ〕
vagus nerve〔Ⅹ〕

左喉返神经
left recurrent laryngeal nerve

迷走神经前干
anterior vagal trunk

迷走神经后干
posterior vagal trunk

食管丛
esophageal plexus

副交感神经根（盆内脏神经）
parasympathetic root
(pelvic splanchnic nerve)

盆神经节
pelvic ganglia

图 550　副交感神经系统（模式图）

Parasympathetic nervous system (diagram)

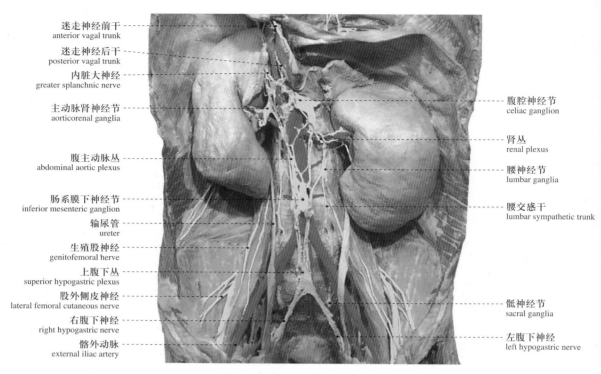

迷走神经前干
anterior vagal trunk

迷走神经后干
posterior vagal trunk

内脏大神经
greater splanchnic nerve

主动脉肾神经节
aorticorenal ganglia

腹主动脉丛
abdominal aortic plexus

肠系膜下神经节
inferior mesenteric ganglion

输尿管
ureter

生殖股神经
genitofemoral nerve

上腹下丛
superior hypogastric plexus

股外侧皮神经
lateral femoral cutaneous nerve

右腹下神经
right hypogastric nerve

髂外动脉
external iliac artery

腹腔神经节
celiac ganglion

肾丛
renal plexus

腰神经节
lumbar ganglia

腰交感干
lumbar sympathetic trunk

骶神经节
sacral ganglia

左腹下神经
left hypogastric nerve

图 551　内脏神经（腹部）
Visceral nerve (abdominal region)

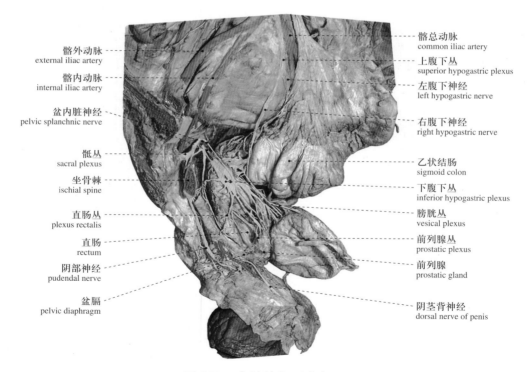

髂外动脉
external iliac artery

髂内动脉
internal iliac artery

盆内脏神经
pelvic splanchnic nerve

骶丛
sacral plexus

坐骨棘
ischial spine

直肠丛
plexus rectalis

直肠
rectum

阴部神经
pudendal nerve

盆膈
pelvic diaphragm

髂总动脉
common iliac artery

上腹下丛
superior hypogastric plexus

左腹下神经
left hypogastric nerve

右腹下神经
right hypogastric nerve

乙状结肠
sigmoid colon

下腹下丛
inferior hypogastric plexus

膀胱丛
vesical plexus

前列腺丛
prostatic plexus

前列腺
prostatic gland

阴茎背神经
dorsal nerve of penis

图 552　内脏神经（盆部）
Visceral nerve (pelvic region)

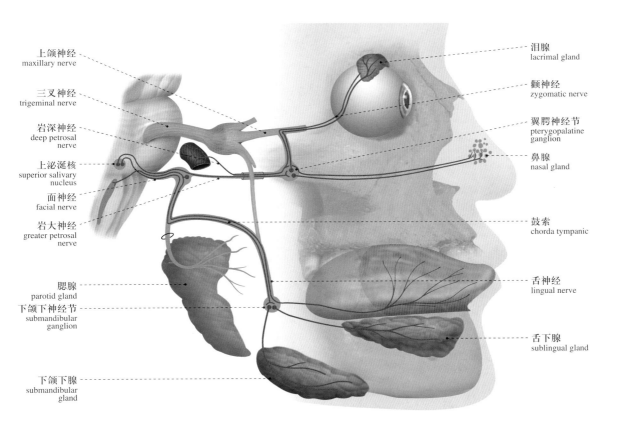

上颌神经
maxillary nerve

三叉神经
trigeminal nerve

岩深神经
deep petrosal
nerve

上泌涎核
superior salivary
nucleus

面神经
facial nerve

岩大神经
greater petrosal
nerve

腮腺
parotid gland

下颌下神经节
submandibular
ganglion

下颌下腺
submandibular
gland

泪腺
lacrimal gland

颧神经
zygomatic nerve

翼腭神经节
pterygopalatine
ganglion

鼻腺
nasal gland

鼓索
chorda tympanic

舌神经
lingual nerve

舌下腺
sublingual gland

图 553　面神经的副交感纤维
Parasympathetic fibers of the facial nerve

第一节

感觉传导通路

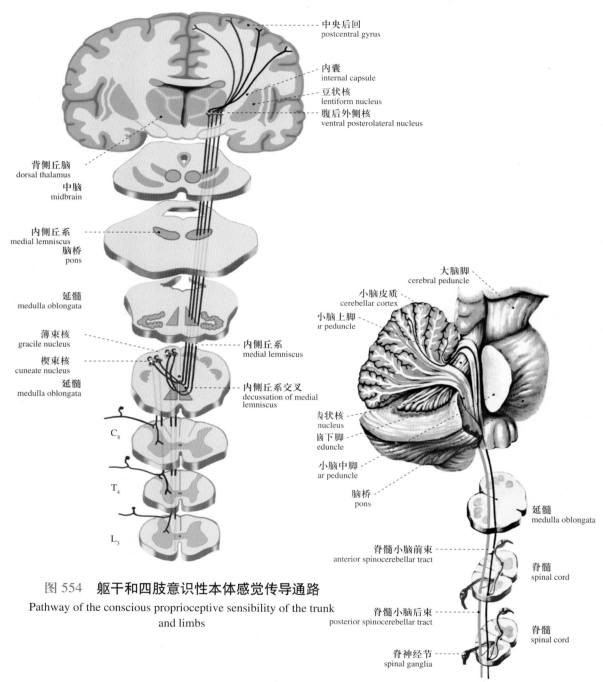

中央后回
postcentral gyrus

内囊
internal capsule

豆状核
lentiform nucleus

腹后外侧核
ventral posterolateral nucleus

背侧丘脑
dorsal thalamus

中脑
midbrain

内侧丘系
medial lemniscus

脑桥
pons

延髓
medulla oblongata

薄束核
gracile nucleus

楔束核
cuneate nucleus

延髓
medulla oblongata

内侧丘系
medial lemniscus

内侧丘系交叉
decussation of medial lemniscus

C_8

T_4

L_3

大脑脚
cerebral peduncle

小脑皮质
cerebellar cortex

小脑上脚
ar peduncle

齿状核
nucleus

齿下脚
eduncle

小脑中脚
ar peduncle

脑桥
pons

延髓
medulla oblongata

脊髓小脑前束
anterior spinocerebellar tract

脊髓小脑后束
posterior spinocerebellar tract

脊神经节
spinal ganglia

脊髓
spinal cord

脊髓
spinal cord

图 554　躯干和四肢意识性本体感觉传导通路
Pathway of the conscious proprioceptive sensibility of the trunk and limbs

图 555　躯干和四肢非意识性本体感觉传导通路
Pathway of the unconscious proprioceptive sensibility of the trunk and limbs

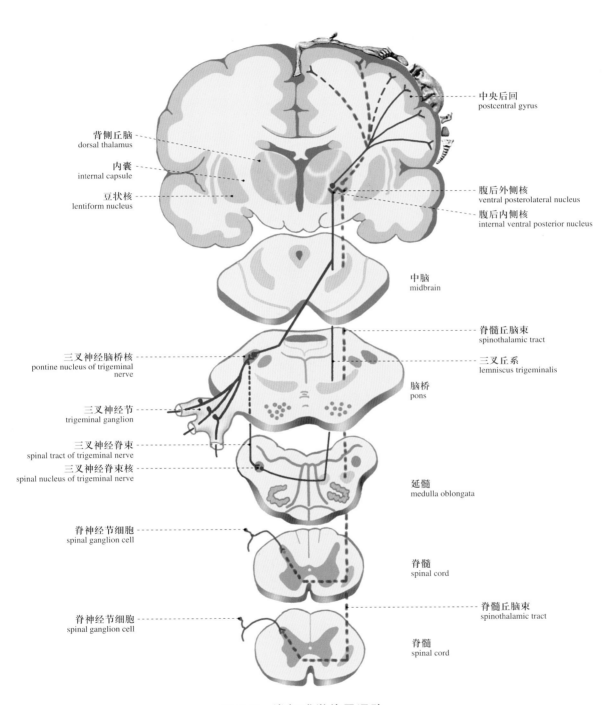

中央后回
postcentral gyrus

背侧丘脑
dorsal thalamus

内囊
internal capsule

豆状核
lentiform nucleus

腹后外侧核
ventral posterolateral nucleus

腹后内侧核
internal ventral posterior nucleus

中脑
midbrain

脊髓丘脑束
spinothalamic tract

三叉神经脑桥核
pontine nucleus of trigeminal nerve

三叉丘系
lemniscus trigeminalis

脑桥
pons

三叉神经节
trigeminal ganglion

三叉神经脊束
spinal tract of trigeminal nerve

三叉神经脊束核
spinal nucleus of trigeminal nerve

延髓
medulla oblongata

脊神经节细胞
spinal ganglion cell

脊髓
spinal cord

脊髓丘脑束
spinothalamic tract

脊神经节细胞
spinal ganglion cell

脊髓
spinal cord

图 556　浅部感觉传导通路
Pathways of the superficial sensory

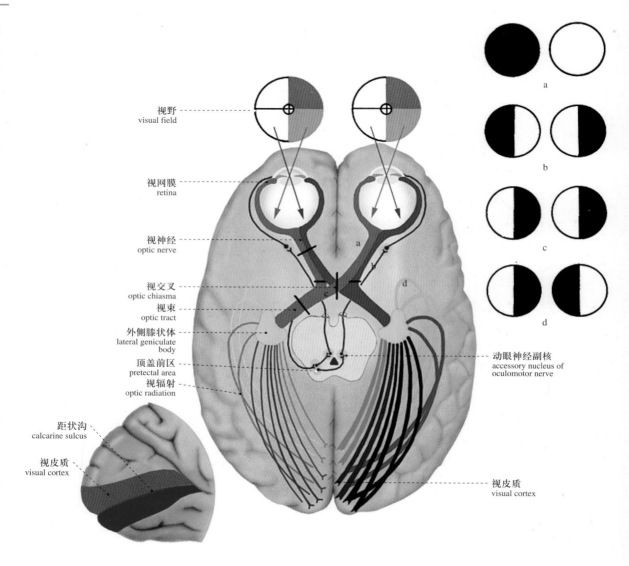

视野
visual field

视网膜
retina

视神经
optic nerve

视交叉
optic chiasma

视束
optic tract

外侧膝状体
lateral geniculate body

顶盖前区
pretectal area

视辐射
optic radiation

距状沟
calcarine sulcus

视皮质
visual cortex

动眼神经副核
accessory nucleus of oculomotor nerve

视皮质
visual cortex

图 557　视觉传导通路和瞳孔对光反射通路
Visual pathway and pupil reflex pathway

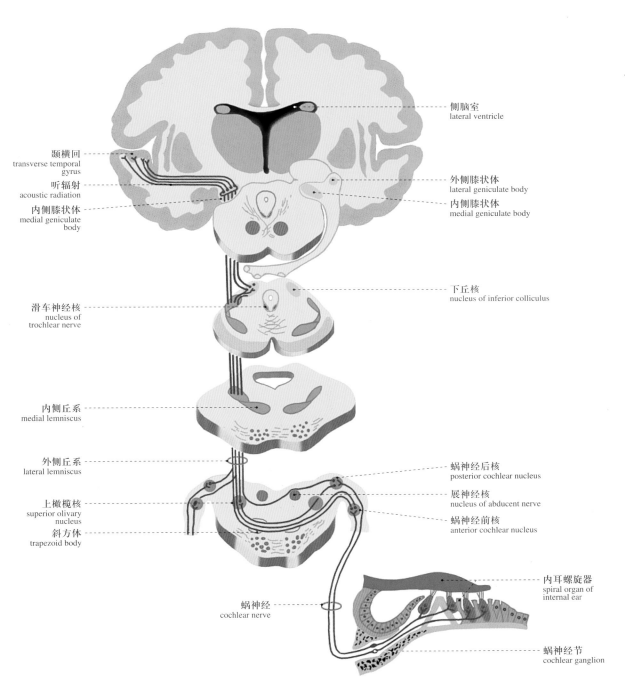

颞横回
transverse temporal gyrus

听辐射
acoustic radiation

内侧膝状体
medial geniculate body

滑车神经核
nucleus of trochlear nerve

内侧丘系
medial lemniscus

外侧丘系
lateral lemniscus

上橄榄核
superior olivary nucleus

斜方体
trapezoid body

蜗神经
cochlear nerve

侧脑室
lateral ventricle

外侧膝状体
lateral geniculate body

内侧膝状体
medial geniculate body

下丘核
nucleus of inferior colliculus

蜗神经后核
posterior cochlear nucleus

展神经核
nucleus of abducent nerve

蜗神经前核
anterior cochlear nucleus

内耳螺旋器
spiral organ of internal ear

蜗神经节
cochlear ganglion

图 558　听觉传导通路
Auditory pathway

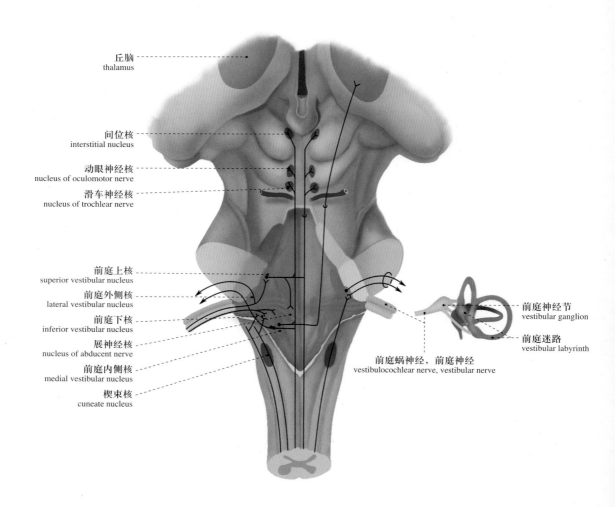

丘脑
thalamus

间位核
interstitial nucleus

动眼神经核
nucleus of oculomotor nerve

滑车神经核
nucleus of trochlear nerve

前庭上核
superior vestibular nucleus

前庭外侧核
lateral vestibular nucleus

前庭下核
inferior vestibular nucleus

展神经核
nucleus of abducent nerve

前庭内侧核
medial vestibular nucleus

楔束核
cuneate nucleus

前庭蜗神经，前庭神经
vestibulocochlear nerve, vestibular nerve

前庭神经节
vestibular ganglion

前庭迷路
vestibular labyrinth

图 559　平衡觉传导通路
Pathway of equilibrium sense

第二节

运动传导通路

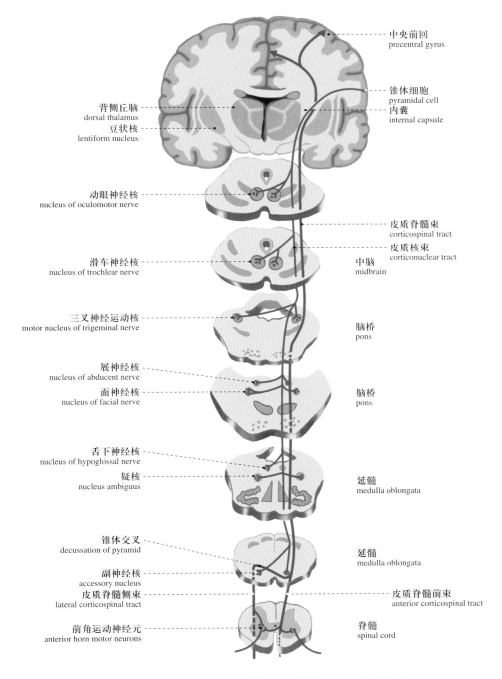

中央前回
precentral gyrus

锥体细胞
pyramidal cell

内囊
internal capsule

背侧丘脑
dorsal thalamus

豆状核
lentiform nucleus

动眼神经核
nucleus of oculomotor nerve

皮质脊髓束
corticospinal tract

皮质核束
corticonuclear tract

中脑
midbrain

滑车神经核
nucleus of trochlear nerve

三叉神经运动核
motor nucleus of trigeminal nerve

脑桥
pons

展神经核
nucleus of abducent nerve

面神经核
nucleus of facial nerve

脑桥
pons

舌下神经核
nucleus of hypoglossal nerve

疑核
nucleus ambiguus

延髓
medulla oblongata

锥体交叉
decussation of pyramid

延髓
medulla oblongata

副神经核
accessory nucleus

皮质脊髓侧束
lateral corticospinal tract

皮质脊髓前束
anterior corticospinal tract

前角运动神经元
anterior horn motor neurons

脊髓
spinal cord

图 560　锥体系中的皮质脊髓束与皮质核束
Corticospinal tracts and corticonuclear tracts in the pyramidal system

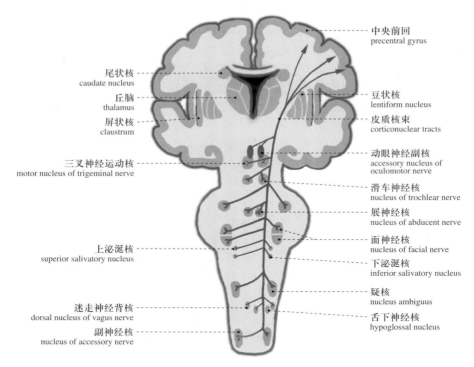

尾状核
caudate nucleus

丘脑
thalamus

屏状核
claustrum

三叉神经运动核
motor nucleus of trigeminal nerve

上泌涎核
superior salivatory nucleus

迷走神经背核
dorsal nucleus of vagus nerve

副神经核
nucleus of accessory nerve

中央前回
precentral gyrus

豆状核
lentiform nucleus

皮质核束
corticonuclear tracts

动眼神经副核
accessory nucleus of oculomotor nerve

滑车神经核
nucleus of trochlear nerve

展神经核
nucleus of abducent nerve

面神经核
nucleus of facial nerve

下泌涎核
inferior salivatory nucleus

疑核
nucleus ambiguus

舌下神经核
hypoglossal nucleus

图 561　脑神经运动核与皮质核束

Motor nuclei of the cranial nerve and the corticonuclear tracts

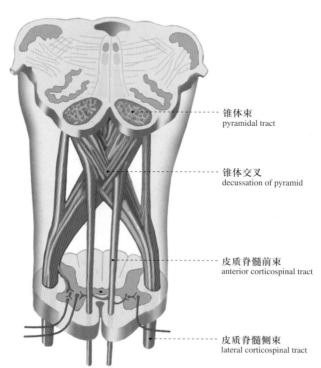

锥体束
pyramidal tract

锥体交叉
decussation of pyramid

皮质脊髓前束
anterior corticospinal tract

皮质脊髓侧束
lateral corticospinal tract

图 562　锥体交叉（模式图）

Pyramidal decussation (diagram)

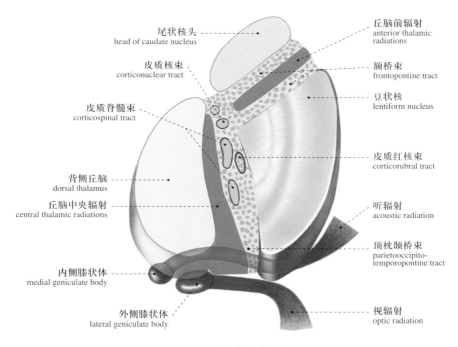

尾状核头
head of caudate nucleus

丘脑前辐射
anterior thalamic radiations

皮质核束
corticonuclear tract

额桥束
frontopontine tract

皮质脊髓束
corticospinal tract

豆状核
lentiform nucleus

皮质红核束
corticorubral tract

背侧丘脑
dorsal thalamus

丘脑中央辐射
central thalamic radiations

听辐射
acoustic radiation

内侧膝状体
medial geniculate body

顶枕颞桥束
parietooccipito-temporopontine tract

外侧膝状体
lateral geniculate body

视辐射
optic radiation

图 563　内囊（模式图）
Internal capsule (diagram)

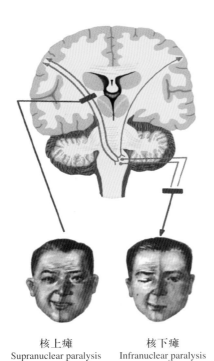

核上瘫
Supranuclear paralysis

核下瘫
Infranuclear paralysis

图 564　面神经瘫
Paralysis of the facial nerve

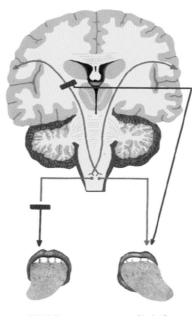

核下瘫
Infranuclear paralysis

核上瘫
Supranuclear paralysis

图 565　舌下神经瘫
Paralysis of the hypoglossal nerve

第一节

脑和脊髓的被膜

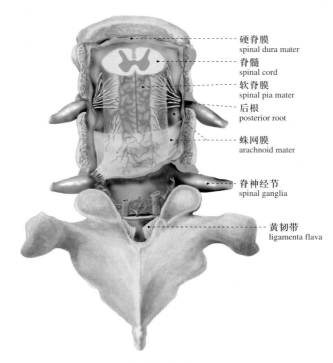

硬脊膜
spinal dura mater

脊髓
spinal cord

软脊膜
spinal pia mater

后根
posterior root

蛛网膜
arachnoid mater

脊神经节
spinal ganglia

黄韧带
ligamenta flava

图 566 脊髓的被膜
Meninges of the spinal cord

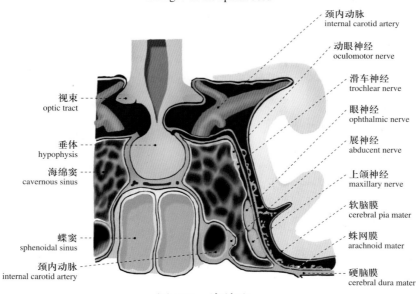

颈内动脉
internal carotid artery

动眼神经
oculomotor nerve

滑车神经
trochlear nerve

眼神经
ophthalmic nerve

展神经
abducent nerve

上颌神经
maxillary nerve

软脑膜
cerebral pia mater

蛛网膜
arachnoid mater

硬脑膜
cerebral dura mater

视束
optic tract

垂体
hypophysis

海绵窦
cavernous sinus

蝶窦
sphenoidal sinus

颈内动脉
internal carotid artery

图 567 海绵窦
Cavernous sinus

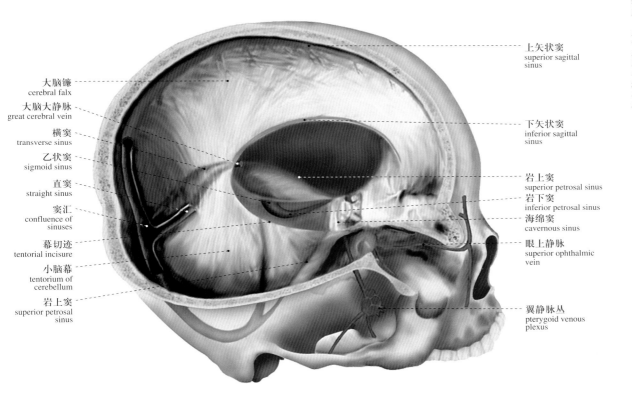

大脑镰
cerebral falx

大脑大静脉
great cerebral vein

横窦
transverse sinus

乙状窦
sigmoid sinus

直窦
straight sinus

窦汇
confluence of sinuses

幕切迹
tentorial incisure

小脑幕
tentorium of cerebellum

岩上窦
superior petrosal sinus

上矢状窦
superior sagittal sinus

下矢状窦
inferior sagittal sinus

岩上窦
superior petrosal sinus

岩下窦
inferior petrosal sinus

海绵窦
cavernous sinus

眼上静脉
superior ophthalmic vein

翼静脉丛
pterygoid venous plexus

图 568　硬脑膜及硬脑膜静脉窦

Cerebral dura mater and the venous sinuses of the dura mater

第二节

脑 血 管

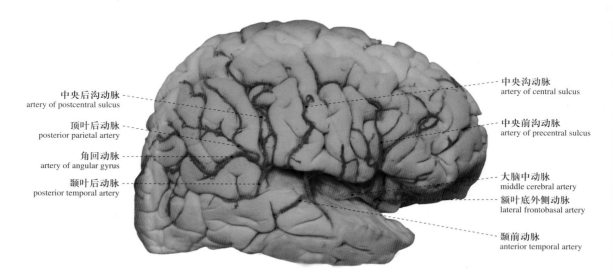

中央后沟动脉
artery of postcentral sulcus

顶叶后动脉
posterior parietal artery

角回动脉
artery of angular gyrus

颞叶后动脉
posterior temporal artery

中央沟动脉
artery of central sulcus

中央前沟动脉
artery of precentral sulcus

大脑中动脉
middle cerebral artery

额叶底外侧动脉
lateral frontobasal artery

颞前动脉
anterior temporal artery

图 569　大脑半球的动脉（外侧面观）
Arteries of the cerebral hemisphere (lateral aspect)

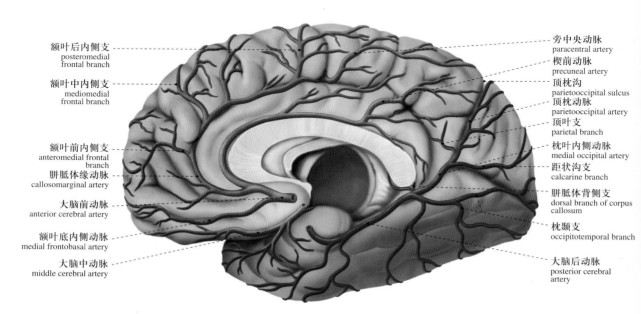

额叶后内侧支
posteromedial frontal branch

额叶中内侧支
mediomedial frontal branch

额叶前内侧支
anteromedial frontal branch

胼胝体缘动脉
callosomarginal artery

大脑前动脉
anterior cerebral artery

额叶底内侧动脉
medial frontobasal artery

大脑中动脉
middle cerebral artery

旁中央动脉
paracentral artery

楔前动脉
precuneal artery

顶枕沟
parietooccipital sulcus

顶枕动脉
parietooccipital artery

顶叶支
parietal branch

枕叶内侧动脉
medial occipital artery

距状沟支
calcarine branch

胼胝体背侧支
dorsal branch of corpus callosum

枕颞支
occipitotemporal branch

大脑后动脉
posterior cerebral artery

图 570　大脑动脉（正中矢状断面观）
Arteries of the cerebrum (midsagittal section aspect)

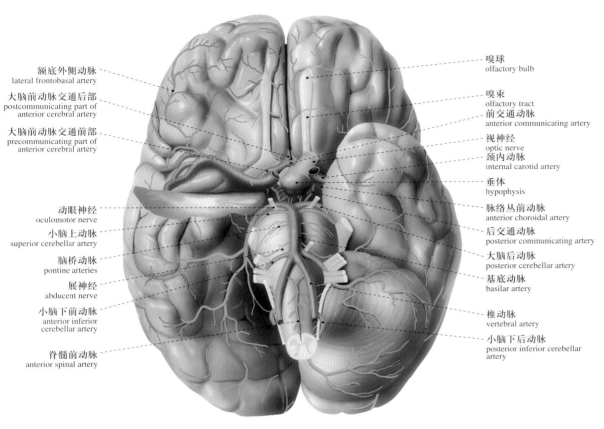

额底外侧动脉
lateral frontobasal artery

大脑前动脉交通后部
postcommunicating part of
anterior cerebral artery

大脑前动脉交通前部
precommunicating part of
anterior cerebral artery

动眼神经
oculomotor nerve

小脑上动脉
superior cerebellar artery

脑桥动脉
pontine arteries

展神经
abducent nerve

小脑下前动脉
anterior inferior
cerebellar artery

脊髓前动脉
anterior spinal artery

嗅球
olfactory bulb

嗅束
olfactory tract

前交通动脉
anterior communicating artery

视神经
optic nerve

颈内动脉
internal carotid artery

垂体
hypophysis

脉络丛前动脉
anterior choroidal artery

后交通动脉
posterior communicating artery

大脑后动脉
posterior cerebellar artery

基底动脉
basilar artery

椎动脉
vertebral artery

小脑下后动脉
posterior inferior cerebellar
artery

图 571　脑的动脉（下面观）
Cerebral arteries (inferior aspect)

尾状核头
head of caudate
nucleus

背侧丘脑
dorsal thalamus

壳
putamen

苍白球
globus pallidus

内囊
internal capsule

皮质支
cortical branches

外侧支
lateral branches

内侧支
medial branches

大脑中动脉
middle cerebral
artery

图 572　大脑动脉的皮质支和中央支
Cortical and the central branches of the cerebral arteries

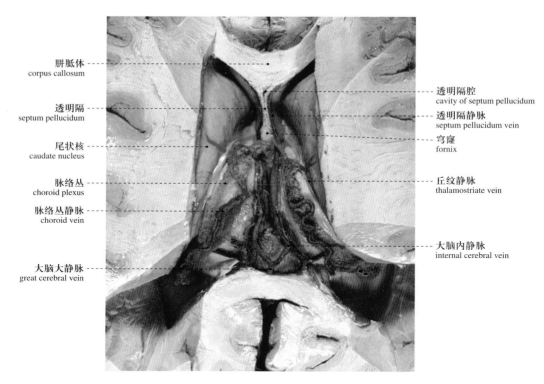

胼胝体
corpus callosum

透明隔
septum pellucidum

尾状核
caudate nucleus

脉络丛
choroid plexus

脉络丛静脉
choroid vein

大脑大静脉
great cerebral vein

透明隔腔
cavity of septum pellucidum

透明隔静脉
septum pellucidum vein

穹窿
fornix

丘纹静脉
thalamostriate vein

大脑内静脉
internal cerebral vein

图 573　大脑大静脉及其属支
Great cerebral vein and its tributaries

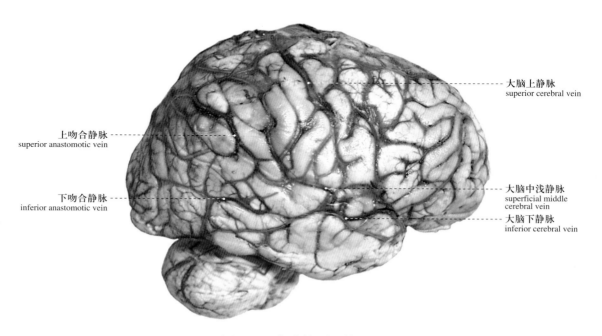

上吻合静脉
superior anastomotic vein

下吻合静脉
inferior anastomotic vein

大脑上静脉
superior cerebral vein

大脑中浅静脉
superficial middle cerebral vein

大脑下静脉
inferior cerebral vein

图 574　大脑外侧面的静脉
Veins of the lateral surface of the cerebrum

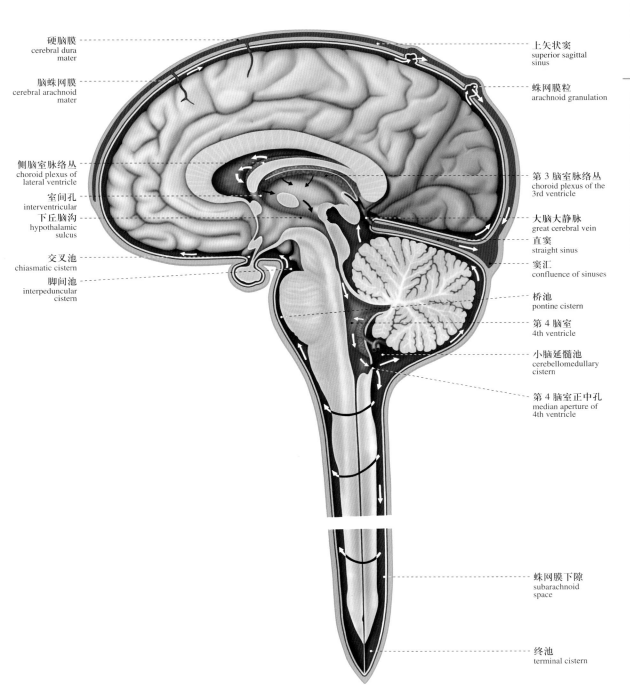

硬脑膜
cerebral dura mater

脑蛛网膜
cerebral arachnoid mater

侧脑室脉络丛
choroid plexus of lateral ventricle

室间孔
interventricular

下丘脑沟
hypothalamic sulcus

交叉池
chiasmatic cistern

脚间池
interpeduncular cistern

上矢状窦
superior sagittal sinus

蛛网膜粒
arachnoid granulation

第 3 脑室脉络丛
choroid plexus of the 3rd ventricle

大脑大静脉
great cerebral vein

直窦
straight sinus

窦汇
confluence of sinuses

桥池
pontine cistern

第 4 脑室
4th ventricle

小脑延髓池
cerebellomedullary cistern

第 4 脑室正中孔
median aperture of 4th ventricle

蛛网膜下隙
subarachnoid space

终池
terminal cistern

图 575　脑脊液循环

Circulation of the cerebrospinal fluid

315

第一节

内分泌系统模式图

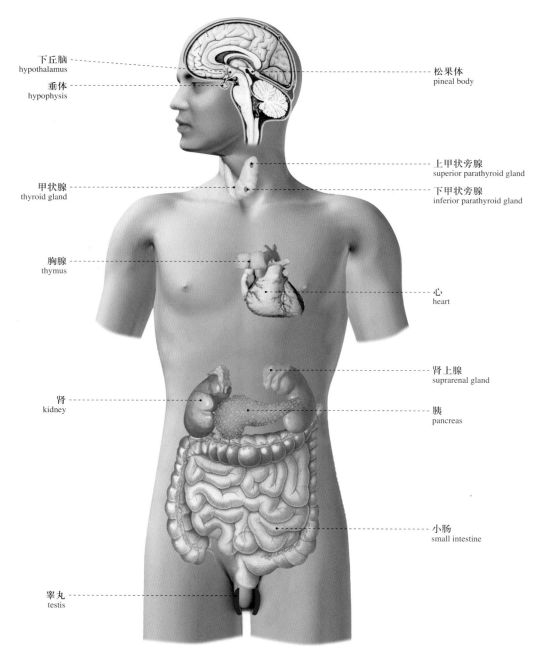

下丘脑
hypothalamus

垂体
hypophysis

甲状腺
thyroid gland

胸腺
thymus

肾
kidney

睾丸
testis

松果体
pineal body

上甲状旁腺
superior parathyroid gland

下甲状旁腺
inferior parathyroid gland

心
heart

肾上腺
suprarenal gland

胰
pancreas

小肠
small intestine

图 576 男性内分泌器官
Male endocrine organs

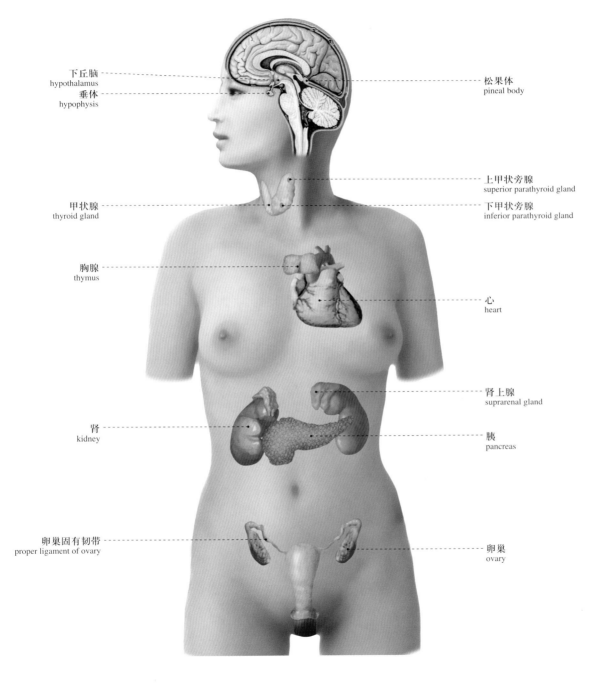

下丘脑
hypothalamus

垂体
hypophysis

松果体
pineal body

上甲状旁腺
superior parathyroid gland

甲状腺
thyroid gland

下甲状旁腺
inferior parathyroid gland

胸腺
thymus

心
heart

肾上腺
suprarenal gland

肾
kidney

胰
pancreas

卵巢固有韧带
proper ligament of ovary

卵巢
ovary

图 577　女性内分泌器官
Female endocrine organs

第二节

内分泌器官

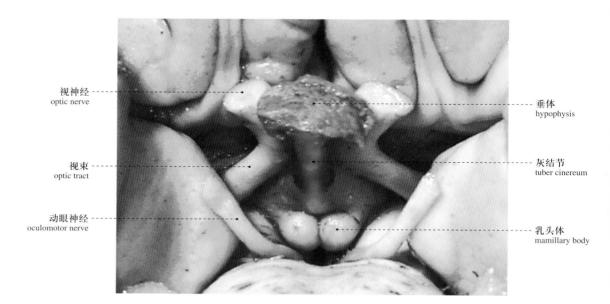

视神经
optic nerve

垂体
hypophysis

视束
optic tract

灰结节
tuber cinereum

动眼神经
oculomotor nerve

乳头体
mamillary body

图 578　垂体
Hypophysis

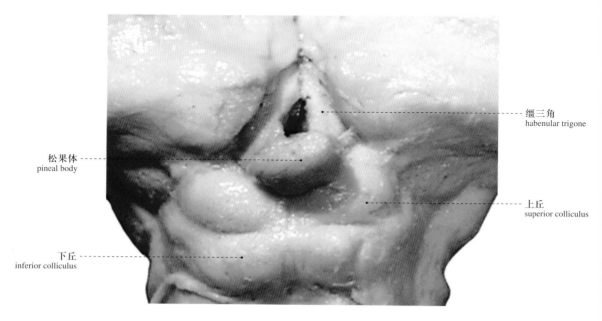

缰三角
habenular trigone

松果体
pineal body

上丘
superior colliculus

下丘
inferior colliculus

图 579　松果体
Pineal body

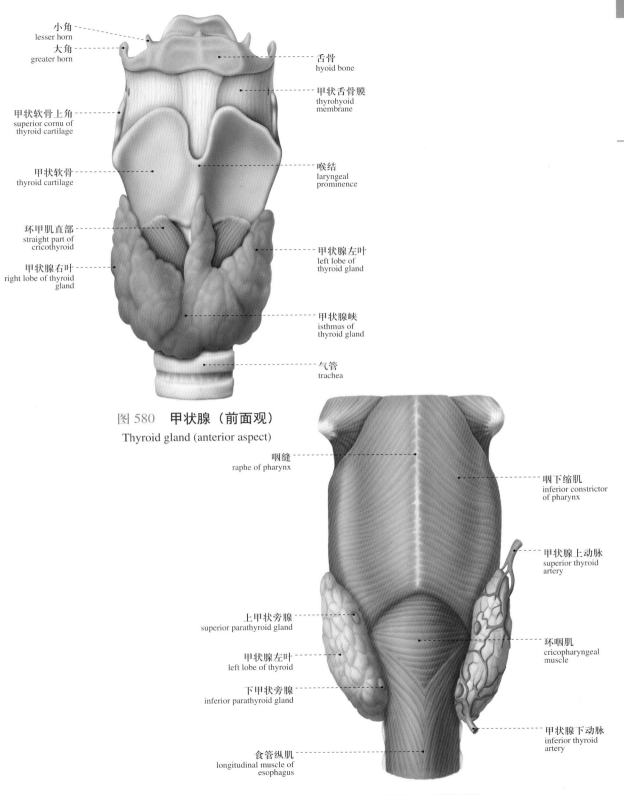

小角
lesser horn

大角
greater horn

甲状软骨上角
superior cornu of
thyroid cartilage

甲状软骨
thyroid cartilage

环甲肌直部
straight part of
cricothyroid

甲状腺右叶
right lobe of thyroid
gland

舌骨
hyoid bone

甲状舌骨膜
thyrohyoid
membrane

喉结
laryngeal
prominence

甲状腺左叶
left lobe of
thyroid gland

甲状腺峡
isthmus of
thyroid gland

气管
trachea

图 580　甲状腺（前面观）
Thyroid gland (anterior aspect)

咽缝
raphe of pharynx

上甲状旁腺
superior parathyroid gland

甲状腺左叶
left lobe of thyroid

下甲状旁腺
inferior parathyroid gland

食管纵肌
longitudinal muscle of
esophagus

咽下缩肌
inferior constrictor
of pharynx

甲状腺上动脉
superior thyroid
artery

环咽肌
cricopharyngeal
muscle

甲状腺下动脉
inferior thyroid
artery

图 581　甲状腺（后面观）
Thyroid gland (posterior aspect)

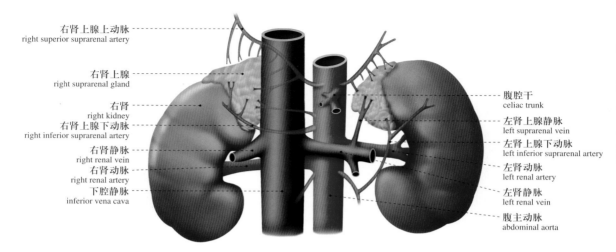

右肾上腺上动脉
right superior suprarenal artery

右肾上腺
right suprarenal gland

右肾
right kidney

右肾上腺下动脉
right inferior suprarenal artery

右肾静脉
right renal vein

右肾动脉
right renal artery

下腔静脉
inferior vena cava

腹腔干
celiac trunk

左肾上腺静脉
left suprarenal vein

左肾上腺下动脉
left inferior suprarenal artery

左肾动脉
left renal artery

左肾静脉
left renal vein

腹主动脉
abdominal aorta

图 582　肾上腺
Adrenal gland

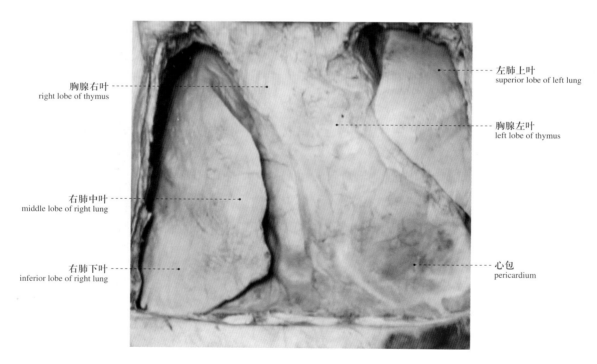

胸腺右叶
right lobe of thymus

右肺中叶
middle lobe of right lung

右肺下叶
inferior lobe of right lung

左肺上叶
superior lobe of left lung

胸腺左叶
left lobe of thymus

心包
pericardium

图 583　胸腺
Thymus

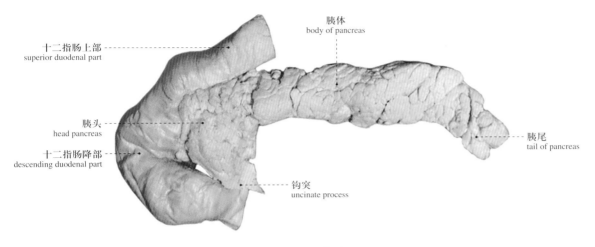

十二指肠上部
superior duodenal part

胰体
body of pancreas

胰头
head pancreas

十二指肠降部
descending duodenal part

钩突
uncinate process

胰尾
tail of pancreas

图 584　胰腺
Pancreas

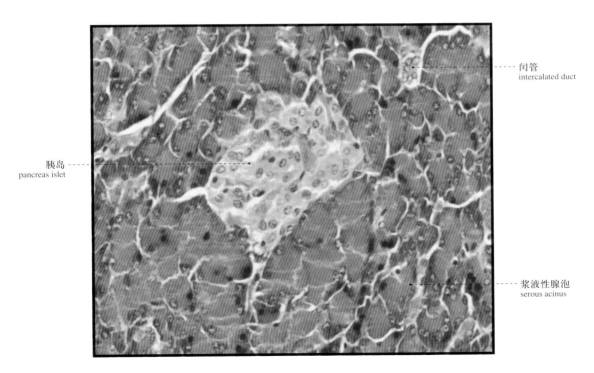

胰岛
pancreas islet

闰管
intercalated duct

浆液性腺泡
serous acinus

图 585　胰岛（人胰腺，×400）
Pancreas islet (human pancreas, ×400)

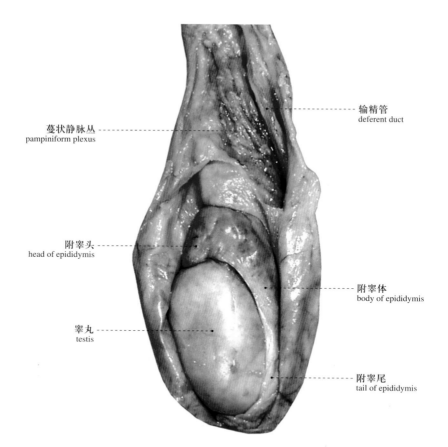

蔓状静脉丛
pampiniform plexus

输精管
deferent duct

附睾头
head of epididymis

附睾体
body of epididymis

睾丸
testis

附睾尾
tail of epididymis

图 586　睾丸
Testis

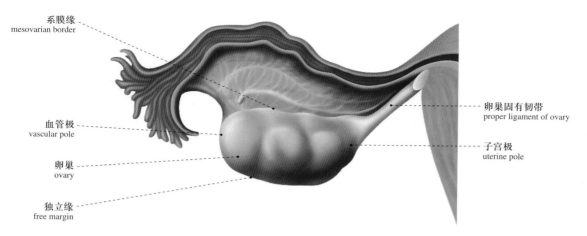

系膜缘
mesovarian border

卵巢固有韧带
proper ligament of ovary

血管极
vascular pole

子宫极
uterine pole

卵巢
ovary

独立缘
free margin

图 587　卵巢
Ovary

参考书目

[1] Schuenke M, Schulte E, Schumacher U. THIEME Atlas of Anatomy, Neck and Internal Organs. Thieme Stuttgart.

[2] Schuenke M, Schulte E, Schumacher U. THIEME Atlas of Anatomy, General Anatomy and Musculoskeletal System. Thieme Stuttgart.

[3] Schuenke M, Schulte E, Schumacher U. THIEME Atlas of Anatomy, Head and Neuroanatomy. Thieme Stuttgart.

[4] Putz R, Sobotta PR. Atlas der Anatomie des Menschen. Band 2, 21st edition. Elsevier, Pte Ltd.

[5] David W, Stoller MR. 廉宗澂译. 关节镜和外科解剖图片集. 天津科技翻译出版公司.

[6] Standring S. GRAY'S Anatomy Susan Standring. Churchill Livingstone Elsevier.

[7] Netter FH. Atlas of Human Anatomy. SAUNDERS Elsevier.

[8] Bontrager KL, Lampignano JP. Radiographic Positioning and Related Anatomy. SAUNDERS Elsevier.

[9] Moore KL, Persaud TVN. The Developing Human. Saunders Elsevier.

[10] Stoller DW. MRI, Arthroscopy, and Surgical Anatomy of the Joints. Lippincott Williams & Wilkins lnc.

[11] Agur AMR. Grant's Atlas of Anatomy. Lippincott Williams & Wilkins Inc.

[12] 高士濂. 实用解剖图谱, 上肢分册. 上海科学技术出版社.

[13] 高士濂. 实用解剖图谱, 下肢分册. 上海科学技术出版社.

[14] 托尼·史密斯. 左焕琛译. 人体. 上海科学技术出版社.

[15] 张朝佑. 人体解剖学. 人民卫生出版社.

[16] 郭光文, 王序. 人体解剖彩色图谱. 人民卫生出版社.

[17] 柏树令, 段坤昌, 陈金宝. 人体解剖学彩色图谱. 上海科学技术出版社.

[18] 石玉秀, 邓纯忠, 孙桂媛, 等. 组织学与胚胎学彩色图谱. 上海科学技术出版社.

[19] 段坤昌, 王振宇, 李庆生. 颅脑颈部应用解剖学彩色图谱. 辽宁科学技术出版社.

[20] 金连弘. 人体断面解剖学彩色图谱. 人民卫生出版社.

[21] 姜树学, 马述盛. 断面解剖与 MRI、CT、ECT 对照图谱. 辽宁科学技术出版社.

[22] 汪忠镐, 舒畅. 血管外科临床解剖学图谱. 山东科学技术出版社.

对提供本页书目的作者和出版社，在此一并表示衷心的感谢。